FREQUENTLY PRESCRIBED MEDICATIONS

Drugs You Need to Know

Michael A. Mancano, PharmD

Associate Chair, Department of Pharmacy Practice
Clinical Professor of Pharmacy Practice
Temple University School of Pharmacy
Philadelphia, Pennsylvania

Jason C. Gallagher, PharmD, BCPS

Clinical Associate Professor of Pharmacy Practice
Temple University School of Pharmacy
Philadelphia, Pennsylvania

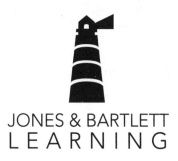

JONES & BARTLETT
LEARNING

World Headquarters

Jones & Bartlett Learning
40 Tall Pine Drive
Sudbury, MA 01776
978-443-5000
info@jblearning.com
www.jblearning.com

Jones & Bartlett Learning
Canada
6339 Ormindale Way
Mississauga, Ontario L5V 1J2
Canada

Jones & Bartlett Learning
International
Barb House, Barb Mews
London W6 7PA
United Kingdom

Jones & Bartlett Learning books and products are available through most bookstores and online booksellers. To contact Jones & Bartlett Learning directly, call 800-832-0034, fax 978-443-8000, or visit our website, www.jblearning.com.

Substantial discounts on bulk quantities of Jones & Bartlett Learning publications are available to corporations, professional associations, and other qualified organizations. For details and specific discount information, contact the special sales department at Jones & Bartlett Learning via the above contact information or send an email to specialsales@jblearning.com.

The authors, editors, and publisher have made every effort to provide accurate information. However, they are not responsible for errors, omissions, or for any outcomes related to the use of the contents of this book and take no responsibility for the use of the products and procedures described. Treatments and side effects described in this book may not be applicable to all people; likewise, some people may require a dose or experience a side effect that is not described herein. Drugs and medical devices are discussed that may have limited availability controlled by the Food and Drug Administration (FDA) for use only in a research study or clinical trial. Research, clinical practice, and government regulations often change the accepted standard in this field. When consideration is being given to use of any drug in the clinical setting, the health care provider or reader is responsible for determining FDA status of the drug, reading the package insert, and reviewing prescribing information for the most up-to-date recommendations on dose, precautions, and contraindications, and determining the appropriate usage for the product. This is especially important in the case of drugs that are new or seldom used.

Production Credits
Publisher: David Cella
Acquisitions Editor: Katey Birtcher
Associate Editor: Maro Gartside
Production Manager: Julie Champagne Bolduc
Production Editor: Jessica Steele Newfell
Marketing Manager: Grace Richards
Manufacturing and Inventory Control Supervisor: Amy Bacus
Composition: Glyph International
Cover Design: Kristin E. Parker
Cover Image: © 350jb/Dreamstime.com
Printing and Binding: Courier Stoughton
Cover Printing: Courier Stoughton

Library of Congress Cataloging-in-Publication Data
Frequently prescribed medications : drugs you need to know /
  Michael A. Mancano and Jason C. Gallagher.
      p. ; cm.
  Includes index.
  ISBN 978-0-7637-8117-0 (pbk. : alk. paper)
  1. Drugs—Handbooks, manuals, etc. I. Mancano, Michael A. II. Gallagher, Jason C.
  [DNLM: 1. Pharmaceutical Preparations—Handbooks. QV 39]
  RM301.12.F74 2012
  615'.1—dc22
                                        2010028829

6048

Printed in the United States of America
14 13 12 11   10 9 8 7 6 5 4 3 2

To the alumni, present students, and future students of Temple University School of Pharmacy

BRIEF CONTENTS

CONTENTS

CHAPTER 5   Cardiovascular Agents. 61

Anna M. Wodlinger Jackson, PharmD, BCPS

CHAPTER 6   Central Nervous System
Agents 79

Christine Fitzgerald, PharmD, BCPS

Susan Kent, PharmD, CGP

Joel Shuster, PharmD, BCPP

The genesis of this text was at the Temple University School of Pharmacy as a resource for students to prepare for their "Top 200 Exam," an exam about highly pertinent facts for frequently prescribed medications that all third professional year students must pass before beginning the fourth professional year. Before writing earlier versions of this book, faculty at Temple reviewed many texts, flash cards, and other resources but found none to be optimal references for our students' needs. Many texts were extraordinarily detailed or did not emphasize important information clearly and concisely. For the past 10 years at Temple, we have used versions of this text, and students and faculty have found them to be very helpful resources. This publication expands on the in-house versions of this text by including review questions and including key points for each drug and drug class. Throughout the text, an asterisk (*) is used to indicate the most common uses of a drug. We hope that it will serve as a useful reference for healthcare students and professionals of various disciplines as they learn the most frequently used medications in clinical practice.

Over the past 10 years, numerous revisions of this text have been undertaken. We are indebted to the many clinicians and faculty who have assisted in developing this text to its final version. We would like to thank all of the section editors and authors and thank the following people. Without their assistance earlier versions of this text could not have been written. These individuals are (in alphabetical order): Christina Ruggia-Check, PharmD; Ina Calligaro, PharmD; Joseph Boullata, PharmD, BCNSP; Karissa Kim, PharmD, CACP; Nisha Mehta, PharmD; Olga M. Klibanov, PharmD; Patrick Scoble, PharmD; Steven Gelone, PharmD; and Tanya Knight-Klimas, PharmD, CGP, FASCP.

5-HT3	Serotonin subtype-3 receptors receptors		HGB	Hemoglobin
ACE	Angiotensin-converting enzyme		HIT	Heparin-induced thrombocytopenia
ACEI	Angiotensin-converting enzyme inhibitor		HIV	Human immunodeficiency virus
ADHD	Attention deficit hyperactivity disorder		HMG-CoA	Hydroxymethylglutaryl-coenzyme A
AIDS	Acquired immune deficiency syndrome		HPA	Hypothalamic–pituitary–adrenal axis
AIHA	Autoimmune hemolytic anemia		IBS	Irritable bowel syndrome
ALL	Acute lymphocytic leukemia		IM	Intramuscular
AML	Acute myeloid leukemia		INR	International normalized ratio
aPTT	Activated partial thromboplastin time		IOP	Intraocular pressure
ARB	Angiotensin receptor blocker		IV	Intravenous
ARDS	Acute respiratory distress syndrome		LDL	Low-density lipoprotein
BAS	Bile acid sequestrant		LFT	Liver function test
BMT	Bone marrow transplant		LMWH	Low molecular weight heparin
BPH	Benign prostatic hyperplasia		MALT	Mucosal-associated lymphoid tissue
BZD	Benzodiazepine		MAO	Monoamine oxidase
CABG	Coronary artery bypass graft		MAOI	Monoamine oxidase inhibitor
cAMP	Cyclic adenosine monophosphate		MDI	Metered-dose inhaler
CBC	Complete blood count		MI	Myocardial infarction
cGMP	Cyclic guanosine monophosphate		MOA	Mechanism of action
ClCrest	Estimated creatinine clearance		MRI	Magnetic resonance imaging
CML	Chronic myelocytic leukemia		NG tube	Nasogastric tube
CNI	Calcineurin inhibitors		NLO	Nasolacrimal occlusion
CNS	Central nervous system		NMS	Neuroleptic malignant syndrome
COPD	Chronic obstructive pulmonary disease		NNRTI	Nonnucleoside reverse transcriptase inhibitor
COX-2	Cyclooxygenase-2		NRTI	Nucleoside reverse transcriptase inhibitor
CPK	Creatinine phosphokinase		NSAID	Nonsteroidal anti-inflammatory drugs
CrCl	Creatinine clearance		NTE	Not to exceed
CRF	Chronic renal failure		NYHA	New York Heart Association
CTZ	Chemoreceptor trigger zone		OCD	Obsessive compulsive disorder
CVA	Cerebrovascular accident		OTC	Over-the-counter
CYP	Cytochrome P450		PBPC	Peripheral blood progenitor cell collection
DHA	Docosahexaenoic acid		PCI	Percutaneous coronary intervention
DIC	Disseminated intravascular coagulopathy		PCOS	Polycystic ovary syndrome
DKA	Diabetic ketoacidosis		PCP	*Pneumocystis carinii* pneumonia
DMARD	Disease-modifying antirheumatic drug		PDE5	Phosphodiesterase 5
DVT	Deep vein thrombosis		PE	Pulmonary embolism
ECG/EKG	Electrocardiogram		PI	Protease inhibitor
EPA	Eicosapentaenoic acid		PPARα	Peroxisome proliferator activated receptors
EPS	Extrapyramidal symptoms		PPI	Proton pump inhibitor
FAP	Familial adenomatous polyposis		PTCA	Percutaneous transluminal coronary angioplasty
FDA	U.S. Food and Drug Administration		PUD	Peptic ulcer disease
GAD	Generalized anxiety disorder		RA	Rheumatoid arthritis
G-CSF	Granulocyte colony-stimulating factor		RDA	Recommended Daily Allowance
GERD	Gastroesophageal reflux disease		RLS	Restless legs syndrome
GFR	Glomerular filtration rate		SAD	Social anxiety disorder
GI	Gastrointestinal		SCN	Severe chronic neutropenia
GLP	Glucagon-like peptide		SIADH	Syndrome of inappropriate antidiuretic hormone
Hct	Hematocrit		SJS	Stevens–Johnson syndrome
HCTZ	Hydrochlorothiazide		SLE	Systemic lupus erythematosus
HDL	High-density lipoprotein			

SLL	Small lymphocytic lymphoma	TLC	Therapeutic lifestyle changes
SNRI	Selective norepinephrine reuptake inhibitor	TMJ	Temporomandibular joint
SrCr	Serum creatinine	TNF	Tumor necrosis factor
SSRI	Selective serotonin reuptake inhibitor	TPA	Tissue plasminogen activator
SUB-Q	Subcutaneous	UFH	Unfractionated heparin
TCA	Tricyclic antidepressant	ULN	Upper limits of normal
TG	Triglyceride	VLDL	Very low-density lipoprotein
TIA	Transient ischemic attack	WM	Waldenstrom macroglobulinemia

CONTRIBUTORS

Rachel Clark-Vetri, PharmD, BCOP
Clinical Associate Professor of Pharmacy Practice
Temple University School of Pharmacy
Clinical Oncology/Palliative Care Pharmacist
Temple University Cancer Center

Deborah DeEugenio, PharmD, BCPS, CACP
Clinical Associate Professor of Pharmacy Practice
Temple University School of Pharmacy
Clinical Pharmacist, Ambulatory Internal Medicine
Temple Group Practice

Christine Fitzgerald, PharmD
Clinical Assistant Professor of Pharmacy Practice
Temple University School of Pharmacy
Clinical Pharmacist in Neurology
Temple University Hospital

Carol Holtzman, PharmD, MSc
Clinical Assistant Professor of Pharmacy Practice
Temple University School of Pharmacy
HIV Pharmacotherapy Specialist
Temple Comprehensive HIV Program

Anna M. Wodlinger Jackson, PharmD, BCPS
Pharmacy Clinical Specialist
Inova Fairfax Hospital

Susan Kent, PharmD, CGP
Clinical Assistant Professor
Temple University School of Pharmacy
Clinical Pharmacist, Ambulatory Care
HealthLink Medical Center

Patrick McDonnell, PharmD
Clinical Associate Professor
Temple University School of Pharmacy
Clinical Pharmacy Consultant
Jeanes Hospital

Nima M. Patel, PharmD, BCPS
Clinical Associate Professor
Temple University School of Pharmacy
Ambulatory Care Clinical Pharmacist
Department of Medicine
Temple University Hospital

Mirza Perez, PharmD, BCPS
Clinical Assistant Professor of Pharmacy Practice
Temple University School of Pharmacy
Clinical Pharmacist in Internal Medicine
Temple University Hospital

Christina Rose, PharmD, BCPS
Clinical Assistant Professor of Pharmacy Practice
Temple University School of Pharmacy
Clinical Pharmacy Specialist, Surgical/Trauma and
    Burn Intensive Care Units
Temple University Hospital

Charles Ruchalski, PharmD, BCPS
Clinical Associate Professor of Pharmacy Practice
Temple University School of Pharmacy
Clinical Pharmacy Consultant, Employee Health Services
Temple University

Joel Shuster, PharmD, BCPP
Clinical Professor of Pharmacy Practice
Temple University School of Pharmacy
Psychiatric Pharmacist Specialist
Episcopal Hospital of the Temple Health System

Sarah Slabaugh, PharmD, RD
Clinical Assistant Professor of Pharmacy Practice
Temple University School of Pharmacy
Ambulatory Care Clinical Pharmacist
Department of Medicine
Temple University

Jamila Stanton, PharmD, BCPS
Clinical Assistant Professor of Pharmacy Practice
Temple University School of Pharmacy
Clinical Pharmacist in Internal Medicine
Temple University Hospital

Analgesics

Rachel Clark-Vetri, PharmD, BCOP

Drug Class: Miscellaneous Analgesics

Introduction

Three commonly used analgesics fall into categories of their own and are discussed here. Acetaminophen, one of the most commonly used analgesics, is generally well-tolerated but noted for its hepatotoxicity when given in doses exceeding daily recommendations. Butalbital combinations are most frequently used to treat headaches. Tramadol, which is used for moderate pain, also has proven efficacy for neuropathic pain.

Members of the Drug Class

In this section: Acetaminophen, butalbital with caffeine and acetaminophen, tramadol

■ Acetaminophen

Mechanism of Action

Inhibits brain prostaglandin synthesis, leading to analgesic and antipyretic activity

Brand Names

Tylenol, Various

Generic Name

Acetaminophen

Dosage Forms

Tablets oral and chewable, capsules, gelcaps, elixir, solutions, suppositories

Usage

- Mild pain such as headaches and arthritis pain*, fever*, combined with other analgesics for moderate–severe pain*

Dosing

- Usual dose: 500–650 mg PO every 4–6 hours as needed; maximum adult dose: 4 g/day
- Children: 10–15 mg/kg per dose every 4–6 hours as needed
- Hepatic dosage adjustment: Limit to 2 g/day in chronic alcoholics

Adverse Reactions: Most Common

- Nontoxic at therapeutic doses

Adverse Reactions: Rare/Severe/Important

- Hepatotoxicity with excessive dosing

Major Drug Interactions

Drugs Affecting Acetaminophen

- Ethanol use: >3 drinks/day may increase risk of hepatotoxicity
- Isoniazid: May increase the risk of hepatotoxicity

Acetaminophen's Effect on Other Drugs

- Warfarin: Increased anticoagulant effect

Counseling Points

- Report unresolved pain or fevers to your doctor
- Adults: Do not use >4 g/day

Key Points

- Use with caution in patients with glucose-6-phosphate dehydrogenase deficiency
- Many OTC cold and pain products contain acetaminophen, and patients should be warned to avoid inadvertently overdosing on acetaminophen by taking them in excessive combinations
- Acetaminophen is the preferred analgesic during pregnancy and breastfeeding

■ Butalbital with Caffeine and Acetaminophen

Mechanism of Action

Butalbital is a barbiturate that depresses the sensory cortex and depresses motor activity producing sedation and drowsiness. Caffeine increase cAMP and acts as a vasoconstrictor and a CNS stimulant. The combination is commonly used to treat headaches.

Brand Names

Fioricet, Zebutal, Dolgic Plus

Generic Names
Butalbital, acetaminophen, caffeine

Dosage Forms
Tablets, capsules, oral liquid; tablets, capsules, and 15 ml of the liquid each contain 50 mg of butalbital, 40 mg of caffeine, and 325–750 mg of acetaminophen

Usage
- Relief of tension or muscle contraction headaches*

Dosing
- Initial: 1–2 tablets or capsules (or 15–30 ml solution) every 4 hours; not to exceed 6 tablets or capsules (or 180 ml solution) daily
- Renal dosage adjustment:
  ◦ Dosing should be reduced
- Hepatic dosage adjustment:
  ◦ Dosing should be reduced

Adverse Reactions: Most Common
- Drowsiness, depression, nervousness, insomnia, nightmares, nausea

Adverse Reactions: Rare/Severe/Important
- Hallucinations, hypotension, respiratory and CNS depression, tachycardia, hepatotoxicity (exceeding acetaminophen dosing recommendations)

Major Drug Interactions
Drugs Affecting Butalbital with Caffeine and Acetaminophen
- CNS depressants: May enhance the adverse/toxic effect of other CNS depressants
- Ethanol use: >3 drinks/day may increase risk of hepatotoxicity
- Isoniazid: May increase the risk hepatotoxicity

Butalbital with Caffeine and Acetaminophen's Effect on Other Drugs
- Calcium channel blockers, contraceptives, corticosteroids, cyclosporine, disopyramide, doxycycline, tricyclic antidepressants, voriconazole, warfarin: Increase the metabolism of these agents

Counseling Points
- Report unresolved headache to your doctor
- Do not use more than the recommended daily dose

Key Point
- Many OTC cold and pain products contain acetaminophen and can increase the risk of hepatotoxicity when taken with butalbital, acetaminophen, and caffeine combinations

■ Tramadol

Mechanism of Action
Binds to µ-opioid receptors altering the perception and response to pain and inhibits reuptake of serotonin and norepinephrine.

Brand Names
Ultram, Ultram ER, Ultracet

Generic Name
Tramadol

Dosage Forms
Immediate-release and extended-release tablets; Ultracet is a combination with acetaminophen

Usage
- Moderate* to severe pain, neuropathic pain

Dosing
- Initial dose: 50 mg PO every 4–6 hours as needed
- Maintenance dose: 50–100 mg every 4–6 hours as needed
- Maximum dose: 400 mg/day; 300 mg/day extended-release products
- Hepatic dosage adjustment:
  ◦ 50 mg every 12 hours
- Renal dosage adjustment:
  ◦ 50–100 mg every 12 hours (200 mg/day maximum)

Adverse Reactions: Most Common
- Sedation, dizziness, constipation, nausea and vomiting, somnolence, euphoria/dysphoria

Adverse Reactions: Rare/Severe/Important
- Hypotension, seizures at ≥500 mg/day, abstinence syndrome with abrupt discontinuation

Major Drug Interactions
Drugs Affecting Tramadol
- Carbamazepine decreases tramadol levels
- MAO inhibitors, TCAs, and SSRIs may increase the risk of seizures and serotonin syndrome
- Naloxone may induce a seizure

Tramadol's Effect on Other Drugs
- CNS depressants: Additive respiratory and CNS depressant effects

Counseling Points
- May cause drowsiness
- Abrupt discontinuation may result in withdrawal symptoms

Key Points
- Serotonin syndrome or seizures can occur when combined with antidepressants
- Use with caution in patients with a seizure history
- Tramadol has the potential for abuse

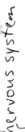

Drug Class: Narcotic Analgesics

Introduction

Narcotic analgesics are common medications used for moderate and severe pain. Given by a variety of different routes of administration and effective for both <u>nociceptive</u> and <u>neuropathic</u> pain symptoms, narcotics are controlled substances with a risk of abuse and <u>diversion.</u>

[handwritten: stimulation of peripheral nerve fibers]

Members of the Drug Class
[handwritten: diverted from lawful purpose into illicit drug]

In this section: Fentanyl, hydromorphone, methadone, morphine, oxycodone

[handwritten: eliminates craving for opiates; once stopped using, cravings will return]

Others: Alfentanil, <u>buprenorphine</u>, butorphanol, levorphanol, meperidine, nalbuphine, opium tincture, oxymorphone, pentazocine, propoxyphene, remifentanil, sufentanil

■ Fentanyl

[handwritten: - the more drug, the more effect at the receptor]

Mechanism of Action

Acts as an μ-opioid receptor <u>agonist</u>, altering the perception and response to pain centrally and peripherally

Brand Names

Actiq, Duragesic, Fentora, Sublimaze, Onsolis

Generic Name

Fentanyl

Dosage Forms

Transdermal patch, buccal tablets, film, lozenges, and injection

Usage

- Severe pain*

Dosing

- Initial dose: 12.5–25 μg/hour transdermal patch every 72 hours; 200 μg buccally every 3 hours as needed; 50–100 μg IV single dose; 1 μg/kg per hour IV infusion
- Maintenance dose: Titrate to response
- Maximum dose: Usually 4 patches for the transdermal system (limited by skin surface area); no maximum dose based on efficacy

Adverse Reactions: Most Common

- Constipation, nausea, vomiting, sedation, dizziness, xerostomia, pruritus (histamine release), skin rash (transdermal)

Adverse Reactions: Rare/Severe/Important

- Hallucinations, hypotension, respiratory and CNS depression

Major Drug Interactions

Drugs Affecting Fentanyl

- Amphetamines: Increase analgesic effects
- Antipsychotic agents: Enhance hypotensive effects
- CNS depressants (including alcohol): Increase sedation and dizziness

- MAO inhibitors: Serotonin syndrome
- Strong and moderate inhibitors of CYP3A4: Decrease metabolism

Fentanyl's Effect on Other Drugs

- CNS depressants: Additive respiratory and CNS depressant effects

Counseling Points

- Wear for 72 hours; then replace with a new patch
- Rotate the application sites of the transdermal system to reduce skin irritation
- Takes 12 hours for onset of effect of the transdermal system
- Never cut patches
- Abrupt discontinuation of fentanyl may result in an abstinence syndrome
- Avoid excessive alcohol use
- May cause drowsiness and impair your ability to operate machinery
- May cause constipation requiring laxatives
- May cause physical or psychological dependence with prolonged use
- Notify your doctor if pain is unrelieved
- A new prescription is required for any refill

Key Points

- Avoid use within 14 days of using an MAO inhibitor
- Do not wear transdermal patches during MRI
- Fever can increase absorption of fentanyl
- Controlled substance schedule II
- Short-acting narcotics should be prescribed concurrently for breakthrough pain
- When converting patients to fentanyl patch from another narcotic, use a recommended equivalent dose
- Do not use buccal and transdermal fentanyl in narcotic naïve patients for acute and postoperative pain
- Use preservative-free solution for epidural and intrathecal use

■ Hydromorphone

Brand Name

Dilaudid

Generic Name

Hydromorphone

Dosage Forms

Liquid oral, immediate-release tablets, injection, suppository

Usage

- Moderate to severe pain*, antitussive

Dosing

- Children:
  - Oral: 0.03–0.08 mg/kg per dose every 4 hours as needed
  - IV, IM, SUB-Q: 0.015 mg/kg per dose every 3–4 hours as needed
  - Antitussive dose: 0.5 mg every 3–6 hours
- Initial adult dose:
  - Oral: 2–4 mg every 4 hours as needed
  - SUB-Q, IV, IM: 0.2–0.6 mg every 2–4 hours as needed
  - Epidural: 1–1.5 mg bolus; 0.04–0.4 mg/hour
- Maintenance adult dose:
  - Oral: 2–8 mg PO every 3–4 hours as needed
  - IV, SUB-Q continuous range: 0.1–0.5 mg/hour
  - Rectal: Every 4 hours
- Maximum dose:
  - Oral, IV, SUB-Q: No maximum dose; titrate to response
- Renal dosage adjustment:
  - None needed

Adverse Reactions: Most Common

- Constipation, nausea, vomiting, sedation, dizziness, xerostomia, pruritis (histamine release)

Adverse Reactions: Rare/Severe/Important

- Hallucinations, agitation, respiratory and CNS depression

Major Drug Interactions

Drugs Affecting Hydromorphone

- CNS depressants: Increase sedation and dizziness

Hydromorphone's Effect on Other Drugs

- CNS depressants: Additive effect
- MAO inhibitors, SSRIs: Serotonin syndrome

Counseling Points

- May cause drowsiness and impair your ability to operate machinery
- May cause constipation requiring laxatives
- Avoid alcohol use
- May cause physical or psychological dependence with prolonged use
- After prolonged use, abrupt discontinuation of hydromorphone may result in an abstinence syndrome
- Notify your doctor if pain is unrelieved
- A new prescription is required for any refill

Key Points

- Controlled substance schedule II
- Very soluble in injectable form; useful for continuous pump and epidural or intrathecal administration

■ Methadone

Brand Names

Methadose, Dolophine

Generic Name

Methadone

Dosage Forms

Tablets, dispersible tablets, injection, oral solution

Usage

- Severe pain*, detoxification for opiate addiction* (as part of a program)

Dosing

- Severe pain:
  - Initial dose: 5 mg PO every 6–8 hours; 2.5–10 mg IV every 8–12 hours
  - Maintenance dose: 15–60 mg daily in divided doses
  - Maximum dose: No maximum dose; titrate to response; no ceiling effect
- Addiction:
  - Initial dose: 20–30 mg single daily dose
  - Maintenance: 40–120 mg single daily dose
- Renal dosage adjustment:
  - CrCl <10 ml/minute: Reduce dose 50–75%
- Hepatic dosage adjustment:
  - Avoid in severe hepatic dysfunction

Adverse Reactions: Most Common

- Constipation, nausea, vomiting, sedation, dizziness, xerostomia, pruritus (histamine release)

Adverse Reactions: Rare/Severe/Important

- Hallucinations, hypotension, respiratory and CNS depression, ECG changes; QT interval prolongation

Major Drug Interactions

Drugs Affecting Methadone

- CNS depressants: Increase sedation and dizziness
- NNRTIs and PIs: Reduce methadone levels
- CYP3A4 inducers: Reduce methadone levels
- CYP3A4 inhibitors: Increase methadone levels
- St. John's wort: Decreases methadone levels
- Grapefruit juice: Decreases absorption

Methadone's Effect on Other Drugs

- CNS depressants: Additive respiratory and CNS depressant effects
- QTc-prolonging agents: Additive risk of ventricular arrhythmias
- Stavudine and didanosine: Decrease bioavailability

Counseling Points

- Abrupt discontinuation of methadone may result in an abstinence syndrome
- Avoid excessive alcohol use
- May cause drowsiness and impair your ability to operate machinery
- May cause constipation requiring laxatives
- May cause physical or psychological dependence with prolonged use
- Notify your doctor if pain is unrelieved
- A new prescription is required for any refill

Key Points

- May prolong QT interval and increase risk for torsade de pointes. Patients should be evaluated for risk. ECG monitoring may be necessary within 1 month of initiation and annually.
- Controlled substance schedule II
- When converting patients to methadone from another narcotic, use a calculated equivalent dose, which is dependent on the daily equivalent dose of morphine
- Accumulation can occur with extended use because of the long half-life
- Monitor for sedation with extended use
- Discontinue slowly after prolonged use

■ Morphine

Brand Names

Astramorph, Avinza, Kadian, MS Contin, Oramorph, Roxanol, Various

Generic Name

Morphine

Dosage Forms

Immediate- and sustained-release tablets, injection, oral solution, suppositories

Usage

- Moderate to severe pain*

Dosing

- Children:
  - Oral: 0.2–0.5 mg/kg per dose every 4 hours as needed
  - IV, IM, SUB-Q: 0.1–0.2 mg/kg per dose every 2–4 hours as needed. Usual maximum: 15 mg/dose
  - IV, SUB-Q continuous: Sickle cell or cancer pain 0.025 mg–2 mg/kg per hour; postoperative pain: 0.01–0.04 mg/kg per hour
- Initial adult dose:
  - Oral immediate release: 10–30 mg PO every 4 hours as needed; controlled release: 15–30 mg PO every 12 hours (opioid naive)
  - SUB-Q, IV, IM: 2.5 mg–10 mg every 2–4 hours as needed
  - IV, SUB-Q continuous: 0.5–1 mg/hour
  - Epidural: 5 mg
- Maintenance adult dose:
  - Oral controlled-release usual range: 60–200 mg/day in divided doses
  - IV, SUB-Q, IM: 10 mg every 4 hours as needed
  - IV, SUB-Q continuous range: 0.5–10 mg/hour up to 80 mg/hour
  - Rectal: 10–20 mg every 4 hours
- Maximum dose:
  - Oral, IV, SUB-Q: No maximum dose; titrate to response
  - Epidural: 10 mg/24 hours
- Renal dosage adjustment:
  - CrCl 10–50 ml/minute: Reduce dose 25%
  - CrCl <10 ml/minute: Reduce dose 50%
  - Dialysis: Administer 50% of normal dose

Adverse Reactions: Most Common

- Constipation, nausea, vomiting, sedation, dizziness, xerostomia, pruritus (histamine release)

Adverse Reactions: Rare/Severe/Important

- Hallucinations, hypotension, respiratory and CNS depression

Major Drug Interactions

Drugs Affecting Morphine

- Alcohol can disrupt the extended-release characteristic of Avinza
- CNS depressants increase sedation and dizziness

Morphine's Effect on Other Drugs

- CNS depressants: Additive effect
- MAO inhibitors and SSRIs can cause serotonin syndrome with morphine

Counseling Points

- May cause drowsiness and impair your ability to operate machinery
- May cause constipation requiring laxatives
- Avoid alcohol use
- May cause physical or psychological dependence with prolonged use
- After prolonged use, abrupt discontinuation of morphine may result in an abstinence syndrome
- Do not crush or chew the controlled-release products
- Notify your doctor if pain is unrelieved
- A new prescription is required for any refill

Key Points

- Controlled substance schedule II
- Avoid use within 14 days of using an MAO inhibitor
- Contraindicated in paralytic ileus
- Avoid in patients with increase intracranial pressure such as head trauma
- The equivalent oral dose is three times more than the IV dose
- Controlled-release products should not be used to treat acute postoperative pain
- Use preservative-free solutions for epidural and intrathecal use

■ Oxycodone

Brand Names

OxyContin, OxyIR, Roxicodone

Generic Name

Oxycodone

Dosage Forms

Capsules, oral liquid, oral concentrate, immediate- and controlled-release tablets

Usage

- Moderate to severe pain*

Dosing

- Initial dose: 10 mg PO every 12 hours (opioid naive)
- Maintenance dose: 20–160 mg PO every 12 hours
- Maximum dose: No maximum dose; titrate to response
- Pediatric dose: 6–12 years: 1.25 mg every 6 hours as needed

Adverse Reactions: Most Common

- Constipation, nausea, vomiting, sedation, dizziness, xerostomia, pruritus (histamine release)

Adverse Reactions: Rare/Severe/Important

- Hallucinations, hypotension, respiratory and CNS depression

Major Drug Interactions

Drugs Affecting Oxycodone

- CNS depressants: Increase sedation and dizziness

Oxycodone's Effect on Other Drugs

- CNS depressants: Additive effect
- MAO inhibitors and SSRIs: Serotonin syndrome

Counseling Points

- May cause drowsiness and impair your ability to operate machinery
- May cause constipation requiring laxatives
- Avoid alcohol use
- May cause physical or psychological dependence with prolonged use
- After prolonged use, abrupt discontinuation of oxycodone may result in an abstinence syndrome
- Do not crush or chew the controlled-release products
- Notify your doctor if pain is unrelieved
- A new prescription is required for any refill

Key Points

- Controlled substance schedule II
- Controlled-release products should not be used to treat acute postoperative pain
- Deaths due to overdose have been reported due to misuse/abuse after crushing the sustained-release tablets

---

Drug Class: Narcotic/Nonnarcotic Combinations

Introduction

Narcotic combinations are common agents prescribed for management of moderate pain. The addition of the nonopioid is commonly ibuprofen or acetaminophen, which works as a coanalgesic. The side effects of the individual components must be considered. These drugs are classified as controlled substances and have the risk of abuse and diversion.

Mechanism of Action for the Drug Class

Narcotic component binds to opioid mu receptors altering the perception and response to pain combined with a nonnarcotic analgesic that inhibits brain prostaglandin synthesis.

Members of the Drug Class

In this section: Codeine/acetaminophen, hydrocodone/acetaminophen, hydrocodone/ibuprofen, oxycodone/acetaminophen, propoxyphene-n/acetaminophen
Others: Pseudoephedrine/hydrocodone/chlorpheniramine

■ Codeine/Acetaminophen

Brand Names

Tylenol 2, Tylenol 3, Tylenol 4, Tylenol with Codeine

Generic Name

Codeine/Acetaminophen

Dosage Forms

Tablets, elixir

Usage

- Moderate pain*

Dosing

- Children: 0.5–1 mg codeine/kg per dose every 4–6 hours or
  - 3–6 years: 5 ml/dose every 6 hours of elixir
  - 7–12 years: 10 ml every 6 hours of elixir
  - >12 years: 15 ml every 4 hours of elixir
- Adult: 30–60 mg codeine every 4–6 hours
- Maximum dose: 4000 mg of acetaminophen component/day (2000 mg in chronic alcoholics)
- Renal dosage adjustment:
  - CrCl 10–50 ml/minute: Reduce dose 25%
  - CrCl <10 ml/minute: Reduce dose 50%

Adverse Reactions: Most Common

- Constipation, nausea, vomiting, sedation, dizziness, xerostomia, pruritus

Adverse Reactions: Rare/Severe/Important

- Hallucinations, hypotension, respiratory and CNS depression, hepatotoxicity (exceeding acetaminophen dosing recommendations)

Major Drug Interactions

Drugs Affecting Codeine/Acetaminophen

- CYP2D6 inhibitors: Prevent conversion of codeine to its active metabolite morphine
- CNS depressants: Increase sedation and dizziness
- Ethanol use: >3 drinks/day may increase risk of hepatotoxicity
- Isoniazid: May increase the risk hepatotoxicity

Codeine/Acetaminophen's Effect on Other Drugs

- Warfarin: Increased anticoagulant effect
- CNS depressants: Additive effect

Counseling Points

- May cause drowsiness and impair your ability to operate machinery
- May cause constipation requiring laxatives
- Avoid alcohol use
- May cause physical or psychological dependence with prolonged use
- After prolonged use, abrupt discontinuation may result in an abstinence syndrome
- Notify your doctor if pain is unrelieved

Key Points

- Differences in individual metabolism mean that some patients will not convert codeine to its active form, necessitating the use of other agents; others may be ultra-rapid metabolizers of codeine, producing higher levels of morphine and leading to higher adverse effects
- Caution during breastfeeding; use lowest possible effective dose
- Controlled substance
- Do not exceed acetaminophen daily dosing recommendations

■ Hydrocodone/Acetaminophen

Brand Names

Lorcet, Lortab, Vicodin, Various

Generic Name

Hydrocodone/Acetaminophen

Dosage Forms

Tablets, elixir, or solution

Usage

- Moderate pain*

Dosing

- Children: <50 kg: 0.1–0.2 mg/kg per dose hydrocodone component every 4–6 hours
- Usual adult dose: 1–2 tablets every 4–6 hours or 5–10 ml elixir every 4–6 hours
- Maximum dose: 4000 mg of acetaminophen component/day (2000 mg in chronic alcoholics)

Adverse Reactions: Most Common

- Constipation, nausea, vomiting, sedation, dizziness, xerostomia, pruritus (histamine release)

Adverse Reactions: Rare/Severe/Important

- Hallucinations, hypotension, respiratory and CNS depression, hepatotoxicity (exceeding acetaminophen dosing recommendations)

Major Drug Interactions

Drugs Affecting Hydrocodone/Acetaminophen

- CNS depressants: Increase sedation and dizziness
- Ethanol use: >3 drinks/day may increase risk of hepatotoxicity
- Isoniazid: May increase the risk hepatotoxicity

Hydrocodone/Acetaminophen's Effect on Other Drugs

- Warfarin: Increases anticoagulant effect
- CNS depressants: Additive effect

Counseling Points

- May cause drowsiness and impair your ability to operate machinery
- May cause constipation requiring laxatives
- Avoid alcohol use
- May cause physical or psychological dependence with prolonged use
- After prolonged use, abrupt discontinuation may result in an abstinence syndrome
- Notify your doctor if pain is unrelieved

Key Points

- Controlled substance schedule III
- Do not exceed acetaminophen daily dosing recommendations

■ Hydrocodone/Ibuprofen

Brand Names

Vicoprofen, Various

Generic Name

Hydrocodone/Ibuprofen

Dosage Forms

Tablets containing 200 mg of ibuprofen and 5, 7.5, or 10 mg of hydrocodone

Usage

- Moderate pain*

Dosing
- Usual adult dose: 1–2 tablets every 4–6 hours
- Maximum dose: 2400 mg ibuprofen (12 tablets/day)

Adverse Reactions: Most Common
- Constipation, nausea, vomiting, sedation, dizziness, xerostomia, pruritus (histamine release), dyspepsia

Adverse Reactions: Rare/Severe/Important
- Hallucinations, hypotension, respiratory and CNS depression, edema, renal impairment, GI bleeding or ulcers, increased blood pressure

Major Drug Interactions
Drugs Affecting Hydrocodone/Ibuprofen
- CNS depressants: Sedation and dizziness

Hydrocodone/Ibuprofen's Effect on Other Drugs
- Anticoagulants: Enhanced anticoagulation
- Antihypertensives: Decreased effects
- Aspirin: Increased bleeding
- CNS depressants: Additive effects
- Lithium: Increased concentration
- MAO inhibitors and SSRIs: Serotonin syndrome

Counseling Points
- May cause drowsiness and impair your ability to operate machinery
- May cause constipation requiring laxatives
- Avoid alcohol use
- May cause physical or psychological dependence with prolonged use
- After prolonged use, abrupt discontinuation may result in an abstinence syndrome
- Notify your doctor if pain is unrelieved

Key Points
- Controlled substance schedule III
- Do not exceed daily dosing recommendations

▇ Oxycodone/Acetaminophen

Brand Names
Endocet, Percocet, Roxicet, Tylox

Generic Name
Oxycodone/Acetaminophen

Dosage Forms
Capsules, tablets, oral liquid; note that various dosage combinations are available

Usage
- Moderate or severe pain*

Dosing
- Initial dose: 1–2 tablets of 5 mg oxycodone/325 mg acetaminophen PO every 4–6 hours or 5–10 ml oral solution every 4–6 hours
- Maximum dose: 4000 mg acetaminophen/day (2000 mg/day in chronic alcoholics)
- Renal dosage adjustment:
  ○ None

Major Drug Interactions
Drugs Affecting Oxycodone/Acetaminophen
- CNS depressants: Increase sedation and dizziness
- Ethanol use: >3 drinks/day may increase risk of hepatotoxicity
- Isoniazid: May increase the risk hepatotoxicity

Oxycodone/Acetaminophen's Effect on Other Drugs
- Warfarin: Increases anticoagulant effect
- CNS depressants: Additive effect

Counseling Points
- May cause drowsiness and impair your ability to operate machinery
- May cause constipation requiring laxatives
- Avoid alcohol use
- May cause physical or psychological dependence with prolonged use
- Notify your doctor if pain is unrelieved
- A new prescription is required for any refill

Key Points
- Multiple combinations of oxycodone/acetaminophen are available in various strengths. The most common dosage is 5 mg oxycodone/325 mg acetaminophen, which was formerly the only available strength. Prescriptions and orders for this drug must include the strength desired.
- Controlled substance schedule II
- Do not exceed acetaminophen daily dosing recommendations

▇ Propoxyphene-n/Acetaminophen

Brand Names
Darvocet-N, Propacet, Various

Generic Name
Propoxyphene-n/Acetaminophen

Dosage Forms
Oral tablets containing 50, 65, or 100 mg of propoxyphene and 325, 500, or 650 mg of acetaminophen

Usage
- Mild to moderate pain*

Dosing
- Maintenance dose: 50–100 mg PO propoxyphene every 4 hours
- Maximum dose: 600 mg PO propoxyphene/day
- Renal dosage adjustment:
  ○ CrCl <10 ml/minute: Avoid use

Adverse Reactions: Most Common
- Hypotension

Absolute Contraindications
- None

Major Drug Interactions
Drugs Affecting Propoxyphene-n/Acetaminophen
- CNS depressants may increase sedation

Propoxyphene-n/Acetaminophen's Effect on Other Drugs
- Carbamazepine level may be increased due to decrease in metabolism

Counseling Points
- Avoid alcohol use
- Do not exceed the recommended dosing

- May cause drowsiness
- May cause physical or psychological dependence with prolonged use

Key Points
- Controlled substance schedule IV

Drug Class: Nonsteroidal Anti-Inflammatory Drug, Selective COX-2 Inhibitor

Introduction
The selective COX-2 inhibitor celecoxib is commonly used for mild pain syndromes such as arthritis with the benefit of a lower incidence of GI ulcers than nonselective NSAIDs. Their use is complicated by a small but significant increase in cardiovascular events such as stroke and myocardial infarction. Although celecoxib has less GI toxicity than nonselective NSAIDs, many of the same warnings, adverse effects, and counseling points still apply to it. Other agents in this class have been removed from the market.

Mechanism of Action for the Drug Class
Inhibits prostaglandin synthesis by decreasing the activity of the enzyme COX-2, which results in decreased formation of prostaglandin precursors. COX-2 inhibitors do not appear to block COX-1 as extensively as nonselective NSAIDs, decreasing the toxicity to the GI mucosa.

Members of the Drug Class
In this section: Celecoxib
   Others: None

■ Celecoxib

Brand Name
Celebrex

Generic Name
Celecoxib

Dosage Forms
Capsules

Usage
- Osteoarthritis*, dysmenorrhea, ankylosing spondylitis, RA*, acute pain, prevention of polyp formation in patients with familial adenomatous polyposis (FAP)

Dosing
- JRA: Children: ≥2 years: 10–25 kg, 50 mg twice daily; >25 kg, 100 mg twice daily
- Adults: 100–200 mg twice daily
- FAP: 400 mg twice daily
- Renal dosage adjustment: No specific dosing recommended; avoid in advanced renal disease
- Hepatic dosage adjustment: Reduce 50% in moderate impairment; not recommended in severe impairment

Adverse Reactions: Most Common
- Nausea, GI ulcers, peripheral edema, hypertension, headache, diarrhea

Adverse Reactions: Rare/Severe/Important
- GI perforation and bleeding, thrombosis, renal toxicity, exfoliative dermatitis, Stevens–Johnson syndrome and toxic epidermal necrolysis, fulminant hepatitis, liver failure, acute renal failure

Major Drug Interactions
Drugs Affecting Celecoxib
- Antacids: Decrease absorption of celecoxib
- Corticosteroids: Increase GI side effects
- Ethanol: Increased GI irritation
- Fluconazole can increase concentrations of celecoxib

Celecoxib's Effect on Other Drugs
- ACE inhibitors and angiotensin II receptor blockers: Decrease antihypertensive effect and increase renal toxicity
- Anticoagulants: Increase bleeding risk
- Aspirin: Increases bleeding risk; diminishes cardioprotective effect
- Cyclosporine: Increases cyclosporine levels
- Diuretics: Decreased effects
- Lithium: Increased concentrations

Counseling Points
- Be informed about signs and symptoms of GI bleeding
- Take with food if GI upset occurs
- Take as directed
- Avoid OTC products unless approved by prescriber
- Do not take with antacids

Key Points

- Use with caution in patients with fluid retention, congestive heart failure, renal insufficiency, or hypertension
- Use of NSAIDs can compromise renal function. Renal toxicity is more likely to occur in patients with impaired renal function, dehydration, heart failure, liver dysfunction, those taking diuretics and ACE inhibitors, and the elderly. Monitor renal function closely. Not recommended for use in patients with advanced renal disease.
- May increase risk for thrombosis, stroke, and myocardial infarction
- Elderly are at increased risk for GI ulcers, CNS and renal toxicities
- Patients with hypersensitivity reactions to sulfonamides (especially nonantibiotic sulfonamides) should avoid celecoxib
- Patients with "aspirin triad" (bronchial asthma, aspirin intolerance, rhinitis) may be at increased risk of hypersensitivity. Do not use in patients who experience bronchospasm, asthma, rhinitis, or urticaria with NSAID or aspirin therapy.
- GI events may occur at any time during therapy and without warning. Use caution with a history of GI disease (bleeding or ulcers), concurrent therapy with aspirin, anticoagulants, and/or corticosteroids, smoking, use of alcohol, the elderly or debilitated patients.

Drug Class: Nonsteroidal Anti-Inflammatory Drugs

Introduction

Nonsteroidal anti-inflammatory drugs are commonly used for mild pain symptoms. They possess both anti-inflammatory and antipyretic effects. The use of these agents is complicated by their GI side effects and cardiovascular risks. Ibuprofen and naproxen are two agents in the class that are available OTC and found in many common cold and headache formulations. NSAIDs have many characteristics in common, and they are listed here.

Mechanism of Action of the Drug Class

Inhibits prostaglandin synthesis by decreasing the activity of COX enzymes 1 and 2, resulting in decreased formation of prostaglandin precursors associated with inflammation and pain.

Members of the Drug Class

In this section: Aspirin, diclofenac, etodolac, ibuprofen, indomethacin, meloxicam, nabumetone, naproxen

Others: Diflunisal, fenoprofen, flurbiprofen, ketoprofen, ketorolac, meclofenamate, mefenamic acid, oxaprozin, piroxicam, sulindac, tolmetin

Major Drug Interactions for the Drug Class

Drugs Affecting NSAIDs

- Corticosteroids: Increase GI side effects
- Ethanol: Increased GI irritation

NSAIDs' Effect on Other Drugs

- ACE inhibitors and angiotensin II receptor blockers: Decrease antihypertensive effect
- Anticoagulants: Increase bleeding risk
- Diuretics: Diminish diuretic effect
- Heparin: Increases anticoagulant effect
- Warfarin: Enhances anticoagulant effect
- Lithium: Increased concentrations, possible toxicity

Adverse Reactions for the Drug Class: Most Common

- Nausea, gastritis, abdominal cramps, GI ulcers, peripheral edema, hypertension, diarrhea

Adverse Reactions for the Drug Class: Rare/Severe/Important

- GI perforation and bleeding, renal toxicity, acute renal failure, angioedema, bronchoconstriction, asthma, rash, tinnitus, hearing loss

Counseling Points for the Drug Class

- Be aware of the signs and symptoms of GI bleeding
- Take with food if GI upset occurs
- Do not take with antacids

Key Points for the Drug Class

- Use with caution in patients with fluid retention, congestive heart failure, renal insufficiency, or hypertension. They are not contraindicated in these disease states but may worsen them in some situations.
- Use of NSAIDs can compromise existing renal function. Renal toxicity can occur in patients with impaired renal function, dehydration, heart failure, liver dysfunction, those taking diuretics and ACE inhibitors, and the elderly. Monitor renal function closely.
- May increase risk for thrombosis, stroke, and myocardial infarction
- Elderly patients are at increased risk for GI ulcers, CNS and renal toxicities
- Patients with "aspirin triad" (bronchial asthma, aspirin intolerance, rhinitis) may be at increased risk of hypersensitivity. Do not use in patients who experience bronchospasm, asthma, rhinitis, or urticaria with NSAID or aspirin therapy.
- GI events may occur at any time during therapy and without warning. Use caution with a history of GI

disease (bleeding or ulcers), concurrent therapy with aspirin, anticoagulants, and/or corticosteroids, smoking, use of alcohol, the elderly or debilitated patients. The concurrent use of proton pump inhibitors or histamine-2 antagonists may reduce the risk of GI ulcers in high-risk patients.

Aspirin

Brand Names
Bayer, Excedrin, Various

Generic Name
Aspirin

Dosage Forms
Enteric coated, buffered, chewable, and controlled-release tablets; gum, suppository

Usage
- Treatment of mild–moderate pain*, inflammation, and fever
- Prevention and treatment of MI*, acute ischemic stroke*, and transient ischemic episodes*
- Management of RA, rheumatic fever, osteoarthritis, and gout (high dose)
- Adjunctive therapy in revascularization procedures (CABG*, PTCA, carotid endarterectomy*), and stent implantation*

Dosing
- Adults:
  - Antiplatelet indications: 50–325 mg daily
  - Pain and inflammation:
    - Oral: 325–650 mg every 4–6 hours up to 4 g/day
    - Rectal: 300–600 mg every 4–6 hours up to 4 g/day
- Pediatrics:
  - Analgesic and antipyretic: Oral, rectal: 10–15 mg/kg/dose every 4–6 hours, up to a total of 4 g/day
  - Anti-inflammatory: Oral: Initial: 60–90 mg/kg per day in divided doses; usual maintenance: 80–100 mg/kg per day divided every 6–8 hours

Adverse Reactions: Rare/Severe/Important
- In addition to the NSAID adverse effects just listed, Reye's syndrome

Major Drug Interactions
Drugs Affecting Aspirin
- Ginkgo biloba: Increases antiplatelet effect
- Other NSAIDs: Diminish cardioprotective effects

Aspirin's Effect on Other Drugs
- Varicella vaccine: Increases risk of Reye's syndrome

Key Points
- Do not use in children for viral infections due to the potential for Reye's syndrome, a rare but life-threatening disorder associated with aspirin use during viral infections
- Contraindicated during pregnancy and in patients with bleeding disorders

Diclofenac

Brand Names
Voltaren, Voltaren-XR, Cataflam, Flector

Generic Name
Diclofenac

Dosage Forms
Tablets, extended-release tablets, transdermal patches, topical gel, ophthalmic solution

Usage
- Acute treatment for mild to moderate pain*, dysmenorrhea*, osteoarthritis*, RA*, ankylosing spondylitis, postoperative inflammation following eye surgery, actinic keratosis

Dosing
- Initial dose: 50 mg three times daily
- Maintenance dose: 150–200 mg daily in divided doses
- Maximum dose: 200 mg daily
- Topical gel: 2–4 g to affected area four times daily
- Topical patch: 1 patch daily to painful site
- Renal dosage adjustment:
  - Use with caution in patients with renal impairment

Etodolac

Brand Name
Lodine

Generic Name
Etodolac

Dosage Forms
Tablets, capsules, extended-release tablets

Usage
- Acute treatment for mild to moderate pain*, osteoarthritis*, RA*

Dosing
- Acute pain: 200–400 mg every 6–8 hours as needed, maximum dose of 1000 mg/day; extended-release tablet dosing needed
- Children (6–16 years) for JRA: 400–1000 mg daily depending on weight using extended-release product
- Renal dosage adjustment:
  - Use with caution in patients with severe impairment; no adjustment for mild–moderate impairment

Ibuprofen

Brand Names
Motrin, Cal dolor, NeoProfen; OTC preparations available as Advil, Motrin, Excedrin IB, Haltran, Ibuprin, Midol 200, Nuprin, Pamprin IB, Trendar, Uni-Pro

Generic Name
Ibuprofen

Dosage Forms
Tablets, chewable tablets, caplets, oral infant drops, oral suspension, injection

Usage
- Acute treatment for mild to moderate pain, acute treatment for gout, osteoarthritis, RA, antipyretic, dysmenorrhea, patent ductus arteriosus, ankylosing spondylitis, cystic fibrosis
- Common uses: Mild to moderate pain and fever

Dosing
- Adults:
  - Initial dose: 200–800 mg three to four times daily
  - Maximum dose: 3200 mg daily
- Children:
  - Antipyretic, analgesic: 5–10 mg/kg/dose every 6–8 hours up to 40 mg/kg per day
  - JRA: 30–50 mg/kg per day
  - Cystic fibrosis: Maintain serum concentration 50–100 µg/ml
  - Patent ductus arteriosus (ibuprofen lysine): 10 mg/kg followed by two doses of 5 mg/kg at 24 and 48 hours

Adverse Reactions: Most Common
- Infant injection: Skin irritation, intraventricular hemorrhage, hypocalcemia, hypoglycemia, anemia, sepsis, apnea

Adverse Reactions: Rare/Severe/Important
- Injection: Electrolyte imbalances, hemorrhage

■ Indomethacin

Brand Names
Indocin, Indocin SR

Generic Name
Indomethacin

Dosage Forms
Capsules, extended-release capsules, injection, suspension, suppository

Usage
- Pain and inflammation associated with rheumatoid disorders, moderate to severe osteoarthritis*, acute gout*, acute bursitis/tendonitis, ankylosing spondylitis, patent ductus arteriosus*

Dosing
- Initial: 25–50 mg 2–3 times daily; sustained-release capsules should be given one to two times daily; maximum dose 200 mg daily

- Pediatric: Patent ductus arteriosus
  - IV: 0.2 mg/kg followed by two doses depending on postnatal age

Adverse Reactions: Most Common
- Infant injection: Skin irritation, intraventricular hemorrhage, hypocalcemia, hypoglycemia, anemia, sepsis, apnea

Adverse Reactions: Rare/Severe/Important
- Injection: Electrolyte imbalances, hemorrhage

■ Meloxicam

Brand Name
Mobic

Generic Name
Meloxicam

Dosage Forms
Tablets, oral suspension

Usage
- Osteoarthritis*, RA*, JRA

Dosing
- Adults: 7.5 mg daily up to 15 mg daily
- Children: 0.125 mg/kg per day; maximum dose 7.5 mg daily
- Renal dosage adjustment:
  - Use with caution in patients with severe impairment; no adjustment for mild to moderate impairment

■ Nabumetone

Brand Name
Relafen

Generic Name
Nabumetone

Dosage Forms
Tablets

Usage
- Osteoarthritis* and RA*

Dosing
- 1000 mg/day; maximum 2000 mg daily
- Renal dosage adjustment:
  - Moderate impairment CrCl 30–49 ml/minute: initial 750 mg up to 1500 mg/day
  - Severe impairment CrCl <30 ml/minute initial 500 mg up to 1000 mg/day

■ Naproxen

Brand Names
Naprosyn, Anaprox, Aleve (OTC)

Generic Name
Naproxen

Dosage Forms
Tablets, capsules, controlled-release tablets, enteric-coated tablets, suspension

Usage
- Acute treatment for mild to moderate pain*, acute treatment for gout, osteoarthritis*, RA, bursitis, tendonitis, dysmenorrhea*, fever, migraine headaches

Dosing
- 250–500 mg every 8–12 hours

Review Questions

1. Which of the following are the most likely potential side effects of Tylenol 3?
   - A. Constipation, nausea, itching
   - B. Diarrhea, nausea, dizziness, myalgias
   - C. Diarrhea, nausea, renal impairment
   - D. Myalgias, constipation, sedation

2. Dilaudid is classified as which of the following?
   - A. Schedule II controlled substance
   - B. Schedule III controlled substance
   - C. Schedule IV controlled substance
   - D. Schedule V controlled substance

3. Which of the following is true regarding OxyContin?
   - A. It can be crushed or chewed if the patient is unable to swallow the tablets.
   - B. It is a short-acting agent and should be dosed every 4–6 hours.
   - C. It is a short-acting analgesic and should be given on an as-needed basis.
   - D. It is a long-acting analgesic and should be dosed every 12 hours.

4. Which of the following is an uncommon potential side effect from oral morphine use?
   - A. Constipation
   - B. Nausea
   - C. Pruritus
   - D. Respiratory depression

5. Which of the following NSAIDs is selective for COX-2 and has a reduced incidence of GI ulcers?
   - A. Celebrex
   - B. Etodolac
   - C. Mobic
   - D. Naproxen

6. Which of the following is a potential side effect from methadone?
   - A. QTc prolongation cardiac arrhythmias
   - B. Renal impairment
   - C. Reye's syndrome
   - D. Steven–Johnson syndrome

7. Fentanyl is available in all the following dosage forms except
   - A. Buccal tablet
   - B. Injection
   - C. Oral tablet
   - D. Transdermal patch

8. Which of the following is an indication for using Fioricet?
   - A. Headache
   - B. Neuropathic pain
   - C. Osteoarthritis
   - D. Rheumatoid arthritis

9. Which of the following drugs can interact with Ultram, potentially causing a seizure?
   - A. Acetaminophen
   - B. Ibuprofen
   - C. Phenytoin
   - D. Tricyclic antidepressants

10. All of the following are potential side effects of NSAIDs except
    - A. Agitation
    - B. Cardiovascular events
    - C. GI ulcers
    - D. Peripheral edema

11. Which of the following is frequently used in the treatment of opioid addiction?
    - A. Codeine
    - B. Methadone
    - C. Morphine
    - D. Naproxen

12. All of the following are indications to use aspirin except
    - A. Analgesic for headache
    - B. Antipyretic for viral infections in children
    - C. Kawasaki disease
    - D. Postmyocardial infarction

13. Excedrin has the potential to interact with all of the following except
    A. Butalbital
    B. Ginkgo biloba
    C. Heparin
    D. Warfarin

14. Which of the following products could lead to hepatic failure if dosing exceeds recommended daily dosing?
    A. Celebrex
    B. Methadose
    C. Ultram
    D. Vicodin

15. Which of the following is used to treat patent ductus arteriosus in neonates?
    A. Celecoxib
    B. Indomethacin
    C. Meloxicam
    D. Nabumetone

Antidiabetic Agents

Charles Ruchalski, PharmD, BCPS

CHAPTER

2

Drug Class: Biguanides

Introduction

The biguanide metformin is the drug of choice as initial therapy for a newly diagnosed patient with type 2 diabetes as an adjunct to diet and exercise. Metformin is contraindicated in certain patients to prevent lactic acidosis, a rare but serious side effect. It is often used in combination with other oral antidiabetic agents and/or insulin in patients who do not reach glycemic goals on those therapies. HbA1c reductions with metformin are generally between 1.5% and 2%.

Mechanism of Action for the Drug Class

Improves glucose tolerance by lowering both basal and postprandial plasma glucose. Decreases hepatic glucose production, decreases intestinal absorption of glucose, and improves insulin sensitivity by increasing peripheral glucose uptake and utilization.

■ Metformin

Brand Names
Fortamet, Glucophage, Glucophage XR, Glumetza, Riomet

Generic Names
Metformin, metformin extended-release

Dosage Forms
Tablets, extended-release tablets, oral solution

Usage
- Type 2 diabetes mellitus*, PCOS, antipsychotic-induced weight gain.

Dosing
- Initial dose:
  - 500 mg twice daily with morning and evening meals, 850 mg once daily with a meal, or 500 mg extended release once daily with a meal

- Maintenance dose:
  - 2000–2550 mg daily in divided doses, or 2000 mg extended-release once daily
- Renal dosage adjustment:
  - Not recommended in patients with renal dysfunction (see Contraindications below)

Adverse Reactions: Most Common
- Diarrhea, vomiting, dyspepsia, flatulence, metallic taste, weight loss

Adverse Reactions: Rare/Severe/Important
- Lactic acidosis, megaloblastic anemia

Major Drug Interactions
Drugs Affecting Metformin
- Alcohol potentiates effect on lactate metabolism
- Iodinated contrast media can lead to acute renal failure and metformin toxicity

Contraindications
- Renal disease (males: SrCr ≥1.5 mg/dl; females: SrCr ≥1.4 mg/dl), heart failure requiring pharmacologic therapy, acute or chronic metabolic acidosis, active liver disease

Counseling Points
- Discontinue immediately and promptly notify healthcare practitioner if unexplained myalgia, malaise, hyperventilation, or unusual somnolence because these are symptoms of lactic acidosis

Key Points
- Temporarily withhold in patients undergoing radiologic procedures involving the parenteral administration of iodinated contrast media because it may result in acute alteration of renal function. Do not restart for at least 48 hours or until renal function appears adequate.

15

Drug Class: Di-Peptidyl Peptidase-4 Inhibitor

Introduction

Sitagliptin is the first di-peptidyl peptidase-4 (DPP-4) inhibitor available. It inhibits the breakdown of active GLP-1 to inactive GLP-1 through the inhibition of the enzyme DPP-4. Active GLP-1 is released from the α cells of the pancreas in response to food intake. GLP-1 plays a role in regulating blood glucose by increasing the secretion of insulin from the pancreas in a glucose-dependent manner. GLP-1 also helps regulate glucagon secretion and decreases hepatic glucose production. Sitagliptin is used as monotherapy as an adjunct to diet and exercise or in combination with other oral antidiabetic agents in patients who do not reach glycemic goals. Average HbA1c reductions are between 0.7% and 1%.

Mechanism of Action for the Drug Class

Inhibition of DPP-4 enhances the activity of active GLP-1, thus increasing glucose-dependent insulin secretion and decreasing levels of circulating glucagon and hepatic glucose production.

Members of the Drug Class

In this section: Sitagliptin
    Other: Saxagliptin

■ Sitagliptin

Brand Name

Januvia

Generic Name

Sitagliptin

Dosage Forms

Tablets

Usage

- Type 2 diabetes mellitus

Dosing

- 100 mg once daily with or without food
- Renal dosage adjustment:
  - 50 mg once daily: CrCl ≥30 to <50 ml/minute
  - 25 mg once daily: CrCl <30 ml/minute

Adverse Reactions: Most Common

- Nasopharyngitis, nausea, diarrhea, vomiting, hypoglycemia, weight loss

Adverse Reactions: Rare/Severe/Important

- Acute pancreatitis, rash (Stevens–Johnson syndrome)

Major Drug Interactions

Sitagliptin's Effect on Other Drugs

- Digoxin: Increased levels

Counseling Points

- Discontinue immediately and promptly notify healthcare practitioner if unexplained persistent nausea and vomiting occur (signs of acute pancreatitis)

Drug Class: Insulin

Introduction

The hormone insulin is endogenously released from the β cells of the pancreas. Patients with type 1 diabetes mellitus have an absolute deficiency of insulin, and patients with type 2 diabetes mellitus may also have a decreased production of endogenous insulin. Insulin is required in all type 1 diabetic patients as a lifelong treatment. Insulin is commonly used in type 2 diabetic patients as either adjunct therapy to oral antidiabetic agents or as monotherapy as the disease progresses. Various substitutions on the insulin molecule and other modifications have led to multiple types of insulins. These are characterized and administered based on their pharmacodynamic and pharmacokinetic characteristics such as onset, peak, and duration of action. Most significantly, they are classified as rapid-acting, short-acting, intermediate-acting, or long-acting types of insulin.

Mechanism of Action for the Drug Class

Insulin lowers blood glucose by stimulating peripheral glucose uptake, especially in skeletal muscle and fat, and by inhibiting hepatic glucose production.

Usage for the Drug Class

- Type 1 diabetes mellitus*, type 2 diabetes mellitus*, hyperkalemia, DKA*/diabetic coma

Dosing for the Drug Class

- Initial dose:
  - 0.5 to 1 unit/kg per day Sub-Q (high interpatient variability)
- Maintenance dose:
  - Adjust doses to achieve premeal and bedtime blood glucose levels of 80–140 mg/dl

- Renal dosage adjustment:
  - CrCl 10–50 ml/minute: Administer 75% of normal dose
  - CrCl <10 ml/minute: Administer 25–50% of normal dose; monitor closely

Adverse Reactions for the Drug Class: Most Common
- Hypoglycemia (anxiety, blurred vision, palpitations, shakiness, slurred speech, sweating), weight gain

Adverse Reactions for the Drug Class: Rare/Severe/Important
- Severe hypoglycemia (seizure/coma), edema, lipoatrophy or lipohypertrophy at injection site

Major Drug Interactions for the Drug Class
Drugs Affecting Insulin (Decreased Hypoglycemic Effect)
- Acetazolamide
- Diuretics
- Oral contraceptives
- Albuterol
- Epinephrine
- Phenothiazines
- Asparaginase
- Estrogens
- Terbutaline
- Corticosteroids
- HIV antivirals
- Thyroid hormones
- Diltiazem
- Lithium

Drugs Affecting Insulin (Increased Hypoglycemic Effect)
- Alcohol
- Fluoxetine
- Anabolic steroids
- Lithium
- β-Blockers
- Sulfonamides
- Clonidine

Contraindications for the Drug Class
- Use during severe hypoglycemia
- Allergy or sensitivity to any ingredient of the product

Counseling Points for the Drug Class
- Follow a prescribed diet and exercise regularly
- Rotate injection sites to prevent lipodystrophy
- Insulin requirements may change during times of illness, vomiting, fever, and emotional stress
- Wear diabetic identification
- Insulin stored at room temperature will be less painful to inject compared to refrigerator-stored insulin
- Mild episodes of hypoglycemia may be treated with oral glucose or carbohydrates

Members of the Drug Class
In this section: Insulin glulisine, insulin lispro, insulin NPH, Insulin (R), insulin glargine, insulin detemir, insulin aspart; various mixtures are also available

---

Types of Insulin

■ Insulin Glulisine
Brand Name
Apidra

Generic Name
Insulin glulisine (rapid-acting insulin)

Dosage Forms
Injection 100 units/ml (10-ml vial and 3-ml cartridge for pen use)

Dosing
- Administer Sub-Q 15 minutes before or immediately after starting a meal

■ Insulin Lispro
Brand Name
Humalog

Generic Name
Insulin lispro (rapid-acting insulin)

Dosage Forms
Injection 100 units/ml (10-ml vial and 3-ml cartridge for pen use)

Dosing
- Administer Sub-Q 15 minutes before or immediately after starting a meal

■ Insulin NPH
Brand Names
Humulin N, Novolin N

Generic Name
Insulin NPH (intermediate-acting insulin)

Dosage Forms

Injection, suspension, 100 units/ml (10-ml vial and 3-ml cartridge for pen use)

Dosing

- NPH should only be mixed with regular insulin
- Draw regular insulin into the syringe first; then add the NPH insulin to the syringe

■ Insulin Regular

Brand Names

Humulin R, Novolin R

Generic Name

Insulin regular (short-acting insulin)

Dosage Forms

Injection 100 units/ml (10-ml vial and 3-ml cartridge for pen use)

Dosing

- Administer Sub-Q 30 minutes before a meal
- Caution: A concentrated 20-ml vial containing 500 units/ml is available

■ 70% NPH and 30% Regular Insulin Mixture

Brand Names

Humulin 70/30, Novolin 70/30

Generic Name

70% NPH and 30% regular insulin mixture

Dosage Forms

Injection, suspension, 100 units/ml (10-ml vial and 3-ml cartridge for pen use)

■ 50% NPH and 50% Regular Insulin Mixture

Brand Name

Humulin 50/50

Generic Name

50% NPH and 50% regular insulin mixture

Dosage Forms

Injection, suspension, 100 units/ml (10-ml vial and 3-ml cartridge for pen use)

■ 75% Intermediate-Acting Lispro Suspension and 25% Rapidacting Lispro Solution

Brand Name

Humalog Mix 75/25

Generic Name

75% intermediate-acting lispro suspension and 25% rapid-acting lispro solution

Dosage Forms

Injection 100 units/ml (10-ml vial and 3-ml cartridge for pen use)

■ Insulin Glargine

Brand Name

Lantus

Generic Name

Insulin glargine (long-acting insulin)

Dosage Forms

Injection 100 units/ml (10-ml vial and 3-ml cartridge for pen use)

Dosing

- When changing to insulin glargine from once-daily NPH, the initial dose of insulin glargine should be the same. When changing to insulin glargine from twice-daily NPH, the initial dose of insulin glargine should be reduced by 20% and adjusted according to patient response.
- Administer once daily
- Starting dose in a type 2 diabetic patient is 10 units at bedtime and titrate according to patient response

■ Insulin Detemir

Brand Name

Levemir

Generic Name

Insulin detemir (long-acting insulin)

Dosage Forms

- Injection 100 units/ml (10-ml vial and 3-ml cartridge for pen use)

Dosing

- Indicated for once-daily or twice-daily dosing
- Once daily is dosed Sub-Q with the evening meal or at bedtime
- Twice daily is dosed every 12 hours

■ Insulin Aspart

Brand Name

NovoLog

Generic Name

Insulin aspart (rapid-acting insulin)

Dosage Forms

Injection 100 units/ml (10-ml vial and 3-ml cartridge for pen use)

Dosing

- Administer Sub-Q 15 minutes before or immediately after starting a meal

TABLE 2-1

Comparison of Insulin Products

Product	Onset, hours	Peak, hours	Duration, hours	Appearance
Rapid-Acting				
Insulin Aspart (NovoLog)	0.25	1–2	3–5	Clear
Insulin Glulisine (Apidra)	0.25	1	3–4	Clear
Insulin Lispro (Humalog)	0.25	0.5–1.5	3–4	Clear
Short-Acting				
Regular Insulin (Humulin R, Novolin R)	0.5–1	2–3	3–6	Clear
Intermediate-Acting				
NPH Insulin (Humulin N, Novolin N)	2–4	6–10	10–16	Cloudy
Long-Acting				
Insulin Detemir (Levemir)	4	N/A	12–24	Clear
Insulin Glargine (Lantus)	4	N/A	24	Clear

■ 70% Intermediate-Acting Insulin Aspart Suspension and 30% Rapid-Acting Aspart Solution

Brand Name
NovoLog Mix 70/30

Generic Name
70% intermediate-acting insulin aspart suspension and 30% rapid-acting aspart solution

Dosage Forms
- Injection 100 units/ml (10-ml vial and 3-ml cartridge for pen use)

■ Comparison of Insulin Products
Refer to Table 2–1.

Drug Class: Sulfonylureas

Introduction

The sulfonylureas are used as adjuncts to diet and exercise in patients with type 2 diabetes mellitus. Although periodically used as monotherapy, sulfonylureas are more commonly used in combination with other oral antidiabetic agents in patients who do not reach glycemic goals, sometimes in the same formulation. General dosing guidelines are to start with a low dose and titrate upward according to patient response while monitoring for signs and symptoms of hypoglycemia, which is a common adverse effect. Use caution in patients with renal or hepatic impairment. HbA1c reductions are between 1% and 2%.

Mechanism of Action for the Drug Class

Lowers blood glucose by stimulating insulin release from the β cells of the pancreatic islets.

Usage for the Drug Class
- Type 2 diabetes mellitus*

Adverse Reactions for the Drug Class: Most Common
- Hypoglycemia, GI distress, dizziness

Adverse Reactions for the Drug Class: Rare/Severe/Important
- SIADH (most commonly with chlorpropamide); disulfiram-like reactions

Major Drug Interactions for the Drug Class
Drugs Affecting Sulfonylureas
- Anticoagulants, azole antifungals, gemfibrozil-enhanced hypoglycemic effects
- β-Blockers: Decreased hypoglycemic effects; also may mask signs and symptoms of hypoglycemia

Sulfonylurea Effects on Other Drugs
- Digoxin: Increased levels

Contraindications for the Drug Class
- Diabetes complicated by ketoacidosis, with or without coma
- Type 1 diabetes mellitus
- Diabetes complicated by pregnancy

Counseling Points for the Drug Class
- Monitor glucose as directed and be aware of the signs and symptoms of hypoglycemia

Members of the Drug Class

In this section: Glimepiride, glipizide, glyburide

Others: Acetohexamide, chlorpropamide, tolazamide, tolbutamide

■ Glimepiride

Brand Name

Amaryl

Generic Name

Glimepiride

Dosage Forms

Tablets

Dosing

- Initial dose:
  - 1–2 mg once daily at breakfast
- Maintenance dose:
  - 1–8 mg once daily

■ Glipizide

Brand Names

Glucotrol, Glucotrol XL

Generic Names

Glipizide, glipizide extended-release

Dosage Forms

Tablets, extended-release tablets

Dosing

- Initial dose:
  - Glucotrol: 2.5–5 mg once daily 30 minutes before breakfast
  - Glucotrol XL: 5 mg extended release once daily with breakfast
- Maintenance dose:
  - Glucotrol: 10–40 mg daily (>15 mg/day should be divided)
  - Glucotrol XL: 5–20 mg extended-release once daily

■ Glyburide

Brand Names

DiaBeta, Micronase, Glynase PresTab

Generic Name

Glyburide

Dosage Forms

Tablets

Dosing

DiaBeta and Micronase

- Initial dose:
  - 1.25–5 mg once daily with breakfast
- Maintenance dose:
  - 1.25–20 mg once daily; may give as single or divided doses

Glynase PresTab

- Initial dose:
  - 1.5–3 mg once daily with breakfast
- Maintenance dose:
  - 1.5–12 mg once daily; may give as single or divided doses

---

Drug Class: Thiazolidinediones

Introduction

The thiazolidinediones, pioglitazone and rosiglitazone, decrease insulin resistance by enhancing insulin-receptor sensitivity. They are used as adjuncts to diet and exercise in patients with type 2 diabetes mellitus. Although periodically used as monotherapy, thiazolidinediones are more frequently used in combination with other oral antidiabetic agents and/or insulin in patients who do not reach glycemic goals. Recent clinical data suggest that patients taking thiazolidinediones may be at an increased risk of myocardial infarction and death, and so they should be used with caution in patients with a history of previous cardiac disease. They are not recommended in patients with NYHA class III and IV heart failure. A structurally similar thiazolidinedione, troglitazone, was removed from the market due to cases of liver failure and death. It is recommended to avoid use in patients with hepatic dysfunction. HbA1c reductions are between 1% and 1.5%.

Mechanism of Action for the Drug Class

Increase insulin sensitivity by affecting the peroxisome proliferator-activated receptor γ (PPAR γ). Acting as an agonist to these receptors, they decrease insulin resistance in adipose tissue, skeletal muscle, and the liver.

Usage for the Drug Class

- Type 2 diabetes mellitus*

Adverse Reactions for the Drug Class: Most Common

- Weight gain, edema, hypoglycemia (when used with insulin or other oral antidiabetic drugs that may cause hypoglycemia)

Adverse Reactions for the Drug Class: Rare/ Severe/Important

- Hepatic failure, heart failure, anemia, ovulation in anovulatory premenopausal women, bone loss

Major Drug Interactions for the Drug Class

Drug Affecting Thiazolidinediones

- Gemfibrozil: Increased levels
- Rifampin: Decreased levels

Thiazolidinedione Effects on Other Drugs

- Oral contraceptives: Decreased efficacy

Contraindications for the Drug Class

- Patients with NYHA class III and IV heart failure
- Active liver disease (alanine aminotransferase [ALT] >2.5 times the upper limit of normal)
- Concurrent insulin or nitrate use with rosiglitazone

Counseling Points for the Drug Class

- Report signs and symptoms of liver dysfunction and/ or shortness of breath immediately

Members of the Drug Class

In this section: Pioglitazone, rosiglitazone

■ Pioglitazone

Brand Name

Actos

Generic Name

Pioglitazone

Dosage Forms

Tablets

Dosing

- Initial dose:
  - 15–30 mg once daily without regard to meals
- Maintenance dose:
  - 15–45 mg once daily

■ Rosiglitazone

Brand Name

Avandia

Generic Name

Rosiglitazone

Dosage Forms

Tablets

Dosing

- Initial dose:
  - 4 mg once daily as a single or divided dose
- Maintenance dose:
  - 4–8 mg once daily

Review Questions

1. Which oral antidiabetic drug works primarily in the pancreas to increase the secretion of insulin?
   A. Avandia
   B. Glucophage
   C. Micronase
   D. Actos

2. What is the correct dose of sitagliptin in a patient with type 2 diabetes and moderate renal dysfunction (CrCl ~40 ml/minute)
   A. 100 mg once daily
   B. 50 mg once daily
   C. 25 mg once daily
   D. Not recommended in patients with moderate renal dysfunction

3. Which of the following insulins should be administered 15 minutes prior to a meal?
   A. Insulin NPH
   B. Insulin glargine
   C. Insulin detemir
   D. Insulin aspart

4. Which antidiabetic mediation has the potential to cause the rare but serious side effect of lactic acidosis?
   A. Metformin
   B. Rosiglitazone
   C. Glyburide
   D. Sitagliptin

5. Which of the following is a contraindication to the use of Glucophage?
   A. Osteoporosis
   B. Obesity
   C. Hyperkalemia
   D. Renal disease

6. Which diabetes medication is contraindicated in patients with NYHA III or IV heart failure?
   A. Sitagliptin
   B. Rosiglitazone
   C. Glimepiride
   D. Insulin lispro

7. Which class of drugs is indicated for both type 1 and type 2 diabetes mellitus?
   A. Biguanide
   B. Sulfonylurea
   C. Insulin
   D. Thiazolidinedione

8. What is the maximum daily dose of Actos?
   A. 8 mg once daily
   B. 12 mg daily
   C. 45 mg once daily
   D. 2550 mg daily

9. What is the average HbA1c reduction expected with sitagliptin?
   A. 0.7–1%
   B. 1–1.5%
   C. 1–2%
   D. 1.5–2%

10. What is the only insulin suspension (cloudy) that is on the market?
    A. Insulin glulisine
    B. Insulin regular
    C. Insulin NPH
    D. Insulin glargine

11. Which oral antidiabetic medication should you temporarily withhold in patients undergoing radiologic procedures involving the parenteral administration of iodinated contrast media?
    A. Pioglitazone
    B. Glyburide
    C. Sitagliptin
    D. Metformin

12. Which antidiabetic medication has the potential to cause acute pancreatitis?
    A. Glucophage
    B. Januvia
    C. Levemir
    D. Amaryl

13. Which medication is available by the brand names DiaBeta, Glynase, and Micronase?
    A. Glimepiride
    B. Glipizide
    C. Glyburide
    D. Metformin

14. Which of the following is used to treat diabetic ketoacidosis?
    A. Metformin
    B. Insulin
    C. Glipizide
    D. Rosiglitazone

15. Which medication works to increase insulin sensitivity by affecting the peroxisome proliferator-activated receptor γ (PPAR γ)?
    A. Insulin lispro
    B. Metformin
    C. Pioglitazone
    D. Sitagliptin

Anti-Infective Agents

Jason C. Gallagher, PharmD, BCPS
Carol Holtzman, PharmD, MSc

Drug Class: Aminoglycosides

Introduction

Aminoglycosides are bactericidal, Gram-negative agents that are used in serious infections. They are notable for their toxicities, namely nephrotoxicity and ototoxicity. They are often used empirically and then transitioned to more safe agents as culture results become available. Gentamicin and tobramycin are extremely similar drugs, with virtually identical pharmacokinetics and dosing. Only minor differences in spectra separate them. Neomycin is combined with polymyxin and used topically for superficial infections.

Mechanism of Action for the Drug Class

Irreversibly bind to the 30S ribosomal subunit, disrupting bacterial protein synthesis and resulting in cell death.

Members of the Drug Class

In this section: Gentamicin, tobramycin, neomycin-polymyxin B
   Others: Amikacin, streptomycin

▪ Gentamicin

Brand Name
Garamycin

Generic Name
Gentamicin

Dosage Forms
Injection

Usage

- Systemic aerobic Gram-negative infections of the bloodstream, lung, skin and soft tissue, bone, CNS, abdomen, heart, including those caused by *Pseudomonas aeruginosa**, systemic infections (in particular those of the bloodstream and/or heart) caused by staphylococci, streptococci, or enterococci (treatment must be in combination with a cell-wall active agent for Gram-positive infections)

Dosing

- Initial dose:
   - Conventional dosing: 1.5–2 mg/kg per dose every 8 hours based on ideal or adjusted body weight
   - Extended-interval dosing: 5–7 mg/kg per day based on ideal or adjusted body weight
- Renal dosage adjustment:
   - Dosing must be individualized based on CrCl and therapeutic drug monitoring
- Pharmacokinetic monitoring:
   - Peaks associated with efficacy range from 5 to 10 µg/ml, with higher concentrations for more severe or resistant infections; troughs associated with decreased nephrotoxicity range from <1 to 2 µg/mL; extended-interval dosing is monitored via nomograms with concentrations measured 6–14 hours from the time of administration. Do not use traditional peak and trough concentrations to monitor aminoglycosides dosed this way.

Adverse Reactions: Most Common

- Electrolyte wasting (particularly potassium and magnesium); nephrotoxicity, manifesting usually as increased SrCr before changes in urine output are seen

Adverse Reactions: Rare/Severe/Important

- Ototoxicity, neuromuscular blockade

Major Drug Interactions

Drugs Affecting Gentamicin

- Concomitant oto- or nephrotoxic agents: Additive oto- or nephrotoxicity

Gentamicin's Effect on Other Drugs

- Neuromuscular blocking agents: Potentiated neuromuscular blockade

Counseling Point

- Report any changes in hearing function or decline in urination to a healthcare practitioner immediately

Key Points

- Monitor serum peak and trough levels to ensure non-toxic levels. Nephrotoxicity is associated with elevated trough concentrations.
- Ototoxicity is irreversible. Patients receiving extended courses of aminoglycosides must have hearing monitored. Aminoglycosides should be discontinued at the first sign of hearing or balance problems.
- Extended-interval dosing may be more effective and less nephrotoxic than traditional dosing. However, it is not ideal for patients with changing renal function.
- Dosage should be based on ideal or adjusted body weight, not total body weight

■ Tobramycin

Brand Names
Tobrex, Tobi (inhalation)

Generic Name
Tobramycin

Dosing
- IV: Same as gentamicin
- Inhalation: 300 mg every 12 hours

Usage
- IV: Same as gentamicin
- Inhalation: Given to improve pulmonary function in cystic fibrosis by decreasing bacterial colony counts

Key Points
- All of the preceding points for gentamicin apply to tobramycin. Tobramycin has slightly better activity against *P. aeruginosa* than gentamicin, and gentamicin has slightly better Gram-positive activity than tobramycin, but they are otherwise nearly identical.
- Inhalation therapy with tobramycin is used to prevent exacerbations in cystic fibrosis patients. It should not be used as monotherapy to treat pneumonia.

■ Neomycin-Polymyxin B

Brand Name
Neosporin

Generic Name
Neomycin-polymyxin B

Dosage Forms
Topical: Ointment, cream

Usage
- Minor skin infections

Dosing
- Apply to affected area three to four times daily

Adverse Reactions: Most Common
- Local irritation

Counseling Points
- Do not use for deep wounds, puncture wounds, animal or human bites, or serious burns
- Do not apply to the eyes
- Cover treated area with a gauze or bandage
- See a healthcare provider if the wound does not begin to heal in a few days

Key Points
- Neomycin is an aminoglycoside antibiotic. It is often coupled with polymyxin B in a topical formulation branded Neosporin. Note that not all products that contain the Neosporin name contain the neomycin/polymyxin B combination.
- Topical antibiotics are not effective in the treatment of skin infections that are any more severe than superficial

---

Drug Class: Antimycobacterial Agents

Introduction

Mycobacteria such as *Mycobacterium tuberculosis* have cell walls with a very different anatomy from other bacteria. Many antibiotics are not active against mycobacteria. Isoniazid and rifampin are both highly active against *M. tuberculosis* and are the two most important drugs in the treatment of tuberculosis. They are often used in combination in the treatment of tuberculosis, frequently with other agents as well.

Mechanism of Action for the Drug Class

Isoniazid inhibits the synthesis of mycolic acids, an essential component of the mycobacterial cell wall. Rifampin inhibits the synthesis of RNA by preventing the action of RNA polymerase. Its activity is not specific to mycobacteria.

Members of the Drug Class
In this section: Isoniazid, rifampin
Others: Ethambutol, pyrazinamide, rifabutin, rifapentine

■ Isoniazid

Brand Names
Laniazid, Nydrazid

Generic Name
Isoniazid

Dosage Forms

Tablets, solution, injection

Usage

- Treatment of active and latent tuberculosis

Dosing

- Active tuberculosis: 5 mg/kg daily (maximum of 300 mg/dose) or 15 mg/kg two to three times weekly (maximum of 900 mg/dose)
- Latent tuberculosis: 5 mg/kg daily (maximum of 300 mg/dose)
- Hepatic impairment:
  ○ In patients with moderate to severe hepatic dysfunction, consider reducing the dose or extending the dosing interval

Adverse Reactions: Most Common

- Peripheral neuropathy, elevated liver function tests, abdominal pain

Adverse Reactions: Rare/Severe/Important

- Hepatitis, hypersensitivity, anemia, thrombocytopenia, systemic lupus erythematosus

Major Drug Interactions

Drugs Affecting Isoniazid

- Cycloserine, ethionamide: Potentiated nervous system toxicity
- Ethanol: Increased hepatotoxicity

Isoniazid's Effect on Other Drugs

- Carbamazepine: Increased levels
- Phenytoin: Increased levels
- Serotonergic agents: Potential serotonin syndrome secondary to the weak MAO-inhibiting effect of isoniazid

Counseling Points

- Avoid alcohol intake while on isoniazid
- Report persistent abdominal pain (≥3 days' duration), dark urine, fever, or fatigue because these may be signs of liver problems

Key Points

- For treatment of active tuberculosis, must be part of a multidrug regimen
- Administer with pyridoxine (vitamin B_6) to prevent peripheral neuropathy
- Common abbreviation is INH

■ Rifampin

Brand Names

Rifadin, Rimactane

Generic Name

Rifampin

Dosage Forms

Capsules, injection

Usage

- Active and latent tuberculosis, treatment of asymptomatic carriers of *Neisseria meningitides*, synergistic therapy for Gram-positive infections (such as endocarditis) with other antibiotics

Dosing

- 600 mg IV or PO every 24 hours
- Hepatic adjustment:
  ○ In patients with moderate to severe hepatic dysfunction, consider reducing the dose or extending the dosing interval

Adverse Reactions: Most Common

- Nausea, vomiting, cramps, rash, fever, drowsiness, elevated liver function tests

Adverse Reactions: Rare/Severe/Important

- Hypersensitivity, hyperbilirubinemia, thrombocytopenia

Major Drug Interactions

Drugs Affecting Rifampin

- Antacids: May reduce absorption of rifampin
- Cotrimoxazole: May increase the levels of rifampin
- Isoniazid or halothane: Potentiate hepatotoxicity

Rifampin's Effect on Other Drugs

- Rifampin is a potent inducer of many hepatic enzymes, particularly of the cytochrome P450 system. Careful monitoring of patients on concomitant drugs that are metabolized via the liver is recommended.
- Examples of drugs that are known to be cleared more rapidly by rifampin include: phenytoin, disopyramide, quinidine, warfarin, azole antifungals, diltiazem, nifedipine, barbiturates, β-blockers, chloramphenicol, clarithromycin, digoxin, oral contraceptive, doxycycline, oral hypoglycemic agents, levothyroxine, methadone, narcotic analgesics, tricyclic antidepressants, tacrolimus, cyclosporine, and theophylline. Decreased therapeutic effects of these drugs are common with coadministration.

Counseling Point

- Drug will turn your bodily fluids orange/red. This includes tears, urine, and sweat. Contact lenses will be stained by this red color and should not be worn during rifampin therapy.

Key Points

- Always screen patients for drug interactions when rifampin therapy is started. If interactions cannot be avoided, careful monitoring is required.
- Rifabutin is a related drug with somewhat less potent enzyme induction that may be used in place of rifampin for some indications
- In the treatment of active tuberculosis, combination therapy is always needed, not rifampin alone

Introduction

Penicillins were the second class of antibiotics to be developed. They make up a very large class of antibiotics and vary between agents with broad antimicrobial spectra and more narrow-spectrum agents. Some of them are able to be given orally.

Mechanism of Action for the Drug Class

Inhibits bacterial cell growth in susceptible bacteria by inhibiting transpeptidase enzymes (also known as penicillin-binding proteins), preventing the cross-linking of peptidoglycan strands and thereby inhibiting the synthesis of the bacterial cell wall

Adverse Reactions for the Drug Class: Most Common

- Nausea, vomiting, diarrhea, rash

Adverse Reactions for the Drug Class: Rare/Severe/Important

- Hypersensitivity, anaphylaxis, seizures, pseudomembranous colitis

Major Drug Interactions for the Drug Class

Drugs Affecting Penicillins

- Probenecid: Decreases the renal tubular secretion of penicillins and will result in increased and prolonged serum concentrations
- Chloramphenicol, macrolides, sulfonamides, and tetracyclines interfere with the bactericidal effects of penicillins

Counseling Points for the Drug Class

- Complete entire prescription. Do not stop taking the medication when you feel better.

Key Points for the Drug Class

- Use with caution in patients allergic to cephalosporin antibiotics

Members of the Drug Class

In this section: Amoxicillin, amoxicillin/clavulanate, penicillin

Others: Ampicillin, cloxacillin, dicloxacillin, nafcillin, oxacillin, piperacillin, piperacillin/tazobactam, ticarcillin/clavulanate

■ Amoxicillin

Brand Names

Amoxil, Trimox

Generic Name

Amoxicillin

Dosage Forms

Capsules, tablets, suspension

Usage

- Upper respiratory tract infections*, urinary tract infections, skin and skin structure infections, *Helicobacter pylori* infection*

Dosing

- Adults:
  - Mild–moderate infections: 250 mg three times daily or 500 mg twice daily
  - Moderate–severe infections: 500 mg three times daily or 875 mg twice daily
- Children:
  - 20–40 mg/kg three times daily or 25–45 mg/kg twice daily
- Renal dosage adjustment:
  - Adjust with a CrCl of <30 ml/minute

Key Point

- Amoxicillin and ampicillin have nearly identical antimicrobial spectra, but amoxicillin has much better oral absorption

■ Amoxicillin/Clavulanate

Brand Name

Augmentin

Generic Name

Amoxicillin/clavulanate

Dosage Forms

Tablets, suspension

Usage

- Upper and lower respiratory tract infections*, skin and skin structure infections*, urinary tract infections, mixed aerobic and anaerobic infections

Dosing

- Dosing is based on the amoxicillin component
- Adults:
  - Mild–moderate infections: 250 mg three times daily or 500 mg twice daily
  - Moderate–severe infections: 500 mg three times daily or 875 mg twice daily
- Children:
  - Otitis media: 45 mg/kg per day in two divided doses or 40 mg/kg per day in three divided doses
  - Less severe infections: 25 mg/kg/day in two divided doses or 20 mg/kg/day in three divided doses
- Renal dosage adjustment:
  - Adjust with a CrCl <30 ml/minute

Counseling Point

- To minimize gastrointestinal-adverse events, take at the start of a meal

Key Points

- Twice-daily dosing is associated with significantly less diarrhea

- The 250- and 500-mg tablets contain the same quantity of clavulanic acid; therefore, do not substitute two 250-mg tablets for one 500-mg tablet
- Amoxicillin/clavulanate has a significantly broader antimicrobial spectrum than amoxicillin alone. This is advantageous in treating some potentially drug-resistant infections but not needed in those likely to be drug susceptible.

■ Penicillin

Brand Names
Beepen-VK, Pen-VK, Veetids

Generic Name
Penicillin

Dosage Forms
Tablets, oral solution

Usage
- Streptococcal infections*, uncomplicated anthrax, necrotizing ulcerative gingivitis, prophylaxis of pneumococcal infections, prophylaxis of recurrent rheumatic fever

Dosing
- 250–500 mg two to three times daily
- Renal dosage adjustment:
  - CrCl <10 or dialysis: Administer twice daily

Drug Class: Cephalosporins

Introduction
Cephalosporins are β-lactam antibiotics and one of the largest classes of antibiotics. They are more resistant to β-lactamase enzymes (enzymes produced by bacteria to destroy β-lactams) than penicillins, although β-lactamases that destroy cephalosporins have since evolved. They have more broad-spectrum antimicrobial activity than penicillins, activity that broadens in spectrum moving "down" the generations from first- to fourth-generation agents. The cephalosporins listed here are among the most frequently used and are representative of the much larger category of drugs.

Mechanism of Action for the Drug Class
Inhibits bacterial cell growth in susceptible bacteria by inhibiting transpeptidase enzymes (also known as penicillin-binding proteins), preventing the cross-linking of peptidoglycan strands and thereby inhibiting the synthesis of the bacterial cell wall

Adverse Reactions for the Drug Class: Most Common
- Hypersensitivity, rash, diarrhea

Adverse Reactions for the Drug Class: Rare/Severe/Important
- Anaphylaxis, bone marrow suppression, *Clostridium difficile*–associated diarrhea

Counseling Points for the Drug Class
- Complete entire prescription
- Report any signs of an allergic reactions such as a rash or hives to your healthcare practitioner immediately

Key Point for the Drug Class
- In patients allergic to a penicillin derivative, caution should be exercised. Cross-reactivity between the two types of β-lactams seems to be lower than initially suggested but is still possible.

Members of the Drug Class
In this section: Cefprozil, ceftriaxone, cefuroxime, cephalexin

Others: Cefaclor, cefadroxil, cefamandole, cefazolin, cefdinir, cefixime, cefonicid, cefoperazone, ceforanide, cefotaxime, cefotetan, cefoxitin, cefprozil, ceftazidime, ceftibuten, ceftizoxime, cephalexin, cephalothin, cephapirin, loracarbef, moxalactam

■ Cefprozil

Brand Name
Cefzil

Generic Name
Cefprozil

Dosage Forms
Tablets, suspension

Usage
- Upper and lower respiratory tract infections*, uncomplicated skin and skin structure infections*, tonsillitis

Dosing
- Adults: 250–500 mg twice daily
- Children: 7.5 mg/kg twice daily or 20 mg/kg daily, depending on the indication
- Renal dosage adjustment:
  - Reduce dose 50% with a creatinine clearance of <30 ml/minute

Adverse Reactions: Most Common
- Nausea, vomiting

Major Drug Interactions

Drugs Affecting Cefprozil
- Probenecid: Increases concentrations of cefprozil through impaired excretion

Key Points
- The oral suspension contains phenylalanine and should be avoided in patients with phenylketonuria
- This is a second-generation cephalosporin

■ Ceftriaxone

Brand Name
Rocephin

Generic Name
Ceftriaxone

Dosage Forms
Injection (IV and IM)

Usage
- Upper and lower respiratory tract infections*, skin and skin structure infections, urinary tract infections*, gonorrhea*, pelvic inflammatory disease, bacteremia, endocarditis, bone and joint infections, intra-abdominal infections, meningitis*, surgical prophylaxis, Lyme disease

Dosing
- Adults:
  - 1–2 g given once or twice daily; maximum daily dose not to exceed 4 g
  - Meningitis: 2 g IV every 12 hours
  - Gonorrhea: 125 mg IM given once
- Pediatrics:
  - 50–75 mg/kg given daily (in one or two divided doses); maximum daily dose should not exceed 2 g
  - Meningitis: 100 mg/kg daily (in one to two divided doses); maximum daily dose should not exceed 4 g

Adverse Reactions: Most Common
- Injection site (local irritation)
- Biliary sludging in neonates

Key Points
- In patients receiving long-term therapy, ceftriaxone-calcium may deposit in the gallbladder. This has been associated with symptoms of gallbladder disease. This salt deposit and the subsequent symptoms are reversible upon discontinuation of ceftriaxone therapy.
- Biliary sludging may lead to jaundice in neonates, and alternative cephalosporins should be used in them
- This is a third-generation cephalosporin
- Patients being treated for gonorrhea should receive concomitant therapy for chlamydia

■ Cefuroxime

Brand Name
Ceftin

Generic Name
Cefuroxime

Dosage Forms
Tablets, suspension, injection

Usage
- Upper and lower respiratory tract infections*, uncomplicated skin and skin structure infections urinary tract infections*, gonorrhea*, tonsillitis, early Lyme disease

Dosing
- Adults: 250–500 mg twice daily
- Pediatrics (under 12 years): 20–30 mg/kg per day divided into two doses (maximum daily dose:1 g)
- Gonorrhea (adults): 1 g given once
- Renal dosage adjustment:
  - Dose every 24 hours with a CrCl of <10 ml/ minute

Key Points
- Available both intravenously and orally, unlike many β-lactam antibiotics
- This is a second-generation cephalosporin and has a similar antimicrobial spectrum to cefprozil
- Patients being treated for gonorrhea should receive concomitant therapy for chlamydia

■ Cephalexin

Brand Names
Keflex, Keftab

Generic Name
Cephalexin

Dosage Forms
Capsules, suspension

Usage
- Upper respiratory tract infections*, uncomplicated skin and soft tissue infections*, urinary tract infections

Dosing
- Adults: 1–4 g daily in divided doses; most commonly 250 mg four times daily
- Pediatrics: 25–50 mg/kg per day in two to four divided doses; in the treatment of acute otitis media, 75–100 mg/kg per day in four divided doses should be given
- Renal dosage adjustment:
  - Interval should be increased with a CrCl <40 ml/ minute

Key Points
- Most commonly used for skin infections, but it is ineffective against methicillin-resistant *Staphylococcus aureus* (MRSA) like all other currently available β-lactams. As MRSA increases, the usefulness of cephalexin decreases for skin infections.
- This is a first-generation cephalosporin

Drug Class: Fluoroquinolones

Introduction

Fluoroquinolones are among the most frequently used antibiotics. Their utility is driven by their relatively broad antimicrobial spectra and their once- or twice-daily dosing strata. All are available both intravenously and orally, making transitional therapy easy in the inpatient setting. Unfortunately, frequent utilization of fluoroquinolones has led to inevitable increases in antimicrobial resistance, particularly in *P. aeruginosa* and *Escherichia coli*.

Mechanism of Action for the Drug Class

Fluoroquinolones inhibit DNA gyrase (topoisomerase II) and topoisomerase IV, which results in an inability for bacterial DNA to supercoil; this results in a bactericidal effect

Adverse Reactions for the Drug Class: Most Common

- Headache, dizziness, confusion, photosensitivity, nausea, diarrhea

Adverse Reactions for the Drug Class: Rare/Severe/Important

- QTc prolongation, hypotension, tremor, seizures, skin reactions, hepatitis, acute interstitial nephritis, arthropathy, tendon rupture (Achilles tendon), hypoglycemia, pseudomembranous colitis

Major Drug Interactions for the Drug Class

Drugs Affecting Fluoroquinolones

- Di- and trivalent cations: Greatly decrease fluoroquinolone absorption

Fluoroquinolone Effects on Other Drugs

- QTc-prolonging drugs: Potentiated QTc prolongation, possibly leading to polymorphic ventricular tachycardia

Counseling Points for the Drug Class

- Complete full prescribed course of therapy
- Separate administration from di- and trivalent cations by at least 2 hours
- Avoid excessive exposure to sunlight; use sunscreen if exposure is unavoidable

Key Points for the Drug Class

- The safety and efficacy of fluoroquinolones in children <18 years of age (except for the use of ciprofloxacin in inhalational anthrax for postexposure and children with cystic fibrosis), pregnant women, and lactating women has not been established. They are generally avoided in these populations for that reason.

Members of the Drug Class

In this section: Ciprofloxacin, levofloxacin, moxifloxacin
Others: Gemifloxacin, ofloxacin

■ Ciprofloxacin

Brand Names

Cipro, Cipro XR

Generic Name

Ciprofloxacin

Dosage Forms

Tablets, extended-release tablets, suspension, injection, ophthalmic solution and ointment, otic suspension

Usage

- Upper and lower respiratory tract infections*, urinary tract infections*, intra-abdominal infections*, skin and soft tissue infections, osteomyelitis, infectious diarrhea, gonorrhea, anthrax

Dosing

- Oral: 250–750 mg twice daily dependent on the location and severity of infection
- Oral extended release: 500–1000 mg daily for urinary tract infections
- IV: 200–400 mg twice or three times daily dependent on the location and severity of infection
- Renal dosage adjustment:
  - Required with CrCl of <30–50 ml/minute

Major Drug Interactions

Drugs Affecting Ciprofloxacin

- NSAIDs: May increase the risk of CNS stimulation and/or seizures

Ciprofloxacin's Effect on Other Drugs

- Theophylline: Concentrations increase on average by 33% but may be much higher
- Phenytoin: Both increased and decreased levels have been reported; close monitoring is recommended
- Warfarin: Enhanced anticoagulant effect

Key Points

- Ciprofloxacin has less Gram-positive activity than other fluoroquinolones, and treatment failures have been reported in streptococcal pneumonia. It is better used in hospital-acquired pneumonia than community-acquired pneumonia.
- Ciprofloxacin is one of two fluoroquinolones with clinically useful activity against *P. aeruginosa*, although resistance to it is high in many hospitals
- Resistance in *Neisseria gonorrhea* to fluoroquinolones has risen to the point that they are no longer preferred agents in the treatment of gonorrhea

■ Levofloxacin

Brand Name

Levaquin

Generic Name

Levofloxacin

Dosage Forms

Tablets and injection

Usage

- Upper and lower respiratory tract infections*, urinary tract infections*, skin and soft tissue infections*

Dosing

- 250–750 mg once daily, depending on indication
- Renal dosage adjustment:
  - Dose adjust with a CrCl <50 ml/minute

Major Drug Interactions

Drugs Affecting Levofloxacin

- NSAIDs: May increase the risk of CNS stimulation and/or seizures

Levofloxacin's Effect on Other Drugs

- Antidiabetic agents: May result in enhanced hypoglycemic effect

Key Points

- Levofloxacin has strong Gram-negative and Gram-positive activity, and it is useful in both hospital-acquired and community-acquired infections such as pneumonia
- Levofloxacin is one of two fluoroquinolones with clinically useful activity against P. aeruginosa, although resistance to it is high in many hospitals
- Some indications for levofloxacin use higher dosing to shorten the course of therapy (e.g., community-acquired pneumonia)
- Levofloxacin has excellent absorption and is given in equivalent doses orally and intravenously

■ Moxifloxacin

Brand Name
Avelox

Generic Name
Moxifloxacin

Dosage Forms
Tablets, injection

Usage

- Upper and lower respiratory tract infections*, skin and soft tissue infections*, intra-abdominal infections

Dosing

- 400 mg once daily
- No renal dose adjustment is necessary

Key Points

- Unlike most other fluoroquinolones (including the two listed here), moxifloxacin is not eliminated by the kidney but is instead excreted via the biliary tract. For this reason, it is not used in the treatment of urinary tract infections.
- Moxifloxacin has potent activity against many Gram-positive organisms and has more activity against anaerobic bacteria than other fluoroquinolones. This increases its utility in intra-abdominal infections.
- Moxifloxacin lacks activity against P. aeruginosa and is more suitable for therapy of community-acquired pneumonia than hospital-acquired pneumonia

---

Drug Class: Glycopeptide

Introduction

The glycopeptides are cell-wall synthesis inhibitors of Gram-positive organisms. The rise of antimicrobial resistance among S. aureus has led to vancomycin becoming one of the most commonly used antibiotics in hospitals. The poor bioavailability of vancomycin necessitates IV therapy for systemic infections, although it is given orally for C. difficile infections of the colon.

Mechanism of Action for the Drug Class

Glycopeptides bind to D-alanyl-D-alanine in the growing bacterial cell wall, preventing the elongation of peptidoglycan strands and halting cell wall synthesis. They are only effective against Gram-positive organisms.

Members of the Drug Class

In this section: Vancomycin

Others: Teicoplanin (outside the United States), telavancin (a lipoglycopeptide)

■ Vancomycin

Brand Name
Vancocin

Generic Name
Vancomycin

Dosage Forms
Injection, capsules

Usage

- Injection: Treatment of systemic infections caused by Gram-positive organisms including those of the respiratory tract*, bloodstream*, skin and skin structure*, gastrointestinal system, and genitourinary tract
- Oral: Treatment of C. difficile infection*

Dosing

- Oral:
  - 125–500 mg every 6 hours

- Injection:
  - Adults: 15–20 mg/kg twice daily
  - Children: 10 mg/kg per dose given every 6 hours
  - Infants: Loading dose of 15 mg/kg followed 10 mg/kg every 12 hours (first week of life) or every 8 hours (>1 week of life up to 1 month of life)
- Renal dosage adjustment:
  - Dose of the intravenous formulation needs to be reduced based on creatinine clearance. Most clinicians reduce doses of vancomycin at a CrCl of 50–60 ml/minute or less.

Pharmacokinetic Monitoring
- Therapeutic troughs are generally considered to be from 10 to 20 mg/liter. Troughs of >15–20 mg/liter may be associated with nephrotoxicity.
- Peaks are no longer routinely monitored but should be <60 mg/liter
- Evidence correlating vancomycin concentrations with efficacy is lacking

Adverse Reactions: Most Common
- Infusion related: "red man's syndrome" (rash, flushing, tachycardia, hypotension), phlebitis, nephrotoxicity (higher doses)

Adverse Reactions: Rare/Severe/Important
- Bone marrow suppression (rare), hypersensitivity (rare)

Major Drug Interactions
Drugs Affecting Vancomycin
- Nephrotoxic or ototoxic agents: Enhanced toxicity

Vancomycin's Effect on Other Drugs
- Anesthesia: May result in enhanced histamine release and rash

Counseling Point
- Nurses: Administer vancomycin at a rate of 1 g/hour to prevent infusion-related toxicity

Key Points
- Vancomycin is a drug of choice for infections caused by MRSA
- Closely monitor patients on concomitant nephrotoxic or ototoxic agents
- Oral therapy is ineffective for the treatment of systemic infection
- Systemic therapy is ineffective for the treatment of enterocolitis or pseudomembranous colitis

---

Drug Class: Lincosamide

Introduction
Clindamycin is the only commonly used lincosamide. Clindamycin has good activity against staphylococci, streptococci, and anaerobic organisms. It is being used more frequently now for the treatment of skin infections due to the increase in MRSA infections seen in the community.

Mechanism of Action for the Drug Class
Clindamycin binds to the 50S subunit of bacterial ribosomes, suppressing protein synthesis.

Members of the Drug Class
In this section: Clindamycin
   Other: Lincomycin

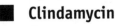 Clindamycin

Brand Name
Cleocin

Generic Name
Clindamycin

Dosage Forms
Capsules, injection

Usage
- Skin and skin structure infections*, aspiration pneumonia, intra-abdominal infections*

Dosing
- Adults:
  - Oral: 150–450 mg every 6–8 hours
  - IV: 300–900 mg every 6–8 hours
- Pediatrics:
  - 8–20 mg/kg per day oral or IV in three to four divided doses
- Hepatic dosage adjustment:
  - In patients with moderate to severe hepatic dysfunction, consider reducing the dose or extending the dosing interval

Adverse Reactions: Most Common
- Abdominal pain, nausea, vomiting, rash, pruritus

Adverse Reactions: Rare/Severe/Important
- Pseudomembranous colitis, hypersensitivity, jaundice, severe skin eruption

Major Drug Interactions
Clindamycin's Effect on Other Drugs
- Neuromuscular blocking agents: Enhanced neuromuscular blockade

Counseling Point

- To avoid esophageal irritation, take clindamycin capsules with a full glass of water

Key Points

- *C. difficile*–associated disease, including pseudomembranous colitis, has been associated with all classes of antibiotics, but clindamycin is perhaps most closely associated with it in the minds of many clinicians. It is a popular exam question.
- Many, but not all, strains of MRSA are susceptible to clindamycin. Community-associated strains are much more likely to be susceptible than hospital-acquired strains.

Drug Class: Macrolides

Introduction

Macrolides are antibiotics commonly used for respiratory tract infections. Clarithromycin and erythromycin in particular are strong inhibitors of the cytochrome P450 enzyme system, and clinicians must be wary of drug interactions with them.

Mechanism of Action for the Drug Class

Macrolides inhibit bacterial protein synthesis by binding to the 50S ribosomal subunit, generally resulting in a bacteriostatic effect.

Adverse Reactions for the Drug Class: Most Common

- Nausea, diarrhea, abdominal pain, pain at injection site (IV), rash, elevated liver function tests

Adverse Reactions for the Drug Class: Rare/Severe/Important

- Allergic reaction

Members of the Drug Class

In this section: Azithromycin, clarithromycin, erythromycin
  Others: Dirithromycin, troleandomycin

■ Azithromycin

Brand Names

Zithromax, Z-pak, Zmax

Generic Name

Azithromycin

Dosage Forms

Capsules, tablets, suspension, injection

Usage

- Community-acquired upper and lower respiratory tract infections*, chlamydia, treatment and prophylaxis of *Mycobacteria avium intracellulare* complex (MAI or MAC)*, skin and skin structure infections, syphilis

Dosing

- Adults:
  - Most indications: 500 or 250 mg once daily
    - Z-pak is 500 mg on day 1, followed by 250 mg on days 2–5
    - Zmax is a single 2-g dose
  - Prevention of MAC: 1200 mg once weekly
  - Treatment of disseminated MAC: 600 mg daily
- Pediatrics:
  - Most indications: 5–12 mg/kg once daily
  - Otitis media can be 30 mg/kg once

Adverse Reactions: Most Common

- Pain at injection site (IV)

Major Drug Interactions

In drug interaction studies, azithromycin has not been reported to result in metabolic interactions associated with other macrolides. However, careful monitoring is suggested in patients receiving digoxin, theophylline, ergotamine derivatives, triazolam, warfarin, and other agents known to be metabolized via the cytochrome P450 enzyme system.

Counseling Points

- Capsules and suspension (bottle) should not be administered with food (at least 1 hour before or 2 hours after a meal)
- Suspension powder packet and tablet may be administered without regard to meals
- Parenteral product should not be given as a bolus injection or intramuscularly
- Patients who vomit immediately after taking azithromycin may need to be re-dosed but should not do this without consulting their healthcare provider

Key Points

- Rising resistance rates to macrolides in *S. pneumoniae* have led to decreased efficacy for azithromycin. It should not be used as monotherapy in severely ill patients with pneumonia.
- Azithromycin has a very long terminal half-life, which allows for short-course therapy for many indications

Clarithromycin

Brand Names
Biaxin, Biaxin-XL

Generic Name
Clarithromycin

Dosage Forms
Tablets, extended-release tablets, suspension

Usage
- Community-acquired upper and lower respiratory tract infections*, skin and skin structure infections, treatment of MAI or MAC*, treatment of *H. pylori* infection (in combination with amoxicillin and omeprazole or lansoprazole)

Dosing
- Adults:
  - Most indications: 250–500 mg every 12 hours
  - Extended release: 1000 mg every 24 hours
- Pediatrics:
  - 7.5 mg/kg every 12 hours
- Renal dosage adjustment:
  - Dose adjusted with a CrCl <60 ml/minute

Adverse Reactions: Most Common
- Altered taste

Adverse Reactions: Rare/Severe/Important
- Prolonged QTc interval (especially when administered with concomitant drugs that prolong the QTc interval); severe hepatic dysfunction

Major Drug Interactions
Drugs Affecting Clarithromycin
- Ritonavir will increase the concentration of clarithromycin by 77% and its metabolite by 100%

Clarithromycin's Effect on Other Drugs
- Theophylline concentrations: Increase by 20% on average
- Carbamazepine levels will increase
- Warfarin: Enhanced anticoagulant effect
- Digoxin levels: Increase significantly
- Ergot derivatives: May result in acute ergot toxicity; combination is contraindicated
- QTc-prolonging drugs: Potentiated QTc prolongation, possibly leading to polymorphic ventricular tachycardia

Contraindications
- Concomitant administration with cisapride, pimozide, or terfenadine

Counseling Point
- Take tablets and suspension without regard to meals; take extended-release tablets with food

Key Points
- Drug interactions reported with erythromycin are likely to occur with clarithromycin
- Patients receiving drugs that are metabolized by the cytochrome P450 enzyme system should be closely monitored

Erythromycin

Brand Names
Ery-Tab, E-Mycin, EES, EryPed, Ilosone

Generic Name
Erythromycin

Dosage Forms
Ophthalmic ointment; topical ointment, gel, and solution; multiple oral formulations; injection

Usage
- Community-acquired upper and lower respiratory tract infections*, skin and skin structure infections, chlamydia, conjunctivitis*, preoperative bowel preparation*

Dosing:
- Adults:
  - Mild–moderate infection: 250–500 mg four times daily
  - Severe infection: 500–1000 mg every 6 hours
- Pediatrics:
  - Mild–moderate infection: 7.5–12.5 mg (base)/kg four times daily
  - Severe infection: 15–25 mg/kg (base) four times daily

Adverse Reactions: Most Common
- Infusion site pain (IV), phlebitis, prolonged QTc interval, diarrhea

Adverse Reactions: Rare/Severe/Important
- Hepatotoxicity (estolate form), ototoxicity (high dose)

Major Drug Interactions
Erythromycin's Effect on Other Drugs
- Carbamazepine, valproic acid: Increased levels
- Cyclosporine: Increased levels
- Ergot derivatives: Increased levels (contraindicated)
- Many HmG-CoA reductase inhibitors: Increased risk of rhabdomyolysis
- Midazolam, triazolam: Decreased clearance, prolonged sedative effect
- Theophylline: Increased concentrations
- Warfarin: Potentiated anticoagulant effect
- QTc-prolonging drugs: Potentiated QTc prolongation, possibly leading to polymorphic ventricular tachycardia

Counseling Points
- Take with a full glass of water
- Report persistent abdominal pain (>3 days duration)
- Report any changes in hearing function

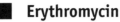

Key Points

- Dosing varies based on the specific salt being used
- Erythromycin is commonly used off-label as a pro-motility agent. This effect also causes more diarrhea with erythromycin than with other macrolides.

- Patients receiving drugs that are metabolized by the cytochrome P450 enzyme system should be closely monitored

---

Drug Class: Nitroimidazole

Introduction

Metronidazole is the only commonly used nitroimidazole. It is unique in that it only has clinically useful activity against anaerobic organisms and is thus frequently used in anaerobic infections. It is also a drug of choice for treating *C. difficile* infections.

Mechanism of Action for the Drug Class

In susceptible organisms, metronidazole is reduced to unidentified polar products, which result in cytotoxic antimicrobial effects.

Members of the Drug Class

In this section: Metronidazole
   Other: Tinidazole

■ Metronidazole

Brand Name
Flagyl

Generic Name
Metronidazole

Dosage Forms
Tablets, extended-release tablets, capsules, injection, topical gel

Usage

- Treatment of anaerobic bacterial infections*, *C. difficile* infection*, trichomoniasis, amebiasis, giardiasis, bacterial vaginosis, pelvic inflammatory disease*, rosacea, *H. pylori* infection (in combination with other drugs), prophylaxis in gastrointestinal surgery

Dosing

- Adults:
  - Most indications: 250–500 mg two to four times daily
  - Trichomoniasis: Can be treated with 2000 mg once

- Pediatrics:
  - 15–50 mg/kg per day in three divided doses
- Hepatic dosage adjustment:
  - In patients with moderate to severe hepatic dysfunction, consider reducing the dose or extending the dosing interval

Adverse Reactions: Most Common

- Nausea, metallic taste, peripheral neuropathy

Adverse Reactions: Rare/Severe/Important

- Pancreatitis, hypersensitivity, stomatitis, confusion, dizziness, seizures

Major Drug Interactions

Drugs Affecting Metronidazole

- Alcohol: May result in a mild disulfiram reaction
- Phenobarbital: Decreased half-life of metronidazole

Metronidazole's Effect on Other Drugs

- Warfarin: Potentiated anticoagulant effect, possibly leading to bleeding events
- Disulfiram: Acute psychosis and confusion
- Lithium: Increased levels

Counseling Points

- Be aware of possible metallic taste
- Minimize alcohol intake due to potential mild disulfiram reaction

Key Points

- Metronidazole is inferior to oral vancomycin for the treatment of severe *C. difficile* infection but equivalent for mild to moderate infection. It is generally used first-line in mild to moderate cases due to its significantly lower cost.
- Metronidazole has excellent bioavailability and is given in similar oral and intravenous doses
- Metronidazole is also given intravaginally to treat bacterial vaginosis

Introduction

The folic acid antagonists, trimethoprim and the sulfonamides, work synergistically to prevent bacterial growth and replication. The sulfonamides were the first antibiotics made available and introduced the antibiotic era. They are still used today, most commonly in trimethoprim/sulfamethoxazole, where the two active ingredients work together in susceptible bacteria.

Mechanism of Action for the Drug Class

Trimethoprim inhibits folate utilization by inhibiting dihydrofolate reductase in bacteria. Sulfamethoxazole and other sulfonamides compete with para-aminobenzoic acid (PABA) in an earlier step in folate synthesis that only exists in bacteria. The two types of drugs have synergistic activity in many bacteria.

Members of the Drug Class

In this section: Trimethoprim/sulfamethoxazole
  Others: Sulfadiazine, sulfisoxazole; topical formulations

■ Trimethoprim/Sulfamethoxazole

Brand Names

Bactrim, Septra

Generic Name

Trimethoprim/Sulfamethoxazole

Dosage Forms

Tablets, suspension, injection

Usage

- Urinary tract infections, upper and lower respiratory tract infections, skin and skin structure infections, treatment and prophylaxis of *Pneumocystis jiroveci* pneumonia, traveler's diarrhea

Dosing

- Adults:
  - Most indications: 1 DS tablet or equivalent (800 mg sulfamethoxazole/160 mg trimethoprim) twice daily
  - *Pneumocystis* prophylaxis: 1 DS tablet daily or three times a week; 1 SS (400 mg sulfamethoxazole/80 mg trimethoprim) daily

  - *Pneumocystis jiroveci* pneumonia: 15–20 mg/kg per/day of trimethoprim component divided in three to four doses
- Children:
  - Most indications: 8–10 mg/kg per day of trimethoprim component divided in three to four doses
  - *Pneumocystis jiroveci* pneumonia: Same as adult dosing
- Renal dosage adjustment:
  - CrCl of 15–30 ml/minute: 50% of the usual dose
  - Listed as contraindicated with CrCl <15 ml/minute but is sometimes still given in lower doses

Adverse Reactions: Most Common

- Nausea, vomiting, anorexia, rash, urticaria, hyperkalemia, arthralgia, myalgias, hepatitis

Adverse Reactions: Rare/Severe/Important

- Toxic epidermal necrolysis, fulminant hepatic necrosis, agranulocytosis, bone marrow suppression, crystalluria, renal failure, anaphylaxis

Major Drug Interactions

Trimethoprim/Sulfamethoxazole's Effect on Other Drugs

- Thiazides: Concomitant use has been associated with thrombocytopenia with purpura in elderly patients
- Phenytoin: Increased half-life by 39%
- Methotrexate: Increased free concentrations
- Oral hypoglycemic agents: Potentiated hypoglycemia
- Digoxin: Serum levels may increase

Counseling Points

- Take oral product with a full glass of water
- Monitor for signs of hypersensitivity

Key Points

- Dosing is based on the trimethoprim component
- The 5:1 ratio of sulfamethoxazole to trimethoprim is consistent among all dosage forms
- Trimethoprim competes with creatinine for renal secretion. SrCr values may increase during therapy that do not reflect true renal dysfunction.

Drug Class: Tetracyclines

Introduction

Tetracyclines are broad-spectrum antibiotics that have most much of their utility due to increases in bacterial resistance. They are still useful for many indications, however, and they are drugs of choice in several tick-borne diseases.

Mechanism of Action for the Drug Class

Tetracyclines inhibit bacterial protein synthesis by reversibly binding to the 30S ribosomal subunit, resulting in a bacteriostatic effect.

Adverse Reactions for the Drug Class: Most Common

- Nausea, vomiting, diarrhea, gastrointestinal pain, rash, photosensitivity reactions, dizziness

Adverse Reactions for the Drug Class: Rare/Severe/Important

- Hypersensitivity, tooth discoloration with prolonged use

Major Drug Interactions for the Drug Class

Drugs Affecting Tetracyclines

- Di- and trivalent cations: Greatly decrease absorption of tetracyclines

Tetracycline Effects on Other Drugs

- Concurrent use of tetracyclines and methoxyflurane has been reported to result in fatal renal toxicity
- Enhances the activity of warfarin
- Diminishes effect of cell-wall active bactericidal antibiotics when used concomitantly (e.g., β-lactams)
- May render oral contraceptives less effective

Counseling Points for the Drug Class

- Administration to children is likely to result in discoloration of the teeth, particularly with prolonged use. Use in children <8 years of age only when the benefit outweighs the risk.
- Dispose of all unused medication because use of outdated tetracycline products may result in Fanconi syndrome, a disorder characterized by kidney damage
- Separate from multivalent cation containing compounds (including milk) by at least 2 hours

Members of the Drug Class

In this section: Doxycycline, minocycline
   Others: Demeclocycline, tetracycline

■ Doxycycline

Brand Name
Vibramycin

Generic Name
Doxycycline

Dosage Forms
Capsules, suspension, injection

Usage

- Community-acquired upper and lower respiratory tract infections*, chlamydia*, Rocky Mountain spotted fever, typhus fever, Q fever, rickettsialpox, and tick fevers caused by rickettsiae, Lyme disease, plague, tularemia

Dosing

- Adults: 100 mg twice daily
- Children <100 lb: 2 mg/lb divided into two doses on the first day, then 1 mg/lb daily thereafter

■ Minocycline

Brand Name
Minocin

Generic Name
Minocycline

Dosage Forms
Capsules, tablets, suspension, injection

Usage

- Community-acquired upper and lower respiratory tract infections*, acne*, skin and soft tissue infections*, Rocky Mountain spotted fever, typhus fever, Q fever, rickettsialpox, Lyme disease, plague, tularemia

[handwritten annotations: carried by ticks; -pneumonia; bacterial infection; from ticks, rodents]

Dosing

- Adults:
  ○ 200 mg once, then 100 mg twice daily
- Children (>8 years of age):
  ○ 4 mg/kg once, then 2 mg/kg twice daily
- Renal dosage adjustment:
  ○ Use not recommended in renal failure

Drug Class: Nitrofuran

Introduction

Nitrofurantoin is the only available nitrofuran. It has one use, the treatment of acute uncomplicated cystitis (a urinary tract infection). Therapeutic concentrations of nitrofurantoin are not reached anywhere in the body but the urinary tract. It is a drug that has become more useful over time as resistance to fluoroquinolones, trimethoprim/sulfamethoxazole, and other first-line drugs has increased, particularly in *E. coli*.

Mechanism of Action for the Drug Class

The mechanism of nitrofurantoin is not exactly known, but it inhibits several bacterial enzyme systems including acetyl coenzyme A, interfering with metabolism and possibly cell-wall synthesis.

■ Nitrofurantoin

Brand Names
Macrodantin, Macrobid

Generic Names
Nitrofurantoin, nitrofurantoin macrocrystals (macrobid)

Dosage Forms
Capsules

Usage
- Urinary tract infections (acute uncomplicated cystitis)

Dosing
- Macrobid: 100 mg twice daily
- Macrodantin: 50–100 mg four times daily

- Renal dosage adjustment:
  - Contraindicated in patients with a CrCl <60 ml/minute

Adverse Reactions: Most Common
- Nausea, headache, diarrhea, rash, dizziness

Adverse Reactions: Rare/Severe/Important
- Chronic, subacute or acute pulmonary hypersensitivity; hepatic toxicity; lupus-like syndrome; exfoliative dermatitis; peripheral neuropathy (may be irreversible), cholestatic jaundice

Major Drug Interactions
Drugs Affecting Nitrofurantoin
- Antacids containing magnesium trisilicate: Decreased absorption of nitrofurantoin
- Probenecid: Increased nitrofurantoin levels

Counseling Point
- Take with food to enhance tolerability and absorption

Key Points
- Nitrofurantoin therapy will produce a false-positive urine glucose test
- Not for use for any infection other than uncomplicated cystitis
- Unlike fluoroquinolones and trimethoprim/sulfamethoxazole, nitrofurantoin is pregnancy category B and often used in pregnant women

Drug Class: Antifungal, Polyene

Introduction

Polyenes are one of the oldest classes of antifungals. There are two agents: amphotericin B, which is given systemically; and nystatin, which is given as topical therapy only. Neither drug can be given orally for systemic fungal infections. Adverse reactions with IV amphotericin B are considerable.

Mechanism of Action for the Drug Class

Polyenes bind to ergosterol in the fungal cell wall causing cell-wall instability and leakage of cytoplasmic contents.

Members of the Drug Class

In this section: Amphotericin B, nystatin

■ Amphotericin B

Brand Names
Amphocin, Fungizone

Generic Name
Amphotericin B deoxycholate

Dosage Forms
Injection

Usage
- Systemic fungal infections caused by yeasts, molds, and dimorphic fungi*; empiric antifungal therapy in febrile neutropenia*; leishmaniasis

Dosing

- 0.3–1.5 mg/kg per day
- Note: Lipid formulations of amphotericin B are available and are given in much higher doses. Fatal overdoses have occurred when the incorrect formulation has been given at the incorrect dose.

Adverse Reactions: Most Common

- Nephrotoxicity, electrolyte wasting (primarily potassium and magnesium), infusion reactions (fever, chills, nausea, flushing, tachycardia, hypotension)

Adverse Reactions: Rare/Severe/Important

- Bronchospasm, hypoxia, arrhythmias, anemia, hypersensitivity

Major Drug Interactions

Drugs Affecting Amphotericin B

- Concomitant nephrotoxic agents potentiate nephrotoxicity (includes, but not limited to, cyclosporine, pentamidine, aminoglycosides, colistin, cisplatin, vancomycin)
- Corticosteroids: may potentiate the potassium wasting effect

Key Points

- Premedicate with diphenhydramine and/or acetaminophen to minimize infusion reactions
- Ensure adequate hydration by providing boluses of saline before and after the infusion to reduce the incidence of nephrotoxicity

- Infuse over at least 2 hours to decrease infusion-related reactions
- Lipid formulations of amphotericin B are commercially available. These agents tend to have a better adverse event profile. Recommended dosing and administration is quite different for these products.

■ Nystatin

Brand Name
Mycostatin

Generic Name
Nystatin

Dosage Forms
Suspension, powder, tablets, cream, ointment

Usage

- Treatment and prophylaxis of cutaneous, mucocutaneous, and superficial candidal infections

Dosing

- 500,000–1 million units three times daily

Adverse Reactions: Most Common

- Mild nausea, vomiting (tablet)

Counseling Point

- Do not apply in large quantity to open wound
- Cover medicated area with a gauze or bandage

Key Point

- Not effective for systemic fungal infection

Drug Class: Antifungal, Triazole

Introduction

The introduction of the azole antifungals changed the way systemic fungal infections were treated. The excellent bioavailability of some of these drugs allows for oral therapy of systemic infections.

Mechanism of Action for the Drug Class

Azole antifungals inhibit the production of ergosterol, a component of the fungal cell membrane, by inhibiting fungal cytochromes P450.

Adverse Reactions for the Drug Class: Most Common

- Vomiting, abdominal pain, nausea, diarrhea, rash
- Drug interactions via cytochrome P450

Adverse Reactions for the Drug Class: Rare/Severe/Important

- Elevated liver function tests (rare severe hepatic toxicity), hypersensitivity

Major Drug Interactions for the Drug Class

- All agents inhibit the cytochrome P450 system and increase concentrations of drugs metabolized via this pathway

Members of the Drug Class

In this section: Fluconazole, itraconazole, voriconazole
    Others: Ketoconazole, numerous topical agents, posaconazole

■ Fluconazole

Brand Name
Diflucan

Generic Name
Fluconazole

Dosage Forms
Tablets, suspension, injection

Usage

- *Candida* infections of the vagina, oropharyngeal cavity, esophagus, bloodstream, and visceral organs*; cryptococcal meningitis*

Dosing

- Adults:
  - Most indications: 200–800 mg once daily
  - Vaginal candidiasis: 150 mg once
- Pediatrics:
  - 3–12 mg/kg once daily
- Renal dosage adjustment:
  - Decrease dose 50% with CrCl <50 ml/minute

Major Drug Interactions

Drugs Affecting Fluconazole

- Hydrochlorothiazide: Increases fluconazole concentrations
- Rifampin: Decreases fluconazole concentrations

Fluconazole's Effect on Other Drugs

- Drugs metabolized via CYP450: Increased concentrations
  - Notable examples: Phenytoin, cyclosporine, tacrolimus, HmG-CoA reductase inhibitors, theophylline
- Warfarin: Potentiated anticoagulant effect

Counseling Point

- Women being treated with fluconazole for vaginal yeast infections should be told that symptoms (such as itching and irritation) are unlikely to subside on day 1 of therapy, even though the infection is successfully treated

Key Points

- Fluconazole has high bioavailability, and oral and intravenous doses are equivalent
- Patients prescribed fluconazole should always be screened for drug interactions
- Unlike other azoles, fluconazole has appreciable renal elimination and needs to be adjusted in renal dysfunction

■ Itraconazole

Brand Name
Sporanox

Generic Name
Itraconazole

Dosage Forms
Capsules, oral solution

Usage

- Candidiasis, mold infections, dimorphic fungal infections, onychomycosis*

Dosing

- 200 mg once daily, sometimes after a loading dose of 200 mg, two or three times daily for 2 or 3 days

Adverse Reactions: Most Common

- Hypokalemia, rash

Adverse Reactions: Rare/Severe/Important

- Negative inotropic effect, especially in patients with underlying congestive heart failure

Major Drug Interactions

Drugs Affecting Itraconazole

- Inducers of CYP450: Decrease itraconazole concentrations
- Inhibitors of CYP450: Increase itraconazole concentrations
- Antacids, H2-receptor antagonists, proton pump inhibitors: Decrease itraconazole absorption

Itraconazole's Effect on Other Drugs

- Drugs metabolized by CYP450: Increased concentrations
- Cisapride, quinidine, dofetilide: QTc prolongation via inhibition of metabolism

Contraindications

- Coadministration with cisapride, pimozide, quinidine, or dofetilide
- Congestive heart failure

Counseling Points

- Oral solution and capsules are not interchangeable
- Take capsules with food; can add a cola beverage to enhance bioavailability

Key Points

- Oral solution has significantly better bioavailability than oral capsules (area under the curve [AUC] increased by 149%)
- Patients prescribed itraconazole should always be screened for drug interactions
- Oral solution does not have to be taken with food; the capsules should be administered with food. In addition, acid-suppressing agents have less of an effect on the bioavailability of the oral solution.

■ Voriconazole

Brand Name
Vfend

Generic Name
Voriconazole

Dosage Forms
Tablets, suspension, injection

Usage

- Primary therapy of invasive aspergillosis*, invasive candidiasis, esophageal candidiasis, mold infections*

Dosing

- IV: 6 mg/kg every 12 hours twice, then 3–4 mg/kg every 12 hours

- Oral: Either same as IV dosage or 400 mg every 12 hours twice, then 200 mg every 12 hours (100 mg every 12 hours for patients <40 kg)
- Renal dosage adjustment:
  - Injection is not recommended for patients with an CrCl <50 ml/minute due to accumulation

Adverse Reactions: Most Common
- Rash, visual events, hepatic enzyme elevations

Adverse Reactions: Rare/Severe/Important
- Hepatic failure, visual hallucinations, gastrointestinal disturbances

Major Drug Interactions
Drugs Affecting Voriconazole
- Inducers of CYP450: Decrease voriconazole concentrations
- Inhibitors of CYP450: Increase voriconazole concentrations

Voriconazole's Effect on Other Drugs
- Drugs metabolized by CYP450: Increased concentrations

Contraindications
- Coadministration with sirolimus, rifampin, rifabutin, efavirenz, ritonavir, long-acting barbiturates, terfenadine, astemizole, cisapride, pimozide, quinidine, ergot alkaloids, carbamazepine

Counseling Points
- Visual effects are common and dose-related. They usually go away after the first few doses.
- Although IV form is relatively contraindicated with a CrCl <50 ml/minute, it may be used when the benefits of therapy outweigh the risks of cyclodextrin accumulation

Key Points
- Injection contains the solubilizer β-cyclodextrin and can accumulate in renal dysfunction
- Patients prescribed voriconazole should always be screened for drug interactions
- Patients on voriconazole should have liver function tests closely monitored

---

Drug Class: Antivirals

Introduction
Acyclovir is a commonly used antiviral agent for many types of herpesvirus infections. Due to the low bioavailability of the oral form and the need for frequent administration, the prodrug valacyclovir was developed. The only other differences between the two drugs are pharmacokinetic.

Mechanism of Action for the Drug Class
Acyclovir is a competitive inhibitor of viral DNA synthesis. Valacyclovir is a prodrug that is rapidly converted to acyclovir in vivo.

Adverse Reactions for the Drug Class: Most Common
- Nausea, vomiting, diarrhea

Adverse Reactions for the Drug Class: Rare/Severe/Important
- Thrombotic thrombocytopenic purpura (immunocompromised host), anaphylaxis, rash, renal failure, dizziness, agitation, crystalluria

Major Drug Interactions for the Drug Class
Drugs Affecting Acyclovir/Valacyclovir
- Probenecid: Increase in the mean half-life and AUC of acyclovir

Counseling Points for the Drug Class
- Initiate therapy as soon as possible; for genital herpes, ideally during the prodromal period; other diseases, at the onset of rash
- Take oral products with a full glass of water to decrease potential for crystallization in the kidney

Members of the Drug Class
In this section: Acyclovir, valacyclovir
   Other: Famciclovir

■ Acyclovir
Brand Name
Zovirax

Generic Name
Acyclovir

Dosage Forms
- Oral: Capsule (200 mg); suspension (200 mg/5 ml); tablet (400 mg, 800 mg)
- Parenteral: Concentrate (25 mg/ml; 50 mg/ml); infusion (500 mg, 1 g)

Usage
- Mucosal, cutaneous, ocular, and systemic herpes simplex infection including genital herpes*; varicella-zoster virus infection including chicken pox and herpes zoster (shingles)*; herpes encephalitis (IV)

Dosing

- Genital herpes:
  - Initial episode: 200 mg five times daily OR 400 mg three times daily for 7–10 days
  - Initial episode (proctitis): 400 mg five times daily for 10 days OR 800 mg three times daily for 7–10 days
  - Severe initial episode: 5–10 mg/kg IV every 8 hours for 2–7 days or until clinical improvement is observed, followed by oral antiviral therapy to complete a total course of at least 10 days of therapy
  - Recurrent episodes: 200 mg five times daily OR 400 mg three times daily OR 800 mg twice daily for 5 days
  - Chronic suppressive therapy: 400 mg twice daily OR 200 mg 3–5 times daily for up to 1 year
- Varicella (chicken pox; initiate therapy within 24–48 hours of the appearance of rash)
  - Immunocompetent children 2 years of age and older <40 kg: 20 mg/kg four times daily for 5 days
  - Immunocompetent patient >40 kg: 800 mg per dose four times daily for 5 days
  - Herpes zoster (shingles; initiate therapy within 24–48 hours of the appearance of rash)
  - Immunocompetent adults and children ≥12 years of age: 800 mg five times daily for 7–10 days
  - HIV-infected patient with dermatomal zoster: 800 mg five times daily for 7–10 days
  - Immunocompromised patients ≥12 years of age: 10 mg/kg IV every 8 hours for 7 days
  - Immunocompromised patients ≤12 years of age: 20 mg/kg IV every 8 hours for 7 days
- Herpes simplex virus infection:
  - Mucosal or cutaneous infection: Adults: 400 mg five times daily for 7–14 days; children: 10 mg/kg/dose three times daily for 7–14 days
  - Parenteral: Adults: 5 mg/kg IV every 8 hours for 7 days; children: 10 mg/kg IV every 8 hours for 7 days
  - Encephalitis: Adults ≥12 years of age: 10 mg/kg IV every 8 hours for at least 10 days; children <12 years of age: 20 mg/kg IV every 8 hours for at least 10 days
- Renal dosage adjustment:
  - Oral therapy: Dose adjust with CrCl <10–25 ml/minute
  - IV therapy: Dose adjust with CrCl <50 ml/minute

■ Valacyclovir

Brand Name
Valtrex

Generic Name
Valacyclovir

Dosage Forms
Caplet

Usage
- Herpes zoster infection*, genital herpes (initial, recurrent, or suppressive therapy)*

Dosing
- Treatment: 500–1000 mg every 8–12 hours
- Suppression: 500–1000 mg daily
- Renal dose adjustment:
  - Decrease dose with a CrCl <30–49 ml/minute

Drug Class: Antiretroviral, Nucleoside/Nucleotide Reverse Transcriptase Inhibitor

Introduction

Nucleoside/nucleotide reverse transcriptase inhibitors (NRTIs) are antiretrovirals for the treatment of HIV. Currently, it is recommended that antiretroviral regimens contain at least two NRTIs in combination with another class of antiretrovirals, such as a nonnucleoside reverse transcriptase inhibitor, a protease inhibitor, an integrase inhibitor, or a CCR5 antagonist. The NRTIs were the first agents to receive the approval of the Food and Drug Administration (FDA) for the treatment of HIV. All NRTIs except abacavir are renally eliminated and require renal dosage adjustments. As such, there are minimal drug–drug interactions. Mitochondrial toxicities causing lactic acidosis, hepatic steatosis, peripheral neuropathy, pancreatitis, and lipoatrophy are less commonly associated with the NRTIs lamivudine, emtricitabine, abacavir, and tenofovir. These NRTIs are now the most commonly used agents.

Mechanism of Action for the Drug Class
NRTIs inhibit reverse transcriptase, an essential enzyme in the HIV life cycle.

Counseling Points for the Drug Class
- Compliance is essential for successful treatment of HIV. Medications are not a cure.

Members of the Drug Class
In this section: Lamivudine, emtricitabine, tenofovir, abacavir
Others: Didanosine, stavudine, zidovudine

■ Lamivudine

Brand Names
Epivir, Epivir-HBV

Generic Name
Lamivudine

Dosage Forms
Tablets, solution; also available in combination with other antiretrovirals

Usage
- HIV infection*, chronic hepatitis B

Dosing
- 300 mg daily or 150 mg twice daily for HIV; 100 mg daily for hepatitis B
- Renal dosage adjustment:
  - Decrease dose with CrCl <50 ml/minute

Adverse Reactions: Most Common
- No common reactions

Adverse Reactions: Rare/Severe/Important
- Lactic acidosis with hepatic steatosis, severe acute exacerbation of hepatitis may occur in HBV-coinfected patients who discontinue lamivudine

Major Drug Interactions
- Concomitant administration with emtricitabine should be avoided because they are chemically related

Contraindications
- Concomitant administration with emtricitabine

Key Points
- Lamivudine or emtricitabine is almost always part of combination antiretroviral therapy
- Although well-tolerated with minimal toxicity, lamivudine has a low genetic barrier to resistance
- Commonly abbreviated as 3TC

Emtricitabine

Brand Name
Emtriva

Generic Name
Emtricitabine

Dosage Forms
Solution, capsules; also available in combination with other antiretrovirals

Usage
- HIV infection

Dosing
- 200 mg capsule daily or 240 mg (24 ml) oral solution daily
- Renal dosage adjustment:
  - Reduce dose with CrCl <50 ml/minute

Adverse Reactions: Most Common
- Hyperpigmentation/skin discoloration

Adverse Reactions: Rare/Severe/Important
- Lactic acidosis with hepatic steatosis; severe acute exacerbation of hepatitis may occur in HBV-coinfected patients who discontinue emtricitabine

Major Drug Interactions
- Concomitant administration with lamivudine should be avoided because they are chemically related

Contraindications
- Concomitant administration with lamivudine

Key Points
- Lamivudine or emtricitabine are almost always part of combination antiretroviral therapy
- Although well-tolerated with minimal toxicity, emtricitabine has a low genetic barrier to resistance
- Commonly abbreviated as FTC

Tenofovir

Brand Name
Viread

Generic Name
Tenofovir

Dosage Forms
Tablets; also available in combination with other antiretrovirals

Usage
- HIV infection*, treatment of chronic hepatitis B

Dosing
- Usual dose: 300 mg daily
- Renal dosage adjustment:
  - Reduce dose with CrCl <50 ml/minute

Adverse Reactions: Most Common
- Asthenia, headache, nausea, vomiting, diarrhea, flatulence

Adverse Reactions: Rare/Severe/Important
- Nephrotoxicity, decreased bone mineral density, lactic acidosis with hepatic steatosis

Major Drug Interactions
Drug Affecting Tenofovir
- Adefovir: Increased nephrotoxicity

Tenofovir's Effect on Other Drugs
- Atazanavir: Decreased concentrations. When given together, ritonavir must be given as well.

Counseling Point
- Adverse effects such as asthenia, headache, nausea, vomiting, diarrhea, and flatulence should subside in 4 weeks

Key Points

- Tenofovir and emtricitabine are the two NRTIs most commonly used in combination antiretroviral therapy
- Avoid the use of tenofovir in patients with baseline renal impairment
- Do not coadminister with adefovir for hepatitis B infection
- Commonly abbreviated as TDF

■ Abacavir

Brand Name
Ziagen

Generic Name
Abacavir

Dosage Forms
Tablets, oral solution; also available in combination with other antiretrovirals

Usage
- HIV infection

Dosing
- Usual dose: 600 mg once daily or 300 mg twice daily
- Hepatic dosage adjustment:
  ○ Decrease dose with Child-Pugh Score 5–6

Adverse Reactions: Most Common
- No common reactions

Adverse Reactions: Rare/Severe/Important
- Hypersensitivity reaction (symptoms may include fever, rash, nausea, vomiting, malaise or fatigue, or respiratory symptoms such as sore throat, cough, or shortness of breath) (increased risk if HLA-B5701 positive), lactic acidosis with hepatic steatosis

Major Drug Interactions
Abacavir's Effect on Other Drugs
- Methadone: Increased clearance, possibly leading to withdrawal
- Ribavirin: Increased risk of lactic acidosis

Contraindications
- Any manifestation of a hypersensitivity reaction; patients who test positive for HLA-B5701 (relative contraindication)
  ○ Rechallenging with abacavir after an initial reaction can be fatal

Counseling Point
- Report the following signs/symptoms because they may be associated with a hypersensitivity reaction: fever, rash, nausea, vomiting, malaise or fatigue, or respiratory symptoms such as sore throat, cough, or shortness of breath

Key Points
- Patients undergo genetic testing for the presence of the HLA-B5701 allele before starting; if positive, do not give because it is predictive of hypersensitivity
- Avoid in patients at high risk of cardiovascular disease; studies have shown an association between abacavir and an increased risk for myocardial infarction
- Commonly abbreviated as ABC

Drug Class: Antiretroviral, Nonnucleoside Reverse Transcriptase Inhibitor

Introduction

The NNRTIs are antiretrovirals for the treatment of HIV. They are often used in combination with nucleoside/nucleotide reverse transcriptase inhibitors. They tend to have a low genetic barrier to resistance, except for second-generation NNRTIs such as etravirine. Drug interactions are common because agents in this class are substrates, as well as inducers and inhibitors of the CYP450 enzyme system.

Mechanism of Action for the Drug Class

Inhibit the essential viral enzyme reverse transcriptase in a noncompetitive manner, preventing viral replication.

Members of the Drug Class

In this section: Efavirenz
    Others: Etravirine, nevirapine

■ Efavirenz

Brand Name
Sustiva

Generic Name
Efavirenz

Dosage Forms
Capsules, tablets; also available in combination with other antiretrovirals

Usage
- HIV infection

Dosing
- 600 mg daily on an empty stomach

- Hepatic dosage adjustment:
  - No recommendations available; use with caution in hepatic impairment

Adverse Reactions: Most Common

- Dizziness, somnolence, insomnia, abnormal dreams, confusion, abnormal thinking, impaired concentration, hallucinations, elevated transaminases, hyperlipidemia, rash

Adverse Reactions: Rare/Severe/Important

- Grade 3 or 4 rash (has rarely progressed to Stevens–Johnson syndrome)

Major Drug Interactions

- CYP 3A4 substrate, inhibitor, and inducer

Medications That Should Not Be Administered with Efavirenz

- Other NNRTIs, oral midazolam, triazolam, cisapride, pimozide, ergot alkaloids, and voriconazole (at standard doses)

Drug Interactions with Efavirenz That May Require Dosage Adjustments or Monitoring

- Itraconazole, ketoconazole, posaconazole, voriconazole, carbamazepine, phenobarbital, phenytoin, clarithromycin, rifabutin, rifampin, calcium channel blockers, St. John's wort, HMG-CoA reductase inhibitors, ethinyl estradiol, methadone, and warfarin

Contraindications

- Concomitant administration with other NNRTIs, oral midazolam, triazolam, cisapride, pimozide, ergot alkaloids, and voriconazole (at standard doses)

Counseling Points

- Take on an empty stomach at bedtime
- Compliance is essential for successful treatment of HIV. Medications are not a cure.

Key Points

- Avoid in women of childbearing potential because efavirenz should not be used in the first trimester of pregnancy
- Avoid in patients with unstable psychiatric disease due to CNS adverse effects
- Commonly abbreviated as EFV

Drug Class: Antiretroviral, Protease Inhibitors

Introduction

The protease inhibitors (PIs) are antiretrovirals for the treatment of HIV. They are often used in combination with nucleoside/nucleotide reverse transcriptase inhibitors. Most PIs have a low oral bioavailability due to hepatic first-pass metabolism. As a result, almost all PIs should be given with ritonavir to pharmacokinetically "boost" levels of the primary PI. Drugs in this class have a high genetic barrier to resistance. Most are substrates and inhibitors of the CYP450 enzyme system and can cause many drug–drug interactions. Because they are metabolized in the liver, all PIs should be used with caution in patients with liver impairment.

Mechanism of Action for the Drug Class

Directly inhibit the viral protease enzyme, preventing viral maturation.

Indication for the Drug Class

- HIV infection

Adverse Reactions for the Drug Class: Most Common

- Nausea, vomiting, diarrhea, flatulence, rash, elevated transaminases

Adverse Reactions for the Drug Class: Rare/Severe/Important

- Metabolic syndrome (lipodystrophy, dyslipidemia, insulin resistance)

Counseling Point for the Drug Class

- Compliance is essential for successful treatment of HIV. Medications are not a cure.

Key Point for the Drug Class

- Patients receiving drugs that are metabolized by the cytochrome P450 enzyme system should be closely monitored for potential drug–drug interactions

Members of the Drug Class

In this section: Ritonavir, lopinavir/ritonavir, atazanavir, darunavir

Others: Fosamprenavir, Indinavir, nelfinavir, saquinavir, tipranavir

Ritonavir

Brand Name
Norvir

Generic Name
Ritonavir

Dosage Forms

Oral solution, capsules, tablets

Usage

- Used as a pharmacokinetic "booster" for other protease inhibitors

Dosing

- Usual dose (as a pharmacokinetic "booster"): 100–400 mg daily in one to two divided doses

Major Drug Interactions

Medications That Should Not Be Administered with Ritonavir

- Simvastatin, lovastatin, cisapride, pimozide, oral midazolam, triazolam, ergot alkaloids, amiodarone, flecainide, propafenone, quinidine, rifampin, St. John's wort, fluticasone

Drug Interactions with Ritonavir That May Require Dosage Adjustment or Monitoring

- Itraconazole, ketoconazole, posaconazole, voriconazole, carbamazepine, lamotrigine, phenobarbital, phenytoin, valproic acid, clarithromycin, rifabutin, alprazolam, diazepam, HMG-CoA reductase inhibitors, methadone, phosphodiesterase type 5 inhibitors, bosentan, digoxin, calcium channel blockers, hormonal contraceptives, and psychiatric medications

Counseling Points

- Gastrointestinal discomfort is likely during the initiation of therapy but should subside within 4 weeks
- Keep ritonavir in the refrigerator
- Take with food to decrease gastrointestinal side effects

Key Points

- Ritonavir is no longer used as a primary PI due to low tolerance at effective doses but is frequently used as a pharmacokinetic "booster" for other PIs via inhibition of the CYP450 system
- Commonly abbreviated as RTV, or "/r" in combination regimens

■ Lopinavir/Ritonavir

Brand Name

Kaletra

Generic Name

Lopinavir/ritonavir

Dosage Forms

Tablets, oral solution

Dosing

- Usual dose:
  - Lopinavir 400 mg + ritonavir 100 mg (2 tablets) twice daily
  - Lopinavir 800 mg + ritonavir 200 mg (4 tablets) once daily in patients with less than 3 lopinavir resistance-associated substitutions and not for pregnant women or patients receiving efavirenz, nevirapine, fosamprenavir, or nelfinavir

- Concomitant administration with efavirenz or nevirapine:
  - Lopinavir 500 mg + ritonavir 125 mg twice daily (combination of different formulations)
  - Lopinavir 533 mg + ritonavir 133 mg (6.7 ml oral solution) twice daily with food
- Hepatic dosage adjustments:
  - Use with caution in patients with hepatic impairment

Adverse Reactions: Most Common

- Asthenia

Adverse Reactions: Rare/Severe/Important

- PR interval prolongation, QT interval prolongation with possible polymorphic ventricular tachycardia

Major Drug Interactions

Medications That Should Not Be Administered with Lopinavir/Ritonavir

- Amiodarone, flecainide, propafenone, quinidine, pimozide, cisapride, oral midazolam, triazolam, rifampin, voriconazole, lovastatin, simvastatin, fluticasone, ergot alkaloids, fluticasone, St. John's wort

Drug Interactions with Lopinavir/Ritonavir That May Require Dosage Adjustment or Monitoring

- Itraconazole, ketoconazole, posaconazole, carbamazepine, lamotrigine, phenobarbital, phenytoin, valproic acid, clarithromycin, rifabutin, alprazolam, diazepam, HMG-CoA reductase inhibitors, methadone, phosphodiesterase type 5 inhibitors, bosentan, digoxin, calcium channel blockers, hormonal contraceptives, and psychiatric medications

Counseling Points

- Gastrointestinal discomfort is likely during the initiation of therapy but should subside within 4 weeks
- Take with food to decrease gastrointestinal side effects

Key Points

- Lopinavir is pharmacokinetically limited as monotherapy and should always be administered in concert with ritonavir
- Once-daily formulation should only be administered to treatment-naive patients without concurrent CYP450 inducers
- Commonly abbreviated as LPV/r or LPV/RTV

■ Atazanavir

Brand Name

Reyataz

Generic Name

Atazanavir

Dosage Forms

Capsules

Dosing

- Boosted, treatment experienced, or with tenofovir: Atazanavir 300 mg + ritonavir 100 mg once daily
- Unboosted and PI naive: Atazanavir 400 mg once daily
- Concomitant administration with efavirenz and treatment naive: Atazanavir 400 mg + ritonavir 100 mg once daily
- Renal dosage adjustment:
  - Adjust for treatment-naive patients on dialysis; avoid for treatment-experienced patients on dialysis
- Hepatic dosage adjustment:
  - Ritonavir boosting is not recommended in patients with hepatic impairment (Child-Pugh Score ≥7)
  - Child-Pugh score 7–9: Atazanavir 300 mg daily
  - Child-Pugh score >9: Not recommended

Adverse Reactions: Most Common

- Indirect hyperbilirubinemia

Adverse Reactions: Rare/Severe/Important

- Nephrolithiasis, PR interval prolongation

Major Drug Interactions

Medications That Should Not Be Administered with Atazanavir

- Etravirine, nevirapine, indinavir, nevirapine, simvastatin, lovastatin, rifampin, cisapride, pimozide, quinidine, oral midazolam, triazolam, ergot alkaloids, irinotecan, St. John's wort, proton pump inhibitors (if unboosted)

Drug Interactions with Atazanavir That May Require Dosage Adjustment or Monitoring

- Acid-reducing agents, itraconazole, ketoconazole, posaconazole, carbamazepine, lamotrigine, phenobarbital, phenytoin, valproic acid, clarithromycin, rifabutin, alprazolam, diazepam, HMG-CoA reductase inhibitors, methadone, phosphodiesterase type 5 inhibitors, bosentan, digoxin, calcium channel blockers, hormonal contraceptives, and psychiatric medications

Atazanavir and Acid-Reducing Agents

Drug-regimen modification is required due to the need for gastric acidity to absorb atazanavir. Specific recommendations are available and differ between acid-reducing agents and the level of treatment experience of the patient.

Counseling Points

- Gastrointestinal discomfort is likely during the initiation of therapy but should subside within 4 weeks
- Take with food and drink plenty of water
- Do not take antacids without first talking to your physician
- You may notice that the color of your skin turns yellow; talk to your physician

Key Points

- Be cautious with patients taking acid-reducing agents. Many of these agents are overused, and it may be possible to discontinue them.
- Commonly abbreviated as ATV

■ Darunavir

Brand Name

Prezista

Generic Name

Darunavir

Dosage Forms

Tablets

Dosing

- Treatment naive: Darunavir 800 mg + ritonavir 100 mg daily with food
- Treatment experienced: Darunavir 600 mg + ritonavir 100 mg twice daily with food
- Hepatic dosage adjustments:
  - Not recommended in patients with severe hepatic impairment

Adverse Reactions: Most Common

- Rash, headache

Adverse Reactions: Rare/Severe/Important

- Hypersensitivity

Major Drug Interactions

Medications That Should Not Be Administered with Darunavir

- Simvastatin, lovastatin, rifampin, cisapride, pimozide, oral midazolam, triazolam, ergot alkaloids, carbamazepine, phenobarbital, phenytoin, amiodarone, lidocaine, quinidine, fluticasone

Drug Interactions with Darunavir That May Require Dosage Adjustment or Monitoring

- Acid-reducing agents, itraconazole, ketoconazole, posaconazole, carbamazepine, lamotrigine, phenobarbital, phenytoin, valproic acid, clarithromycin, rifabutin, alprazolam, diazepam, HMG-CoA reductase inhibitors, methadone, phosphodiesterase type 5 inhibitors, bosentan, digoxin, calcium channel blockers, hormonal contraceptives, and psychiatric medications

Counseling Points

- Gastrointestinal discomfort is likely during the initiation of therapy but should subside within 4 weeks
- Take with food to decrease gastrointestinal side effects and for increased absorption of the drug

Key Points

- Use caution in patients with sulfa allergies due to sulfa moiety in darunavir
- Do not give without ritonavir
- Commonly abbreviated as DRV

Drug Class: Antiretroviral, Integrase Inhibitor

Introduction

The integrase inhibitor raltegravir stands alone in its own class of antiretrovirals. As such, it is useful in patients who have failed other antiretroviral treatment. Its lack of metabolism by CYP450 is a significant advantage in a therapeutic area where drug interactions are common and problematic.

Mechanism of Action for the Drug Class

Inhibition of HIV integrase enzyme, preventing integration of proviral gene into human DNA.

■ Raltegravir

Brand Name
Isentress

Generic Name
Raltegravir

Dosage Forms
Tablets

Usage
- HIV infection

Dosing
- 400 mg twice daily
- Concomitant administration with rifampin: 800 mg twice daily
- Hepatic dosing adjustment:
  ◦ May require adjustment in severe hepatic impairment

Adverse Reactions: Most Common
- No common reactions

Adverse Reactions: Rare/Severe/Important
- Creatine phosphokinase elevation

Major Drug Interactions

Drugs Affecting Raltegravir
- Rifampin: Decreases raltegravir concentrations, necessitating dose increases of raltegravir

Counseling Point
- Compliance is essential for successful treatment of HIV. Medications are not a cure.

Key Point
- Although well tolerated with minimal drug interactions, raltegravir has a low genetic barrier to resistance

---

Review Questions

1. Which of the following drugs is a drug of choice for methicillin-resistant *Staphylococcus aureus* infections?
   - A. Amoxicillin
   - B. Neosporin
   - C. Rifampin
   - D. Vancomycin

2. Which drug is a nonnucleoside reverse transcriptase inhibitor?
   - A. Abacavir
   - B. Epivir
   - C. Sustiva
   - D. Tenofovir

3. Which drug is useful in the treatment of tuberculosis?
   - A. Bactrim
   - B. Cleocin
   - C. Isoniazid
   - D. Vancocin

4. Which drug can be given twice a day in the treatment of genital herpes in a patient with normal kidney function?
   - A. Abacavir
   - B. Acyclovir
   - C. Epivir
   - D. Valacyclovir

5. Which of the following drugs is closely associated with severe allergic reactions that can be largely prevented by genetic screening?
   - A. Acyclovir
   - B. Bactrim
   - C. Clindamycin
   - D. Ziagen

6. Which of the following antiretrovirals should always be given with ritonavir?
   - A. Atazanavir
   - B. Darunavir
   - C. Efavirenz
   - D. Raltegravir

7. Which antifungal works by binding to ergosterol in the fungal cell wall?
   A. Fluconazole
   B. Fungizone
   C. Itraconazole
   D. Vfend

8. Which of these drugs should not be used for the treatment of urinary tract infections?
   A. Avelox
   B. Cipro
   C. Macrobid
   D. Septra

9. Which of the following drugs is associated with the "red man's syndrome?"
   A. Abacavir
   B. Doxycycline
   C. Fluconazole
   D. Vancomycin

10. Which of these drugs works by inhibiting protein synthesis?
    A. Amoxil
    B. Bactrim
    C. Minocin
    D. Nitrofurantoin

11. Which drug is commonly associated with dizziness, confusion, and other CNS disturbances?
    A. Levaquin
    B. Metronidazole
    C. Septra
    D. Vancomycin

12. Which of the following drugs is ototoxic?
    A. Clindamycin
    B. Doxycycline
    C. Gentamicin
    D. Nitrofurantoin

13. Which antiretroviral should never be added to a regimen containing lamivudine?
    A. Abacavir
    B. Emtricitabine
    C. Kaletra
    D. Raltegravir

14. Which of the following drugs cannot be given concurrently with calcium carbonate?
    A. Acyclovir
    B. Avelox
    C. Cleocin
    D. Vfend

15. Which of the following drugs decreases the metabolism of many other drugs, increasing their concentrations?
    A. Amoxicillin
    B. Doxycycline
    C. Rifampin
    D. Ritonavir

Antineoplastics

Rachel Clark-Vetri, PharmD, BCOP

Drug Class: Alkylating Agents

Introduction

Cyclophosphamide is a common chemotherapeutic agent used in adults and children to treat a number of malignant and nonmalignant diseases. The most notable side effects are bone marrow suppression, nausea, and hemorrhagic cystitis. There is a wide dosing range of this agent depending on the indication and route of administration.

Mechanism of Action for the Drug Class

Forms strong covalent bonds with DNA inhibiting replication and causing bond breaks and cell death.

Members of the Drug Class

In this section: Cyclophosphamide

Others: Busulfan, carmustine, chlorambucil, dacarbazine, ifosfamide, lomustine, mechlorethamine, melphalan, procarbazine, temozolomide, thiotepa

■ Cyclophosphamide

Brand Name

Cytoxan

Generic Name

Cyclophosphamide

Dosage Forms

Injection, tablets

Usage

- Oncologic:
  - Hodgkin and non-Hodgkin lymphoma*, chronic lymphocytic leukemia (CLL)*, acute myelogenous leukemia (AML)*, acute lymphocytic leukemia*, multiple myeloma, neuroblastoma, breast cancer*, testicular cancer, ovarian cancer, lung cancer, stem cell immobilization, Ewing sarcoma, rhabdomyosarcoma, mycosis fungoides, Wilms' tumor
- Non-oncologic:
  - Severe rheumatoid disorders, Wegener's granulomatosis, myasthenia gravis, multiple sclerosis, systemic lupus erythematosus, lupus nephritis, autoimmune hemolytic anemia, idiopathic thrombocytic purpura (ITP), antibody-induced pure red cell aplasia, and nephrotic syndrome in children

Dosing

- Individual protocols specify dosing for specific indications and institutions
- Usual doses:
  - Oral: 50–100 mg/m^2/day up to 14 days continuous therapy
  - IV single doses 400–1800 mg/m^2, which may be repeated at 2- to 4-week intervals
- Juvenile Rheumatoid Arthritis: IV 10 mg/kg every 2 weeks
- High dose: IV 1.8 g/m^2 per day for 4 days (total of 7.2 g/m^2) or 50 mg/kg per day for 4 days
- Renal dosage adjustment:
  - CrCl <10 ml/minute: Administer 75% of normal dose
  - Hemodialysis: Administer 50% of dose posthemodialysis
- Hepatic dosage adjustment:
  - Bilirubin 3.1–5 mg/dl: Administer 75% of dose
  - Bilirubin >5 mg/dl: Avoid use

Adverse Reactions: Most Common

- Leucopenia, nausea and vomiting, alopecia, diarrhea, mucositis, amenorrhea

Adverse Reactions: Rare/Severe/Important

- Hemorrhagic cystitis, sterility, secondary malignancies, SIADH, cardiac necrosis, renal tubular necrosis, skin rash

Major Drug Interactions

Drugs Affecting Cyclophosphamide

- Antineoplastics: Enhance bone marrow suppression

Cyclophosphamide's Effect on Other Drugs

- Succinylcholine: Decreased metabolism
- Vaccines: Diminished therapeutic effect of vaccines via immunosuppression
- Warfarin: Increased bleeding risk

Counseling Points

- Drink plenty of fluids (3–4 liters/day) for at least 24 hours after an intravenous dose
- Report any painful urination; discolored or bloody urine
- Take oral doses early in the day

Key Points

- Doses >1 g/m^2 are likely to require mesna uroprotection to prevent hemorrhagic cystitis
- Monitor patients for signs of leucopenia and infection
- Give patient antiemetics to prevent nausea and vomiting

Drug Class: Anthracyclines

Introduction

Anthracyclines are a group of antineoplastic drugs used to treat a variety of malignant diseases both hematologic and solid tumors. Given only as an IV treatment, they are most notably known for their risk of causing cardiotoxicity. In addition, they are vesicants and cause severe skin necrosis if extravasation occurs.

Mechanism of Action for the Drug Class

Inhibition of DNA and RNA synthesis by intercalation of DNA base pairs and inhibition of DNA repair by topoisomerase.

Members of the Drug Class

In this section: Doxorubicin

Others: Daunorubicin, epirubicin, idarubicin, mitoxantrone

■ Doxorubicin

Brand Name

Adriamycin

Generic Name

Doxorubicin

Dosage Forms

Injection

Usage

- Treatment of ALL, AML, Hodgkin disease, malignant lymphoma*, soft tissue and bone sarcomas, thyroid cancer, small cell lung cancer, breast cancer*, gastric cancer, ovarian cancer, bladder cancer, neuroblastoma, Wilms tumor, multiple myeloma

Dosing

- Individual protocols specify dosing for specific indications and institutions
- Children:
  - 30–75 mg/m^2 per dose every 3–4 weeks; 20–30 mg/m^2 per dose once weekly; 60–90 mg/m^2 given as a continuous infusion over 96 hours every 3–4 weeks

- Adults:
  - 60–75 mg/m^2 per dose every 3–4 weeks; 20–30 mg/m^2 per day for 3 days every 4 weeks; 60 mg/m^2 per dose every 2 weeks (dose dense)
- Hepatic dosage adjustment:
  - Transaminases two to three times; ULN: Administer 75% of dose
  - Bilirubin 1.2–3 mg/dl or transaminases more than three times; ULN: Administer 50% of dose
  - Bilirubin 3.1–5 mg/dl: Administer 25% of dose
  - Bilirubin >5 mg/dl: Do not administer

Adverse Reactions: Most Common

Leucopenia, anemia, thrombocytopenia, nausea and vomiting, alopecia, diarrhea, mucositis, amenorrhea

Adverse Reactions: Rare/Severe/Important

- Acute and delayed cardiotoxicity, sterility, secondary malignancy

Major Drug Interactions

Drugs Affecting Doxorubicin

- Cyclosporine: May increase doxorubicin levels
- Paclitaxel: Reduces the clearance of doxorubicin
- Trastuzumab: May increase cardiotoxicity of doxorubicin

Doxorubicin's Effect on Other Drugs

- Digoxin: Levels may be decreased
- Phenytoin: Levels may be decreased
- Radiation: Severe skin reactions are possible

Counseling Points

- This drug may darken your urine for 24–48 hours
- Watch for fever, malaise, sore mouth or throat, pain or swelling at injection site

Key Points

- Dose adjustments may be needed for patients with inadequate marrow reserve
- No live virus vaccines should be given during therapy

- Doxorubicin is a vesicant. Extravasation should be treated with topical dimethylsulfoxide and cold compresses or dexrazoxane.
- Patients should have ejection fraction measured before starting therapy

- Monitor patients for signs of infection and mucositis
- Premedicate with antiemetics to prevent nausea and vomiting

Drug Class: Antimetabolites

Introduction
The agents of this class of antineoplastics are all similar in structure to naturally occurring compounds. All these agents cause gastrointestinal side effects to varying degrees depending on the agent, dose, and route of administration. Unique side effects can also be seen with each agent.

Mechanism of Action for the Drug Class
These compounds kill tumor cells by inhibiting DNA synthesis by a specific mechanism or they incorporate themselves into DNA, causing apoptosis. They generally have greater toxicity in rapidly growing cancer cells than normal cells of the host, but many of their toxicities arise from host cell effects.

Members of the Drug Class
In this section: Capecitabine, cytarabine, 5-fluorouracil, gemcitabine, mercaptopurine, methotrexate

Others: Cladribine, fludarabine, floxuridine, hydroxyurea, nelarabine, pemetrexed, thioguanine

■ Capecitabine

Brand Name
Xeloda

Generic Name
Capecitabine

Dosage Forms
Tablets

Usage
- Treatment of metastatic colorectal cancer*; adjuvant therapy of colon cancer*; metastatic breast cancer*, gastric cancer*, pancreatic cancer*, esophageal cancer, ovarian cancer, metastatic renal cell cancer, neuroendocrine tumors, metastatic CNS lesions

Dosing
- Individual protocols specify dosing for specific indications and institutions
- Usual dose: 1000–1250 mg/m^2 orally twice daily
- Renal dosage adjustment:
  ○ CrCl 30–50 ml/minute: Administer 75% of dose
  ○ CrCl <30 ml/minute: Contraindicated

- Hepatic dosage adjustment:
  ○ Avoid in severe impairment

Adverse Reactions: Most Common
- Leucopenia, anemia, thrombocytopenia, nausea and vomiting, diarrhea, mucositis, skin discoloration, palmar-plantar erythrodysesthesias, eye irritation

Adverse Reactions: Rare/Severe/Important
- Chest pain, venous thrombosis

Major Drug Interactions
Drugs Affecting Capecitabine
- Leucovorin: Enhances the toxic effect

Capecitabine's Effect on Other Drugs
- Phenytoin: Increases serum concentration of phenytoin

Counseling Points
- Report any fever, mouth sores, rashes, or diarrhea
- Avoid sunlight exposure and use sunscreen when exposure cannot be avoided
- Take with food
- Avoid use of antacids within 2 hours of taking medicine
- Do not crush, chew, or dissolve tablets

Key Points
- No live virus vaccines should be given during therapy
- Food reduces the rate and extent of absorption of capecitabine
- May cause a painful rash on the hands and feet

■ Cytarabine
Brand Name
ARA-C

Generic Name
Cytarabine

Dosage Forms
Injection

Usage
- Treatment of AML*, ALL*, CML (blast phase)*, and lymphomas; prophylaxis and treatment of meningeal leukemia

Dosing

- Individual protocols specify dosing for specific indications and institutions
- Usual IV doses:
  - Children: 75–200 mg/m² for 5- to 10-day therapy
  - Adults: 100–200 mg/m² per day for 5–10 days or 100 mg/m² per day for 7 days or 100 mg/m² per dose every 12 hours for 7 days or high dose 1–3 g/m² every 12 hours for up to 12 doses
- Usual intrathecal doses:
  - Adults: 5–75 mg/m² per dose every 2–7 days
  - Children: 30 mg/m² per dose; children <3 years of age: dose based on age
- Renal dosage adjustment:
  - No adjustment needed for 100–200 mg/m²
  - High dose: CrCl 46–60 ml/minute: Administer 60% of dose
  - High dose: CrCl 31–45 ml/minute: Administer 50% of dose
  - High dose: CrCl <30 ml/minute: Avoid use
- Hepatic dosage adjustment:
  - Reduce dose in severe dysfunction

Adverse Reactions: Most Common

- Mucositis, diarrhea, nausea and vomiting, leucopenia, anemia, thrombocytopenia, conjunctivitis, alopecia

Adverse Reactions: Rare/Severe/Important

- Chest pain, tumor lysis syndrome, neurotoxicity, coma, rash, skin desquamation, ocular toxicity

Major Drug Interactions

None

Counseling Points

- No live virus vaccines should be given during therapy
- Watch for fever, mouth sores, and diarrhea
- Stay well hydrated by drinking lots of fluids during therapy
- Report any changes in mental status
- May cause nausea and vomiting
- Increased risk of infection

Key Points

- Monitor for mental status changes during therapy
- Patients require aggressive hydration and antiemetic therapy
- May require prophylaxis for tumor lysis syndrome
- Myelosuppression can be severe and prolonged
- Patients require steroid eye drops to prevent ocular toxicities

■ 5-Fluorouracil

Brand Names
5-FU, Efudex

Generic Name
5-Fluorouracil

Dosage Forms
Injection, topical cream, topical solution

Usage

- Treatment of carcinomas of the breast*, colon*, rectum*, pancreas*, stomach; head and neck cancer, anal cancer and cervical cancer; topically for the management of actinic or solar keratoses and superficial basal cell carcinomas*

Dosing

- Individual protocols specify dosing for specific indications and institutions:
  - IV bolus: 500–600 mg/m² per day weekly OR 425 mg/m² per day on days 1–5 every 4 weeks
  - Continuous IV infusion: 1000 mg/m² per day for 4–5 days every 3–4 weeks or 300–400 mg/m² per day OR 225 mg/m² per day for 5–8 weeks (with radiation therapy)
  - Topical: Apply to lesions twice daily for 2–4 weeks
- Renal dosage adjustment:
  - No dose adjustment
  - Dose after dialysis: Administer 50% of dose
- Hepatic dosage adjustment:
  - Bilirubin ≥5 mg/dl: Avoid use

Adverse Reactions: Most Common

- Leucopenia, anemia, thrombocytopenia, nausea and vomiting, diarrhea, mucositis, skin discoloration, palmar-plantar erythrodysesthesias, eye irritation; skin irritation with topical

Adverse Reactions: Rare/Severe/Important

- Chest pain

Major Drug Interactions

Drugs Affecting 5-Fluorouracil
- Leucovorin: Increases both toxic effects and efficacy

5-Fluorouracil's Effect on Other Drugs
- Carvedilol: Increases serum concentrations
- Natalizumab: Increases toxicities
- Phenytoin: Increases serum concentration
- Warfarin: Increases bleeding risk

Counseling Points

- No live virus vaccines should be given during therapy
- Watch for fever, mouth sores, and diarrhea
- Avoid sunlight exposure and use sunscreen when exposure cannot be avoided
- Wash hands after using topical formulation
- Avoid drinking alcohol while taking this medication

Key Points

- Patients with a genetic deficiency of dihydropyrimidine dehydrogenase have increased systemic toxicities
- May be an irritant if it extravasates from the vein
- May cause severe diarrhea and mucositis

■ Gemcitabine

Brand Name

Gemzar

Generic Name

Gemcitabine

Dosage Forms

Injection

Usage

- Treatment of metastatic breast cancer*; locally advanced or metastatic non–small cell lung cancer (NSCLC) or pancreatic cancer*; advanced, relapsed ovarian cancer, bladder cancer, cervical cancer, Hodgkin disease, non-Hodgkin lymphomas, small cell lung cancer*, hepato-biliary cancers*

Dosing

- Individual protocols specify dosing for specific indications and institutions
- 1000 mg/m^2 per day IV weekly up to 7 weeks followed by 1 week rest
- Renal dosage adjustment:
  ○ Caution with severe impairment although no specific recommendations on dose reductions are available

Adverse Reactions: Most Common

- Leucopenia, thrombocytopenia, anemia, diarrhea, skin rash, nausea, flulike symptoms, peripheral edema, proteinuria

Adverse Reactions: Rare/Severe/Important

- Hematuria, hepatotoxicity

Major Drug Interactions

Gemcitabine's Effect on Other Drugs

- Bleomycin: Increases risk of pulmonary toxicity
- Fluorouracil: Increases serum concentration
- Warfarin: Increases bleeding risk

Counseling Points

- Watch for fever, bleeding, and bruising
- Flu symptoms can be severe; analgesics may be used to decrease these effects

Key Points

- No live virus vaccines should be given during therapy
- Rash is usually self-limiting
- Thrombocytopenia is common
- Flulike symptoms may require the use of acetaminophen or NSAIDs
- Gemcitabine is a radiosensitizer and will increase the toxicity of radiation therapy if used concurrently

■ Mercaptopurine

Brand Name

Purinethol

Generic Name

Mercaptopurine

Dosage Forms

Tablets

Usage

- Treatment (maintenance and induction) of ALL*, steroid-sparing agent for corticosteroid-dependent Crohn's disease (CD) and ulcerative colitis (UC); maintenance of remission in CD; fistulizing CD

Dosing

- Individual protocols specify dosing for specific indications and institutions
- Oncologic indications:
  ○ Induction: 2.5–5 mg/kg per day
  ○ Maintenance: 1.5–2.5 mg/kg per day or 80–100 mg/m^2 per day given once daily
- Reduction of steroid use in CD or UC, maintenance of remission in CD or fistulizing disease (unlabeled uses):
  ○ Oral: Initial: 50 mg daily; may increase by 25 mg/day every 1–2 weeks as tolerated to target dose of 1–1.5 mg/kg per day
- Renal dosage adjustment:
  ○ CrCl <50 ml/minute: Administer every 48 hours
  ○ Hemodialysis: Administer every 48 hours
- Hepatic dosage adjustment:
  ○ Reduced dosage may be required

Adverse Reactions: Most Common

- Leucopenia, thrombocytopenia, anemia, hepatotoxicity, drug fever, hyperpigmentation and rash

Adverse Reactions: Rare/Severe/Important

- Encephalopathy, ascites

Major Drug Interactions

Drugs Affecting Mercaptopurine

- Allopurinol: Increases mercaptopurine levels

Mercaptopurine's Effect on Other Drugs

- Warfarin: Effects may be inhibited

Counseling Points

- Watch for fever, malaise, bleeding, and bruising
- Take on an empty stomach

Key Points

- No live virus vaccines should be given during therapy
- Administration in the evening (versus morning administration) may lower the risk of relapse
- Dosage adjustment with concurrent allopurinol: Reduce mercaptopurine dosage by a quarter to a third of the usual dose
- TPMT genotyping may identify individuals at risk for toxicity
- Do not use the terms *6-mercaptopurine* or *6-MP* when writing prescriptions. The use of these terms has been associated with sixfold overdosage.

■ Methotrexate

Brand Name
Rheumatrex

Generic Names
Methotrexate

Dosage Forms
Injection, tablets

Usage
- Non-oncologic: Treatment of psoriasis (severe, recalcitrant, disabling) and severe RA*, including polyarticular-course JRA; ectopic pregnancy*; CD
- Oncologic: Treatment of trophoblastic neoplasms (gestational choriocarcinoma, chorioadenoma destruens, and hydatidiform mole)*, ALL*, meningeal leukemia*, breast cancer, head and neck cancer (epidermoid), cutaneous T-cell lymphoma (advanced mycosis fungoides), lung cancer (squamous cell and small cell), advanced non-Hodgkin lymphomas, osteosarcoma

Dosing
- Adults:
  - Individual protocols specify dosing for specific indications and institutions
  - Antineoplastic dosage range: IV: Range is wide from 30–40 mg/m² per week to 100–12,000 mg/m² with leucovorin rescue
  - RA: Oral: 7.5 mg once weekly or 2.5 mg every 12 hours for 3 doses/week, not to exceed 20 mg/week
  - Psoriasis: Oral: 2.5–5 mg/dose every 12 hours for 3 doses given weekly or oral, IM: 10–25 mg/dose given once weekly
  - Ectopic pregnancy and abortion: 50 mg/m², IM once
  - Note that doses for oncologic indications are frequently much higher than for other uses
- Pediatrics:
  - JRA: Oral, IM: 10 mg/m² once weekly, then 5–15 mg/m² per week as a single dose or as three divided doses given 12 hours apart
- Antineoplastic dosage range:
  - Oral, IM: 7.5–30 mg/m² per week or every 2 weeks
  - IV: 10–18,000 mg/m² bolus dosing or continuous infusion over 6–42 hours
- Meningeal leukemia: Intrathecal: 6–12 mg/dose based on age up to a maximum of 12 mg/dose
- Renal dosage adjustment:
  - CrCl 61–80 ml/minute: Administer 75% of dose
  - CrCl 51–60 ml/minute: Administer 70% of dose
  - CrCl 10–50 ml/minute: Administer 30–50% of dose
  - CrCl <10 ml/minute: Avoid use
  - Hemodialysis: Not dialyzable (0–5%); supplemental dose is not necessary
  - Peritoneal dialysis effects: Supplemental dose is not necessary
- Hepatic dosage adjustment:
  - Bilirubin 3.1–5 mg/dl or transaminases more than three times ULN: Administer 75% dose
  - Bilirubin >5 mg/dl: Do not administer

Adverse Reactions: Most Common
- Dependent on dose and route of administration
- Intrathecal 12 mg/m²: Headache, myelosuppression, nausea
- Low oral dose (<50 mg/week): Hepatotoxicity
- Moderate IV dose (50–100 mg/m²): Leukopenia, nausea, vomiting, thrombocytopenia, anemia, diarrhea, mucositis
- High IV dose (>100 mg/m²): Severe nausea and vomiting, alopecia, hepatotoxicity, renal toxicity, life-threatening myelosuppression and mucositis (must give with leucovorin rescue)

Adverse Reactions: Rare/Severe/Important
- Renal failure, arachnoiditis, encephalopathy (intrathecal administration), demyelinating encephalopathy, hepatotoxicity, sterility

Major Drug Interactions
Drugs Affecting Methotrexate
- Ciprofloxacin: May increase the serum concentration of methotrexate
- Cyclosporine: May increase the serum concentration of methotrexate
- NSAIDs: May reduce the excretion of methotrexate
- Penicillin: May decrease the excretion of methotrexate
- Proton pump inhibitors: May reduce the excretion of methotrexate
- Salicylates: Reduce methotrexate renal clearance and may displace methotrexate from binding sites
- Sulfonamides: Reduce methotrexate renal clearance and may displace methotrexate from binding sites

Methotrexate's Effect on Other Drugs
- Cyclosporine: Levels may be increased

Counseling Points
- Watch for fever, malaise, bleeding, bruising, sore mouth and throat, and flank pain
- Avoid prolonged exposure to sunlight

Key Points
- No live virus vaccines should be given during therapy
- Cannot be administered with radiation therapy
- Use preservative-free solution when preparing methotrexate for intrathecal administration
- Doses between 100 and 500 mg/m² may require leucovorin rescue. Doses >500 mg/m² require leucovorin rescue: IV, IM, Oral: Leucovorin 10–15 mg/m² every 6 hours for 8 or 10 doses, starting 24 hours after the start of methotrexate infusion. Continue until the methotrexate level is ≤0.1 micromolar (10^{-7} M). Leucovorin calcium must be given when using high doses of methotrexate to avoid severe life-threatening myelosuppression and mucositis.
- Avoid use in patients with third spacing such as ascites and effusions because of the reservoir effect

Introduction

These agents are cell-cycle nonspecific agents that are directly toxic to DNA by causing strand breaks to form. They are used in a variety of malignant diseases. All of them cause some degree of neurotoxicity but also possess unique toxicities.

Mechanism of Action for the Drug Class

Forms strong covalent bonds with DNA inhibiting replication and causing cell death.

Members of the Drug Class

In this section: Carboplatin, cisplatin
   Others: oxaliplatin

 ## Carboplatin

Brand Name

Paraplatin-AQ

Generic Name

Carboplatin

Dosage Forms

Injection

Usage

- Treatment of ovarian cancer*, lung cancer*, head and neck cancer*, endometrial cancer, esophageal cancer, bladder cancer*, breast cancer, cervical cancer, CNS tumors, germ cell tumors, osteogenic sarcoma, and high-dose therapy with stem cell/bone marrow support

Dosing

- Individual protocols specify dosing for specific indications and institutions
- Children:
  ○ Solid tumor: 300–600 mg/m² once every 4 weeks
  ○ Brain tumor: 175 mg/m² weekly for 4 weeks every 6 weeks, with a 2-week recovery period between courses
- Adults:
  ○ 300–360 mg/m² IV every 3–4 weeks or target area under the curve (AUC) of 5–7 mg given every 3 weeks dosed by the Calvert equation
    - Calvert equation: Dose = AUC (glomerular filtration rate [GFR] + 25)
  ○ Autologous BMT: IV: 1600 mg/m² (total dose) divided over 4 days
- Renal dosage adjustment:
  ○ Dosing based on renal dosing using the Calvert equation: Dose = AUC (GFR + 25)
  ○ CrCl 41–59 ml/minute; initiate at 250 mg/m²
  ○ CrCl 16–40 ml/minute; initiate at 200 mg/m²

Adverse Reactions: Most Common

- Leucopenia, anemia, thrombocytopenia, nausea and vomiting, peripheral neuropathies and alopecia

Adverse Reactions: Rare/Severe/Important

- Ototoxicity, hypersensitivity

Major Drug Interactions

Drugs Affecting Carboplatin

- Aminoglycosides: Increase risk of ototoxicity

Carboplatin's Effect on Other Drugs

- Taxanes: Increase bone marrow suppression

Counseling Points

- This drug may cause severe fetal defects; avoid pregnancy and breastfeeding during therapy
- Drink plenty of fluids after chemotherapy
- Severe nausea and vomiting could occur for several days after chemotherapy
- Contact your healthcare practitioner if you are unable to keep food or fluids down
- Contact your healthcare practitioner if there is any hearing loss

Key Points

- No live virus vaccines during therapy
- May be an irritant if it extravasates from the vein
- Hypersensitivity risk increases with more than six treatments

Cisplatin

Brand Names

Platinol, Platinol-AQ

Generic Names

Cisplatin, CDDP

Dosage Forms

Injection

Usage

- Treatment of bladder, testicular, and ovarian cancer*, head and neck cancer*, breast cancer*, gastric cancer, esophageal cancer, cervical cancer*, prostate cancer, NSCLC*, small cell lung cancer*; Hodgkin and non-Hodgkin lymphoma; neuroblastoma; sarcomas, myeloma, melanoma, mesothelioma, osteosarcoma

Dosing

- Individual protocols specify dosing for specific indications and institutions
- Pediatrics:
  ○ 37–100 mg/m² every 21–28 days or 15–20 mg/m² per day for 5 days every 3–4 weeks
- Adults:
  ○ 10–20 mg/m² per day for 5 days every 3–4 weeks; 50–120 mg/m² every 3–4 weeks; maximum dose: 120 mg/m² per cycle
  ○ High-dose BMT: 55 mg/m² per day for 3 days: 165 mg/m² total

- Renal dosage adjustment:
  - CrCl 46–60 ml/minute: Administer 75% of dose
  - CrCl 31–45 ml/minute: Administer 50% of dose
  - CrCl <30 ml/minute: Consider use of alternative drug
  - Hemodialysis: Administer 50% of normal dose postdialysis

Adverse Reactions: Most Common
- Nausea and vomiting, peripheral neuropathies, anemia, alopecia, nephrotoxicity, electrolyte imbalances

Adverse Reactions: Rare/Severe/Important
- Ototoxicity

Major Drug Interactions
Drugs Affecting Cisplatin
- Aminoglycosides: Increase nephrotoxicity
- Amifostine: Can *reduce* nephrotoxicity
- Taxanes: Increase bone marrow suppression

Cisplatin's Effect on Other Drugs
- Topotecan: Reduced clearance
- Vinorelbine: Increased risk of neutropenia

Counseling Points
- This drug may cause severe fetal defects; avoid pregnancy and breastfeeding during therapy
- Drink plenty of fluids after chemotherapy
- Severe nausea and vomiting could occur for several days after chemotherapy
- Contact your healthcare practitioner if you are unable to keep food or fluids down
- Contact your healthcare practitioner if there is any hearing loss

Key Points
- Verify any dose >100 mg/m^2
- Assess renal function prior to cisplatin administration
- Assess electrolytes, particularly potassium and magnesium, and replace as needed
- IV hydration should be given before and after cisplatin therapy
- Mannitol or furosemide can be given to reduce nephrotoxicity
- Highly emetogenic; premedicate to prevent nausea and vomiting
- Patients should also receive antiemetics after chemotherapy to prevent delayed emesis
- Ototoxicity is more pronounced in children

Drug Class: Targeted Therapy

Introduction
This class of drugs kills tumor cells by targeting abnormal genetic signaling proteins specific to the cancer. Each one works by a specific mechanism and has unique side effects. Many of these agents are used in combination with other cytotoxic drugs.

Mechanism of Action for the Drug Class
Imatinib inhibits tyrosine kinase needed for cell proliferation and targets the Philadelphia fusion gene. Rituximab and trastuzumab are monoclonal antibodies that target CD-20 antigen on B-cells and the HER2/neu oncogene, respectively.

Members of the Drug Class
In this section: Imatinib, rituximab, trastuzumab

Others: Alemtuzumab, bevacizumab, cetuximab, dasatinib, gemtuzumab, lapatinib, nilotinib, panitumumab, sorafenib, sunitinib, temsirolimus

■ Imatinib
Brand Name
Gleevec

Generic Name
Imatinib

Dosage Forms
Tablets

Usage
- Gastric stromal cell tumor*, chronic myelogenous leukemia*, Ph+ acute lymphoblastic leukemia, dermatofibrosarcoma protuberans, hypereosinophilic syndrome, myelodysplastic disease, desmoid tumors

Dosing
- Adults:
  - 400 mg daily; up to 800 mg daily in divided doses
- Pediatrics:
  - 260–340 mg/m^2 per day; maximum of 600 mg/day
- Renal dosage adjustment:
  - Mild impairment: No adjustment
  - Moderate impairment CrCl 20–39 ml/minute: Administer 50% of dose
  - Severe impairment CrCl <20 ml/minute: Not recommended
- Hepatic dosage adjustment:
  - Mild–moderate impairment: No adjustment
  - Severe impairment: Reduce dose by 25%

Adverse Reactions: Most Common
- Fluid retention, nausea, diarrhea, rash, leucopenia, thrombocytopenia, anemia, myalgias, arthralgias, muscle cramps

Adverse Reactions: Rare/Severe/Important

- Hepatotoxicity, heart failure, severe bullous dermatologic reactions, hemorrhage

Major Drug Interactions

Drugs Affecting Imatinib

- Azole antifungals: Increase the serum concentration of imatinib
- Lansoprazole: Enhances the dermatologic adverse effects of imatinib; monitoring is necessary

Imatinib's Effect on Other Drugs

- Carbamazepine: Inhibition of carbamazepine metabolism, resulting in increased carbamazepine concentrations and toxicity
- Digoxin: Decreased absorption
- Codeine: Diminished therapeutic effect due to inhibition of codeine conversion to active metabolite
- Colchicine, cyclosporine, fentanyl: Serum levels may increase
- Fludarabine: Therapeutic effects may be diminished
- Simvastatin: Metabolism may be reduced
- Tamoxifen: Therapeutic effects may be diminished
- Tramadol: Therapeutic effects may be diminished
- Warfarin: Bleeding effects may be increased

Counseling Points

- Take with food and/or large glass of water
- Report any fevers, bleeding, bruising, or flank pain
- Report any shortness of breath

Key Points

- Edema can progress to pulmonary edema
- Edema is worse in the elderly
- Food may reduce gastrointestinal irritation

■ Rituximab

Brand Name
Rituxan

Generic Name
Rituximab

Dosage Forms
Injection

Usage

- B-cell non-Hodgkin lymphoma*, CLL*, RA*, Burkitt's lymphoma, CNS lymphoma, Hodgkin lymphoma (lymphocyte predominant); MALT lymphoma (gastric and nongastric), splenic marginal zone lymphoma, SLL; WM; AIHA in children; chronic ITP; refractory pemphigus vulgaris, treatment of systemic autoimmune diseases (other than RA); treatment of steroid-refractory chronic graft-versus-host disease

Dosing

- Usual dosing: 375 mg/m^2 IV weekly
- RAs: 1000 mg on days 1 and 15 in combination with methotrexate
- Infusion notes:
  - Initial infusion: Start rate of 50 mg/hour; if there is no reaction, increase the rate 50 mg/hour every 30 minutes, to a maximum of 400 mg/hour
  - Subsequent infusions: If patient did not tolerate initial infusion well, follow initial infusion guidelines. If patient tolerated initial infusion, start at 100 mg/hour; if there is no reaction, increase the rate by 100 mg/hour every 30 minutes, to a maximum of 400 mg/hour.
  - Note: If a reaction occurs, slow or stop the infusion. If the reaction abates, restart the infusion at 50% of the previous rate.

Adverse Reactions: Most Common

- Infusion reaction, tumor lysis syndrome, lymphopenia, rash, nausea, myalgias and arthralgias

Adverse Reactions: Rare/Severe/Important

- Severe and sometimes fatal mucocutaneous, reactions (lichenoid dermatitis, paraneoplastic pemphigus, Stevens–Johnson syndrome, toxic epidermal necrolysis, and vesiculobullous dermatitis), anaphylaxis, progressive multifocal leukoencephalopathy, bowel obstruction and perforation

Major Drug Interactions

Rituximab's Effect on Other Drugs

- Antihypertensives: Hypotension may be increased

Counseling Points

- Report immediately any shortness of breath or chest tightness, fever and chills during treatments
- There is an increased risk of infection while on treatment

Key Points

- No live virus vaccines during therapy
- Infusion-related reactions are common. Monitor the patient during the infusion.
- Pretreatment with acetaminophen and diphenhydramine is recommended
- Reactivation of hepatitis B and other serious viral infections (possibly new or reactivated) have been reported

■ Trastuzumab

Brand Name
Herceptin

Generic Name
Trastuzumab

Dosage Forms

Injection

Usage

- Early stage and metastatic breast cancer*

Dosing

- IV 4 mg/kg loading dose, then 2 mg/kg weekly or 6 mg/kg every 3 weeks

Adverse Reactions: Most Common

- Infusion-related reactions, rash, nausea, diarrhea

Adverse Reactions: Rare/Severe/Important

- Cardiotoxicity, pulmonary toxicity

Major Drug Interactions

Trastuzumab's Effect on Other Drugs

- Anthracyclines: Increased cardiotoxicity
- Myelosuppressive chemotherapy: Increases infection risk

Counseling Point

- Report immediately any shortness of breath or chest tightness, fever and chills during treatments

Key Point

- Patient should have ejection fraction measured before starting therapy

---

Drug Class: Taxanes

Introduction

This class of antineoplastics is used to treat a wide range of malignancies. They can be used alone as monotherapy or in combination with other antineoplastics. They are most notable for causing bone marrow suppression and peripheral neuropathies.

Mechanism of Action for the Drug Class

Taxanes stabilize the microtubule bundles by promoting assembly and preventing depolymerization, thereby inhibiting cell replication.

Members of the Drug Class

In this section: Docetaxel, paclitaxel

▪ Docetaxel

Brand Name

Taxotere

Generic Name

Docetaxel

Dosage Forms

Injection

Usage

- Treatment of breast cancer*; locally advanced or metastatic NSCLC*; hormone-refractory metastatic prostate cancer*; advanced gastric adenocarcinoma; locally advanced squamous cell head and neck cancer, bladder cancer, ovarian cancer, small cell lung cancer, soft tissue sarcoma

Dosing

- Individual protocols specify dosing for specific indications and institutions
- Dosing range: 60–100 mg/m^2/dose every 3–4 weeks or 35 mg/m^2 weekly
- Hepatic dosage adjustment:
  - Avoid use if either of the following are present: Total bilirubin greater than the ULN or aspartate aminotransferase/alanine aminotransferase >1.5 times ULN concomitant with alkaline phosphatase >2.5 times ULN

Adverse Reactions: Most Common

- Fluid retention syndrome, leucopenia, anemia, thrombocytopenia, alopecia, peripheral neuropathies, myalgias, arthralgias, diarrhea, stomatitis, mild nausea

Adverse Reactions: Rare/Severe/Important

- Skin desquamation, hypersensitivity, oncolysis

Major Drug Interactions

Drugs Affecting Docetaxel

- Azole antifungals: Decrease the metabolism of docetaxel, raising concentrations
- Carboplatin, cisplatin: Increase myelosuppression

Counseling Points

- No live virus vaccines during therapy
- Watch for fever, malaise
- Risk of infection is increased; report any fever or infection to your healthcare practitioner

Key Points

- Extravasation can cause tissue necrosis
- Must premedicate with a corticosteroid to reduce fluid retention
- Administer taxane derivatives before platinum derivative when given as sequential infusions to limit toxicity

■ Paclitaxel

Brand Name
Taxol

Generic Name
Paclitaxel

Dosage Forms
Injection

Usage

- Treatment of breast cancer*; NSCLC*; locally advanced squamous cell head and neck cancer*, bladder cancer, ovarian cancer*, small cell lung cancer, adenocarcinomas of unknown primary and AIDS-related Kaposi sarcoma

Dosing

- Individual protocols specify dosing for specific indications and institutions
- Dosing range: 135–200 mg/m^2 per dose every 3–4 weeks OR 80–100 mg/m^2 weekly
- Hepatic dosage adjustment: (3-hour infusion):
  - Transaminase levels <10 times ULN and bilirubin level 1.26–2 times ULN: 135 mg/m^2
  - Transaminase levels <10 times ULN and bilirubin level 2.01–5 times ULN: 90 mg/m^2
  - Transaminase levels ≥10 times ULN and bilirubin level >5 times ULN: Avoid use

Adverse Reactions: Most Common

- Bradycardia, flushing, leucopenia, anemia, thrombocytopenia, alopecia, peripheral neuropathies, myalgias, arthralgias, diarrhea, stomatitis, mild nausea

Adverse Reactions: Rare/Severe/Important

- Hypersensitivity, skin rashes

Major Drug Interactions

Drugs Affecting Paclitaxel

- Azole antifungals: Decrease the metabolism of paclitaxel, increasing concentrations
- Carboplatin, cisplatin: Increase myelosuppression
- Trastuzumab: Enhances neutropenia

Paclitaxel's Effect on Other Drugs

- Anthracyclines: Increase cardiotoxicity

Counseling Points

- No live virus vaccines during therapy
- Peripheral neuropathies can occur with continued use
- Risk of infection is increased; report any fever or infection to your healthcare practitioner

Key Points

- Severe bone marrow suppression is possible and may require dose reduction
- Monitor blood pressure regularly while drug is infusing
- Extravasation can cause tissue necrosis
- Must premedicate with a corticosteroid, diphenhydramine, and histamine-2 blocker to prevent hypersensitivity
- Paclitaxel is a radiosensitizer and will increase effect and toxicity of radiation therapy
- Administer a taxane derivative before a platinum derivative when given as sequential infusions to limit toxicity

---

Review Questions

1. Which of the following kills tumors by causing strand breaks in DNA resulting in cell death?
   A. Capecitabine
   B. Cyclophosphamide
   C. Docetaxel
   D. Mercaptopurine

2. Which of the following causes apoptosis to tumor cells by inhibiting cell mitosis?
   A. Paraplatin
   B. Gemcitabine
   C. Gleevec
   D. Taxol

3. Which of the agents is associated with a high incidence of nephrotoxicity?
   A. Carboplatin
   B. Cisplatin
   C. Doxorubicin
   D. Fluorouracil

4. Mercaptopurine has a significant drug interaction requiring dose modification with which of the following drugs?
   A. Allopurinol
   B. Corticosteroids
   C. Ibuprofen
   D. Leucovorin

5. Use of which of the following drugs is contraindicated during therapy with rituximab?
   A. Dexamethasone
   B. Diphenhydramine
   C. FluMist nasal vaccine
   D. Attenuated influenza vaccine

6. Which of the following is an important counseling point for patients taking Xeloda?
   A. Report any fever or sign of infection to your physician
   B. Stop using if nausea occurs
   C. Take orally once a day
   D. Take on empty stomach

7. A patient receiving cytarabine should be monitored frequently during therapy for which of the following side effects?
   A. Electrocardiogram for cardiotoxicity
   B. Liver function tests for hepatotoxicity
   C. Mental status for neurotoxicity
   D. Physical exam for alopecia

8. Which of the following chemotherapy drugs can be administered intrathecally?
   A. Cisplatin
   B. Gemcitabine
   C. Mercaptopurine
   D. Methotrexate

9. Which of the following is used to treat breast cancers that specifically overexpress the oncogene HER2/neu?
   A. Gemcitabine
   B. Imatinib
   C. Docetaxel
   D. Trastuzumab

10. Cytarabine is commonly used to treat which of the following cancers?
    A. Acute myelogenous leukemia
    B. Breast cancer
    C. Colon cancer
    D. Lung cancer

11. Doxorubicin, commonly used to treat breast cancer is dosed based on body surface area at a dose of:
    A. 6 mg/m^2
    B. 60 mg/m^2
    C. 600 mg/m^2
    D. 6000 mg/m^2

12. Which of the following chemotherapy agents should be dose-reduced for hepatic dysfunction?
    A. Carboplatin
    B. Paclitaxel
    C. Rituximab
    D. Trastuzumab

13. Imatinib (Gleevec) could potentially interact with all of the following except
    A. Acetaminophen
    B. Carbamazepine
    C. Lansoprazole
    D. Fluconazole

14. Which of the following antineoplastic agents is also commonly used for rheumatoid arthritis?
    A. Capecitabine
    B. Cytoxan
    C. Purinethol
    D. Methotrexate

15. The following antineoplastic agent is also used topically to treat basal cell skin cancers:
    A. Cytarabine
    B. Doxorubicin
    C. Fluorouracil
    D. Methotrexate

CHAPTER 5

Cardiovascular Agents

Anna M. Wodlinger Jackson, PharmD, BCPS

Drug Class: α-1 Adrenergic Blockers

Introduction

The α-1 adrenergic blockers are used for the treatment of hypertension, although usually not as a first-line agent of choice because there are more effective agents available. More commonly they are used for the treatment of benign prostatic hyperplasia (BPH).

Mechanism of Action for the Drug Class

These drugs selectively block postsynaptic α-1 adrenergic receptors, dilating both peripheral arterioles and veins. They also relax smooth muscles in the prostate and bladder neck. Tamsulosin is selective for the α receptors in the prostate and does not have a therapeutic effect on blood pressure, although orthostatic hypotension is still possible as with other members of this class.

Usage for the Drug Class

- Treatment of hypertension (not first-line) and BPH*

Adverse Reactions for the Drug Class: Most Common

- Dizziness, headache, orthostatic hypotension, syncope, flushing (tamsulosin)

Adverse Reactions for the Drug Class: Rare/Severe/Important

- Intraoperative floppy iris syndrome (in patients undergoing cataract surgery), priapism

Major Drug Interactions for the Drug Class

Drugs Affecting α-1 Adrenergic Blockers

- Concomitant antihypertensive agents and phosphodiesterase-5 inhibitors: Additive hypotension

α-1 Adrenergic Blocker's Effect on Other Drugs

- Antihypertensive agents: Additive hypotension

Counseling Points for the Drug Class

- These drugs may cause dizziness or drowsiness (take at night to avoid)
- Use caution when getting up from a sitting or lying position
- May require 1–2 weeks of therapy before improved symptoms of BPH are seen

Members of the Drug Class

In this section: Doxazosin, tamsulosin, terazosin

Others: Alfuzosin, phenoxybenzamine, phentolamine, prazosin, silodosin

■ Doxazosin

Brand Names

Cardura, Cardura XL

Generic Name

Doxazosin

Dosage Forms

Tablets, extended-release tablets

Dosing

- Initial dose:
  - 1 mg daily
- Dose titration:
  - Up to 16 mg daily (maximum for BPH usually 8 mg)

Key Points

- Although indicated for the treatment of hypertension, doxazosin is not often used first-line. It is more commonly used for the treatment of BPH. Counsel patients about the risk of orthostatic hypotension and signs of dizziness.
- The extended-release formula is a nondeformable matrix that is expelled in the stool

■ Tamsulosin

Brand Name

Flomax

Generic Name

Tamsulosin

Dosage Forms

Capsules

Dosing

- Initial dose:
  - 0.4 mg daily
- Dose titration:
  - Can increase in 2–4 weeks to maximum of 0.8 mg daily

Key Points

- This is a selective α-agonist and therefore has minimal effect on blood pressure and is used only for the treatment of BPH
- Do not crush, chew, or open capsule
- Avoid concomitant use of phosphodiesterase-5 inhibitors (sildenafil, tadalafil, vardenafil)

■ Terazosin

Brand Name

Hytrin

Generic Name

Terazosin

Dosage Forms

Capsules

Dosing

- Initial dose:
  - 1 mg daily
- Dosing adjustments:
  - Up to 20 mg daily

Key Point

- Although indicated for the treatment of hypertension, terazosin is not often used first-line. It is more commonly used for the treatment of BPH. Watch for orthostatic hypotension and signs of dizziness.

Drug Class: α-2 Adrenergic Agonists

Introduction

The α-2 adrenergic agonists are used for the treatment of hypertension, although usually not a first-line agent of choice. They also have several unlabeled uses.

Mechanism of Action for the Drug Class

Stimulation of α-2 adrenergic receptors in the brainstem results in reduced sympathetic outflow from the CNS and a decrease in peripheral resistance, renal vascular resistance, heart rate, and blood pressure.

Members of the Drug Class

In this section: Clonidine

Others: Dexmedetomidine, guanabenz, guanfacine, methyldopa

■ Clonidine

Brand Names

Catapres, Catapres-TTS, Duraclon

Generic Name

Clonidine

Dosage Forms

Tablets, transdermal patches, injection (epidural solution)

Usage

Hypertension*, alcohol withdrawal, attention deficit hyperactivity disorder, cancer pain (intraspinal administration), diabetes-associated diarrhea, dysmenorrhea, glaucoma, heroin or nicotine withdrawal, impulse control disorder, menopausal flushing, migraine prophylaxis, severe pain

Dosing

- Initial dose:
  - Capsule: 0.1 mg twice daily
  - Transdermal: Start with TTS 1
- Dosing adjustments:
  - Capsule: Can increase in weekly intervals by 0.1 mg to maximum dose of 2.4 mg daily. Can give in 2–4 daily doses.
  - Transdermal: Increase in 1- to 2-week intervals
- Renal dosage adjustment:
  - CrCl <10 ml/minute: Administer 50–75% of normal dose initially, then titrate to blood pressure control

Adverse Reactions: Most Common

- CNS depression, constipation, dry mouth, dizziness, drowsiness, orthostatic hypotension

Adverse Reactions: Rare/Severe/Important

- AV block, bradycardia, contact dermatitis (transdermal)

Major Drug Interactions

Drugs Affecting Clonidine

- Concomitant antihypertensive agents: Additive hypotension
- Tricyclic antidepressants: Decreased hypotensive effects
- β-Blockers: Additive bradycardia
- β-Blockers: Discontinuation of clonidine during concurrent use of a β-blocker may increase the risk of clonidine-withdrawal hypertensive crisis. It is preferred to discontinue the β-blocker several days prior to clonidine discontinuation.
- CNS depressants: Additive CNS effects

Clonidine's Effect on Other Drugs

- Cyclosporine: Increases levels

Counseling Points

- Do not stop clonidine abruptly because it may cause rebound hypertension

- Apply transdermal patch weekly to clean hairless area of upper outer arm or chest and rotate sites weekly
- Oral therapy and transdermal therapy may overlap for 1–2 days until the full effect of transdermal therapy occurs
- The transdermal patch may contain metal; must remove before MRI

Key Points

- Clonidine is a very effective blood pressure lowering agent. It is often added to other antihypertensive therapies in patients with resistant hypertension. The risk of rebound hypertension is high if patient discontinues abruptly.
- Transdermal route takes 2–3 days for full therapeutic effect

---

Drug Class: Angiotensin-Converting Enzyme (ACE) Inhibitors

Introduction

The ACE inhibitors are widely used for various cardiovascular diseases. They are effective for the treatment of hypertension and are the foundation of therapy for heart failure and left ventricular dysfunction. In addition, they are used for the prevention and treatment of diabetic nephropathy.

Mechanism of Action for the Drug Class

These agents act primarily through suppression of the renin–angiotensin–aldosterone system. They inhibit ACE, thereby inhibiting the conversion of angiotensin I to angiotensin II, a potent vasoconstrictor.

Usage for the Drug Class

- Diabetic nephropathy*, heart failure*, hypertension*, left ventricular dysfunction after myocardial infarction

Adverse Reactions for the Drug Class: Most Common

- Hypotension, hyperkalemia, cough

Adverse Reactions for the Drug Class: Rare/ Severe/Important

- Angioedema (contraindication for use), azotemia, and renal failure in susceptible patients (e.g., volume depleted), neutropenia/agranulocytosis (captopril), avoid use in patients with bilateral renal artery stenosis; contraindicated in pregnancy

Major Drug Interactions for the Drug Class

Drugs Affecting ACE Inhibitors

- Concomitant antihypertensive agents: Additive hypotension
- Angiotensin II receptor blockers, potassium-sparing diuretics, trimethoprim/sulfamethoxazole: Increased risk of hyperkalemia
- Diuretics: May potentiate renal insufficiency in volume-depleted patients
- NSAIDs: Reduced hypotensive effect of ACE inhibitors

ACE Inhibitor Effects on Other Drugs

- Antihypertensive agents: Additive hypotension
- Cyclosporine: Increased nephrotoxicity
- Lithium: Increased serum levels
- Potassium-sparing diuretics, potassium supplements: May cause elevated potassium levels

Counseling Points for the Drug Class

- Some laboratory work will be needed periodically to monitor therapy (potassium, serum creatinine)
- Seek help immediately if swelling in face, lips, tongue, or throat occurs
- Avoid salt substitutes containing potassium
- Women: Notify your physician if pregnancy is suspected

Key Point for the Drug Class
- ACE inhibitors are widely used for the treatment of hypertension, heart failure, and other cardiovascular diseases. There are some potentially fatal adverse effects associated with their use, so appropriate monitoring and patient counseling is necessary.

Members of the Drug Class
In this section: Benazepril, captopril, enalapril, fosinopril, lisinopril, quinapril, ramipril

Others: Moexipril, perindopril, trandolapril

■ Benazepril
Brand Name
Lotensin

Generic Name
Benazepril

Dosage Forms
Tablets

Dosing
- Initial dose:
  - 10 mg daily
- Dose titration:
  - Up to 40 mg/day in 1–2 divided doses
- Renal dosage adjustment:
  - CrCl <30 ml/minute: Consider starting at lower doses (5 mg daily)

■ Captopril
Brand Name
Capoten

Generic Name
Captopril

Dosage Forms
Tablets

Dosing
- Initial dose:
  - 6.25–25 mg two to three times daily
- Dose titration:
  - Up to 450 mg/day in 3 divided doses
- Renal dosage adjustment:
  - Consider starting at lower doses

Key Point
- The use of captopril is often limited to the inpatient setting because it is administered three times a day, and there are other ACE inhibitors with more convenient dosing regimens (once or twice daily)

■ Enalapril
Brand Name
Vasotec

Generic Name

Enalapril

Dosage Forms
Tablets, injection (as enalaprilat)

Dosing
- Initial dose:
  - 2.5 mg PO two times daily (can be given daily for hypertension)
- Dose titration:
  - Up to 40 mg PO per day in 2 divided doses
- Renal dosage adjustment:
  - Consider starting at lower doses

■ Fosinopril
Brand Name
Monopril

Generic Name
Fosinopril

Dosage Forms
Tablets

Dosing
- Initial dose:
  - 10 mg daily
- Dose titration:
  - Up to 40 mg daily in 1–2 doses

■ Lisinopril
Brand Names
Prinivil, Zestril

Generic Name
Lisinopril

Dosage Forms
Tablets

Dosing
- Initial dose:
  - 5–10 mg daily
- Dose titration:
  - Up to 40 mg/day
- Renal dosage adjustment:
  - Consider starting at lower doses (2.5 mg)

■ Quinapril
Brand Name
Accupril

Generic Name
Quinapril

Dosage Forms
Tablets

Dosing
- Initial dose:
  - 10–20 mg/day (in 1–2 doses)

- Dose titration:
  - Up to 40 mg/day in 2 divided doses
- Renal dosage adjustment:
  - Consider starting at lower doses

■ Ramipril

Brand Name
Altace

Generic Name
Ramipril

Dosage Forms
Capsules, tablets

Dosing
- Initial dose:
  - 2.5 mg/day
- Dose titration:
  - Up to 20 mg/day in 1–2 divided doses
- Renal dosage adjustment:
  - Consider starting at lower doses

Key Point
- Ramipril is also indicated to reduce the risk of myocardial infarction, stroke, and death from cardiovascular causes in patients who are at increased risk of these events.

Drug Class: Angiotensin II Receptor Blockers (ARBs)

Introduction
The ARBs are widely used for the treatment of cardiovascular diseases. They are primarily used for the treatment of hypertension and as an alternative to ACE inhibitors for the treatment of heart failure and diabetic nephropathy. One advantage that they hold over ACE inhibitors is that they do not cause ACE inhibitor-related cough.

Mechanism of Action for the Drug Class
These agents suppress the renin–angiotensin–aldosterone system. They block the binding of angiotensin II to the AT1 receptor, thereby inhibiting the effects of angiotensin II.

Usage for the Drug Class
- Hypertension*, diabetic nephropathy*, heart failure* (select ARBs), myocardial infarction

Adverse Reactions for the Drug Class: Most Common
- Hyperkalemia, hypotension

Adverse Reactions for the Drug Class: Rare/Severe/Important
- Increased SCr, contraindicated in pregnancy

Major Drug Interactions for the Drug Class
Drugs Affecting Angiotensin II Receptor Blockers
- Potassium supplements and potassium-sparing diuretics: Potential additive increases in potassium

Angiotensin II Receptor Blocker Effects on Other Drugs
- Lithium: May reduce elimination

Counseling Points for the Drug Class
- Some laboratory work will be needed periodically to monitor therapy (potassium, serum creatinine)

- Women: Notify your physician if pregnancy is suspected

Key Point for the Drug Class
- ARBs are used widely for the treatment of cardiovascular diseases. They are often used in patients intolerant of ACE inhibitors who have heart failure (candesartan, losartan, valsartan only).

Members of the Drug Class
In this section: Irbesartan, losartan, valsartan
  Others: Candesartan, eprosartan, olmesartan, telmisartan

■ Irbesartan

Brand Name
Avapro

Generic Name
Irbesartan

Dosage Forms
Tablets

Dosing
- Initial dose:
  - 75–150 mg daily
- Dose titration:
  - Up to 300 mg daily

Key Points
- Also indicated for treatment of diabetic nephropathy in patients with diabetes mellitus and hypertension
- Not recommended for heart failure

■ Losartan

Brand Name
Cozaar

Generic Name

Losartan

Dosage Forms

Tablets

Dosing

- Initial dose:
  - 25–50 mg/day
- Dose titration:
  - Up to 100 mg/day in 1–2 divided doses

■ **Valsartan**

Brand Name

Diovan

Generic Name

Valsartan

Dosage Forms

Tablets

Dosing

- Initial dose:
  - 80–160 mg/day
- Dose titration:
  - Up to 320 mg/day in 1–2 divided doses

Key Point

- Preferred ARB in patients with heart failure

Drug Class: Antiarrhythmics, Amiodarone

Introduction

Amiodarone is the most commonly used antiarrhythmic agent. It is used for rate and rhythm control of atrial fibrillation and to treat and prevent ventricular arrhythmias. It has a very long terminal half-life of approximately 2 months and a large volume of distribution and thus requires large loading doses administered over several weeks.

Mechanism of Action for the Drug Class

Amiodarone is considered a class III antiarrhythmic medication; however, it exhibits characteristics of all four Vaughn–Williams antiarrhythmic medication classes. Amiodarone slows intraventricular conduction by blocking sodium channels, slows the heart rate, and impedes AV node conduction by blocking β-adrenergic receptors and calcium channels, and prolongs atrial and ventricular repolarization by inhibiting potassium channels.

■ **Amiodarone**

Brand Names

Cordarone, Pacerone

Generic Name

Amiodarone

Dosage Forms

Tablets, injection

Usage

- Atrial arrhythmias*, life-threatening ventricular arrhythmias*, prevention of postoperative atrial fibrillation in cardiothoracic surgery, prevention of ventricular arrhythmias in patients with internal cardioverter-defibrillators

Dosing

- Loading dose (oral): 800–1600 mg/day in divided doses for 1–3 weeks until adequate arrhythmia control is achieved (usually up to 10 g total)
- Loading dose (IV): 150–300 mg in 20–30 ml NS followed by 1 mg/minute for 6 hours, then 0.5 mg/minute for 18 hours. Infusion can be continued for up to 4 weeks. Should switch to oral as soon as possible.
- Maintenance dose (oral): 200–400 mg/day

Adverse Reactions: Most Common

Bradycardia, corneal microdeposits, hypotension (more common with IV), hypothyroidism, nausea, vomiting (especially with higher doses), phlebitis (IV form), photosensitivity, prolonged QTc interval

Adverse Reactions: Rare/Severe/Important

Blue/gray skin discoloration, hyperthyroidism, liver toxicity, pulmonary toxicity

Major Drug Interactions

Drugs Affecting Amiodarone

- Drugs that prolong the QTc interval: May increase the QTc prolonging effect of amiodarone
- β-Blockers, diltiazem, digoxin, and verapamil: May cause excessive atrioventricular block
- Cimetidine: Decreased metabolism

Amiodarone's Effect on Other Drugs

- Cyclosporine: Decreased metabolism
- Lovastatin, simvastatin: Increased risk of myopathy
- Digoxin: Increased levels
- Warfarin: Increased effects

Counseling Points

- Take with food to decrease gastrointestinal adverse effects
- Use sunscreen or stay out of sun to prevent burns
- Schedule regular blood work for thyroid and liver function

Key Points

- Although amiodarone is the most commonly used antiarrhythmic agent for atrial and ventricular arrhythmias, it should be reserved for patients with life-threatening arrhythmias due to its substantial toxicity. Patients should be hospitalized for initiation of therapy and need to be monitored and counseled appropriately to limit toxicity.
- IV admixtures must be made in glass or non-PVC containers (for all infusions expected to run >1 hour)

Drug Class: Antiarrhythmics, Digitalis Glycosides

Introduction

Digoxin is the only available digitalis glycoside, and is one of the oldest medications used for the treatment of heart failure. Although it is still frequently utilized in heart failure, it is no longer a first-line choice because other agents (ACE inhibitors, β-blockers) have been proven more effective at reducing morbidity and mortality. Digoxin also has a role as a rate-control agent in the treatment of atrial fibrillation.

Mechanism of Action for the Drug Class

Inhibits sodium-potassium ATPase, leading to an increase in the intracellular concentration of sodium and thus, by stimulation of sodium-calcium exchange, an increase in the intracellular concentration of calcium leading to increased contractility. Enhances vagal tone to directly suppress the atrioventricular node, which increases effective refractory period and decreases conduction velocity resulting in decreased ventricular rate.

■ Digoxin

Brand Name
Lanoxin

Generic Name
Digoxin

Dosage Forms
Tablets, capsules, solution, injection

Usage
- Heart failure (stage C)*, supraventricular arrhythmias*

Dosing
- Loading dose: 8–12 μg/kg ideal body weight (adjust for renal function). Average loading dose: 0.75–1 mg.
  - Administration recommendations: Roughly half of the total loading dose administered as the first dose, with the remaining portion divided and administered every 6–8 hours initially
- Maintenance dose: 0.125 mg–0.5 mg daily

- Renal dosage adjustment: Both loading and maintenance doses should be adjusted
  - CrCl 10–50 ml/minute: Administer 25–75% of dose or full dose every 36 hours
  - CrCl <10 ml/minute: Administer 10–25% of dose or full dose every 48 hours
  - End-stage renal disease: Reduce dose by 50%

Pharmacokinetic Monitoring
- Monitor levels after at least 6 hours following administration (usually prior to next dose)
- Obtain within 12–24 hours of initiating therapy if a loading dose is given or 3–5 days following initiation if no loading dose is given
- Usual range 0.5–0.8 ng/dl for heart failure, 0.8–2 ng/dl for arrhythmias

Adverse Reactions: Most Common
- Anorexia, diarrhea, dizziness, headache, nausea

Adverse Reactions: Rare/Severe/Important
- Atrial tachycardia, AV dissociation, blurred or yellow vision, hallucinations, heart block, ventricular fibrillation/tachycardia

Major Drug Interactions

Drugs Affecting Digoxin
- Increased digoxin serum levels:
  - Amiodarone (reduce digoxin dose by 50%)
  - Clarithromycin
  - Cyclosporine
  - Diltiazem
  - Dronedarone (reduce dose by 50%)
  - Erythromycin
  - Fluconazole
  - Itraconazole
  - Quinidine, quinine
  - Tetracyclines
  - Verapamil

- Decreased digoxin therapeutic effects:
  - Cholestyramine
  - Colestipol
  - Kaolin-pectin
  - Sucralfate
- Diuretic-induced electrolyte decreases (potassium, magnesium) may predispose patients to digitalis-induced arrhythmias

Digoxin's Effect on Other Drugs
- Although β-blockers or calcium channel blockers and digoxin may be useful in combination to control atrial fibrillation, their additive effects on AV node conduction may result in advanced or complete heart block

Counseling Points
- Take digoxin at the same time every day
- Notify your healthcare practitioner if any signs of toxicity occur (e.g., nausea, vomiting, blurry vision)

Key Points
- Although digoxin is not a first-line choice, it is often used in the treatment of symptomatic heart failure and atrial fibrillation
- Digoxin has a narrow therapeutic index, and dosing must be adjusted for renal function, weight, and heart failure status. Appropriate monitoring of renal function is necessary to avoid toxicity.

Drug Class: Antiarrhythmics, Sotalol

Introduction
Sotalol has activity as both a β-blocker and class III antiarrhythmic. It is used for rate and rhythm control in patients with atrial fibrillation.

Mechanism of Action for the Drug Class
Sotalol has both nonselective β-adrenergic blockade and class III antiarrhythmic actions that prolong cardiac action potential duration by inhibiting potassium channels.

■ Sotalol

Brand Names
Betapace, Betapace AF, Sorine

Generic Name
Sotalol

Dosage Forms
Tablets

Usage
- Atrial fibrillation*, life-threatening ventricular arrhythmias

Dosing
- Initial dose:
  - Treatment should be initiated in a setting where continuous electrocardiographic (ECG) monitoring is possible
  - Initial dose based on CrCl:
    - CrCl >60 ml/minute: 80 mg twice daily
    - CrCl 40–60 ml/minute: 80 mg daily
    - CrCl <40 ml/min: Contraindicated
- Maintenance dose: Up to 160 mg twice daily
  - Renal dosage adjustment of maintenance dose:
    - CrCl 40–60 ml/minute: Administer daily
    - Contraindicated if CrCl <40 ml/minute

Adverse Reactions: Most Common
- Bradycardia, dizziness, dyspnea, fatigue, QT interval prolongation (avoid if baseline QTc >450 milliseconds; discontinue or decrease dose if QTc >500 milliseconds during therapy)

Adverse Reactions: Rare/Severe/Important
- Bronchospasm, heart block, torsades de pointes

Major Drug Interactions
Drugs Affecting Sotalol
- Calcium channel blockers: Increased bradycardia
- Digoxin: Increased proarrhythmic risk
- Drugs that prolong the QTc interval: Increase the QTc-prolonging effect of sotalol
- Antacids containing aluminum oxide or magnesium hydroxide: Reduced absorption

Sotalol's Effect on Other Drugs
- Although calcium channel blockers and digoxin may be useful in combination with sotalol to control atrial fibrillation, their additive effects on AV node conduction may result in advanced or complete heart block

Counseling Point
- Patient must have routine blood tests to monitor renal function

Key Points
- Initiation of therapy and dose titrations should occur in a hospital setting with continuous monitoring
- Betapace and Betapace AF should not be substituted for each other
- Renal function and QTc interval must be monitored closely and dosing adjustments made accordingly
- Electrolyte abnormalities (hypokalemia, hypomagnesemia) should be corrected prior to initiation
- Should be avoided in heart failure

Introduction

β-Blockers are one of the most widely used cardiovascular medications. They are very effective at preventing morbidity and mortality for several disease states.

Mechanism of Action for the Drug Class

β-Blockers competitively block response to β-adrenergic stimulation, which results in decreases in heart rate, myocardial contractility, blood pressure, and myocardial oxygen demand. β-1 selective agents selectively block β-1 receptors with little or no effect on β-2 receptors.

Usage for the Drug Class

- Angina*, arrhythmias*, heart failure (bisoprolol, carvedilol and metoprolol XL only)*, hypertension*, myocardial infarction*, premature ventricular contractions, adjunctive management of pheochromocytoma
- Noncardiovascular uses: Essential tremors, migraine prophylaxis, adjunctive therapy in the treatment of Parkinson disease, alcohol withdrawal syndrome, aggressive behavior, treatment of antipsychotic-induced akathisia, prevention of esophageal varices rebleeding, treatment of anxiety, adjunctive treatment in schizophrenia and acute panic, prevention of gastric bleeding in portal hypertension, and treatment of thyrotoxicosis symptoms

Adverse Reactions for the Drug Class: Most Common

- Bradycardia, decreased sexual ability, dizziness, hypotension, fatigue, lethargy

Adverse Reactions for the Drug Class: Rare/Severe/Important

- Heart block, worsening heart failure symptoms, bronchoconstriction (nonselective or selective at higher doses), exacerbations of Raynaud disease

Major Drug Interactions for the Drug Class

Drugs Affecting β-Blockers

- Digoxin, diltiazem, verapamil: Enhanced AV nodal inhibition

β-Blocker Effects on Other Drugs

- Oral antidiabetic agents, insulin: May mask the symptoms of hypoglycemia

Counseling Points for the Drug Class

- Do not abruptly stop taking medication. β-Blockers should be gradually tapered when stopping to avoid tachycardia, hypertension, and/or ischemia.
- These medications may increase blood glucose. They may also mask the symptoms of hypoglycemia.
- May decrease heart rate and blood pressure. Tell your healthcare provider if you experience any dizziness or lightheadedness.

Key Point for the Drug Class

- β-Blockers are one of the most widely used cardiovascular agents because they are very effective for the treatment of many cardiovascular diseases. They are also used for some off-label uses not associated directly with cardiovascular disease.

Members of the Drug Class

In this section: Atenolol, carvedilol, labetalol, metoprolol, propranolol

Others: Betaxolol, bisoprolol, esmolol, nadolol, nebivolol, timolol

■ Atenolol

Brand Name
Tenormin

Generic Name
Atenolol (β-1 selective)

Dosage Forms
Tablets

Dosing
- 25–100 mg daily
- Renal dosage adjustment:
  - CrCl 15–35 ml/minute: Maximum dose of 50 mg once daily
  - CrCl <15 ml/minute: Maximum dose 50 mg every other day

■ Carvedilol

Brand Names
Coreg, Coreg CR

Generic Name
Carvedilol (nonselective with α-1 blockade)

Dosage Forms
Tablets, extended-release capsules

Dosing
- Nonextended release: 3.125–50 mg twice daily
- Extended release: 10–80 mg daily

Key Points
- Recommended for heart failure
- Conversion from immediate-release to extended-release is not 1:1
- Inhibits α-1-receptors as well, unlike most other β-blockers

■ Labetalol

Brand Name
Trandate

Generic Name
Labetalol (nonselective with α-1 blockade)

Dosage Forms
Tablets, injection

Dosing
- 100 mg PO twice daily, can be given up to 2400 mg PO daily in divided doses

Key Points
- Often used for hypertension and hypertensive emergencies
- Inhibits α-1-receptors as well, unlike most other β-blockers

■ Metoprolol
Brand Names
Lopressor, Toprol XL

Generic Names
Metoprolol tartrate, metoprolol succinate (β-1 selective)

Dosage Forms
Tablets, injection

Dosing
- Initial dose:
  - Oral: 25–50 mg twice daily (once daily if XL formulation)
  - IV: 1.25–5 mg every 6–12 hours
- Dosing adjustments:
  - Oral: Up to 450 mg in divided daily doses (once daily if XL formulation)
  - IV: Up to 15 mg every 3–6 hours

Key Point
- Only the extended-release formulation (metoprolol succinate) is recommended for use in heart failure patients

■ Propranolol
Brand Names
Inderal, Inderal LA, InnoPran XL

Generic Name
Propranolol (nonselective)

Dosage Forms
Tablets, sustained-release capsules, oral solution, injection

Dosing
- Initial dose:
  - Oral: 40 mg twice daily (once daily if long-acting [LA] formulation)
- Dosing adjustments:
  - Oral: Up to 640 mg in 2–4 divided daily doses (once daily if LA formulation)

Drug Class: Calcium Channel Blockers, Benzothiazepines

Introduction
Diltiazem is the only member of the benzothiazepine class of calcium channel blockers. It is commonly used for the treatment of hypertension and heart rate control in patients with atrial fibrillation due to its effects on both blood pressure and cardiac conduction.

Mechanism of Action for the Drug Class
These drugs inhibit the movement of calcium ions across the cell membranes. The effects on the cardiovascular system include relaxation of coronary vascular smooth muscle and coronary vasodilation. They also increase myocardial oxygen delivery and depress both impulse formation and conduction velocity in the atrioventricular node.

■ Diltiazem
Brand Names
Cardizem, Cardizem CD, Cardizem LA, Cartia XT, Dilacor XR, Dilt-CD, Dilt-XR, Diltia XT, Taztia XT, Tiazac

Generic Name
Diltiazem

Dosage Forms
Tablets, extended-release tablets, extended-release capsules, injection

Usage
- Atrial arrhythmias*, chronic stable angina, hypertension*, paroxysmal supraventricular tachycardias, variant angina

Dosing
- 120–540 mg/day (in 1–4 divided doses depending on drug formulation)

Adverse Reactions: Most Common
- Bradycardia, dizziness, lightheadedness, flushing, headache, hypotension, edema

Adverse Reactions: Rare/Severe/Important

- Third degree AV block, decreased heart contractility (worsening symptoms of heart failure)

Major Drug Interactions

Drugs Affecting Diltiazem

- Diltiazem effects may be increased if given with drugs that inhibit CYP3A4
- Azole antifungal agents: Increased hypotensive effects
- Carbamazepine: Decreased hypotensive effect
- Clarithromycin, erythromycin: Decreased metabolism
- Rifampin: Decreased hypotensive effect
- Sildenafil: Increased hypotensive effect

Diltiazem's Effect on Other Drugs

- Antihypertensive medications: Additive hypotensive effects
- Amiodarone, β-blockers, and digoxin: Enhanced decrease in AV node conduction; increased risk of bradycardia

- Increased concentration of drugs metabolized by CYP3A4 (cyclosporine, HMG-CoA reductase inhibitors, tacrolimus)
- Phenytoin: Decreased metabolism

Counseling Points

- Take on an empty stomach if possible
- Do not crush long-acting formulations
- You may open capsules and sprinkle them on applesauce, which you then swallow without chewing

Key Points

- Diltiazem is used for the treatment of hypertension, angina, and atrial fibrillation. It should be avoided in patients with myocardial infarction and/or heart failure because it is a negative inotrope.
- Extended-release formulations are either daily or twice-daily dosing. Check with specific manufacturer recommendations.

Drug Class: Calcium Channel Blockers, Dihydropyridines

Introduction

The dihydropyridine calcium channel blockers are widely used for the treatment of hypertension. They do not affect heart rate or contractility to the same extent as diltiazem and verapamil.

Mechanism of Action for the Drug Class

These drugs inhibit movement of calcium ions across the cell membranes. The effects on the cardiovascular system include relaxation of coronary vascular smooth muscle and coronary vasodilation. They also increase myocardial oxygen supply.

Usage for the Drug Class

- Chronic stable angina*, hypertension*, pulmonary hypertension, vasospastic angina*

Adverse Reactions for the Drug Class: Most Common

- Dizziness/lightheadedness, flushing, headache, hypotension, peripheral edema

Adverse Reactions for the Drug Class: Rare/Severe/Important

- Orthostasis

Major Drug Interactions for the Drug Class

Drugs Affecting Dihydropyridines

- Increased effects if given with a CYP3A4 inhibitor
- Carbamazepine: Decreased hypotensive effect

- Sildenafil: Increased hypotensive effect
- Azole antifungal agents: Increased hypotensive effects
- Rifampin: Decreased hypotensive effect

Dihydropyridine Effects on Other Drugs

- Antihypertensive agents: Additive hypotension

Counseling Points for the Drug Class

- You may take these medications without regard to meals
- Do not stop therapy abruptly

Key Points for the Drug Class

- The dihydropyridine calcium channel blockers are used primarily for the treatment of hypertension. They also have a role in the treatment of chronic stable angina.
- Immediate-release formulations of nifedipine are no longer recommended due to increased mortality compared to extended-release formulations, although both forms are still available.

Members of the Drug Class

In this section: Amlodipine, felodipine, nifedipine
Others: Clevidipine, isradipine, nicardipine, nimodipine, nisoldipine

■ Amlodipine

Brand Name

Norvasc

Generic Name
Amlodipine

Dosage Forms
Tablets

Dosing
- 2.5–10 mg daily

■ Felodipine

Brand Name
Plendil

Generic Name
Felodipine

Dosage Forms
Extended-release tablets

Dosing
- 2.5–20 mg daily

■ Nifedipine

Brand Names
Adalat CC, Afeditab CR, Nifediac CC, Nifedical XL, Procardia, Procardia XL

Generic Name
Nifedipine

Dosage Forms
Capsules, extended-release tablets

Dosing
- 30–180 mg/day (in 3 doses or daily, depending on formulation)

Key Points
- Immediate-release formulation is not recommended for use
- Nifedipine has negative inotropic effects and may worsen heart failure symptoms

---

Drug Class: Calcium Channel Blockers, Phenylalkylamines

Introduction
Verapamil is the only available member of the phenylalkylamine class of calcium channel blockers. It is used for the treatment of hypertension and heart rate control in patients with atrial fibrillation.

Mechanism of Action for the Drug Class
Verapamil inhibits the movement of calcium ions across the cell membranes. The effects on the cardiovascular system include relaxation of coronary vascular smooth muscle, coronary vasodilation, and decreased myocardial contractility. It also increases myocardial oxygen delivery and depresses both impulse formation and conduction velocity in the atrioventricular node.

■ Verapamil

Brand Names
Calan, Calan SR, Covera-HS, Isoptin SR, Verelan, Verelan PM

Generic Name
Verapamil

Dosage Forms
Tablets, extended- and sustained-release tablets and capsules, injection

Usage
- Atrial fibrillation and flutter*, chronic stable angina, hypertension*, unstable angina, variant angina
- Noncardiovascular uses: Manic manifestations of bipolar disorder, migraine prophylaxis

Dosing
- 120–360 mg/day (given daily or in divided doses depending on formulation)
- Renal dosage adjustment:
  - CrCl <10 ml/minute: Administer 50–75% of normal dose

Adverse Reactions: Most Common
- Bradycardia, constipation (up to 42%), dizziness/lightheadedness, gingival hyperplasia, headache, hypotension, peripheral edema

Adverse Reactions: Rare/Severe/Important
- Worsening of heart failure

Major Drug Interactions
Drugs Affecting Verapamil
- Amiodarone, β-blockers: Increased risk of bradycardia
- Carbamazepine: Decreased hypotensive effect
- Clarithromycin, erythromycin: Increased levels
- Fluconazole, itraconazole: Increased verapamil effects

Verapamil's Effect on Other Drugs
- Digoxin: Increased levels
- Dofetilide: Increased levels leading to ventricular arrhythmias (contraindicated)
- Cyclosporine, tacrolimus: Increased levels

- Phenytoin: Decreased metabolism
- Theophylline: Increased levels
- Lovastatin, simvastatin, atorvastatin: Increased levels

Counseling Points
- Administer sustained-release product with food or milk; other formulations may be taken without regard to food
- Sprinkling contents of capsules onto food does not affect absorption
- Do not crush sustained-release products

Key Point
- Verapamil is used for the treatment of hypertension and atrial fibrillation. It should be avoided in patients with acute myocardial infarction and/or heart failure because it is a negative inotrope. Patients must be counseled on the side effects, particularly constipation.

Drug Class: Loop Diuretics

Introduction
The loop diuretics are very effective at reducing edema in patients who are volume overloaded. They are used to treat symptoms of congestion in patients with heart failure and other diseases that cause fluid retention/overload. They have been supplanted by more effective agents in the treatment of hypertension.

Mechanism of Action for the Drug Class
Loop diuretics are named such because they primarily inhibit the reabsorption of sodium and chloride at the thick ascending limb of the loop of Henle, increasing the excretion of sodium, water, chloride, calcium, and magnesium.

Members of the Drug Class
In this section: Furosemide
  Others: Bumetanide, ethacrynic acid, torsemide

■ Furosemide

Brand Name
Lasix

Generic Name
Furosemide

Dosage Forms
Tablets, oral solution, injection

Usage
- Edema*, hypertension

Dosing
- Initial dose:
  - 20–40 mg PO once or twice daily
- Dosing adjustments:
  - Up to 600 mg/day PO in 2–4 divided doses

Adverse Reactions: Most Common
- Electrolyte depletion, hyperuricemia, hypochloremic alkalosis, hypotension, orthostasis

Adverse Reactions: Rare/Severe/Important
- Renal function impairment, ototoxicity, skin rash

Major Drug Interactions
Drugs Affecting Furosemide
- NSAIDs: Decreased diuresis

Furosemide's Effect on Other Drugs
- Aminoglycosides: Increased ototoxicity
- Lithium: Increased lithium levels
- Digoxin: Increased risk of toxicity due to furosemide-induced hypokalemia

Counseling Points
- Avoid taking before bedtime
- Take with food or milk to reduce GI irritation
- With the possibility of hypokalemia there may be a need for additional potassium in the diet; do not change diet without first checking with your health-care professional
- Use caution when getting up suddenly from a lying or sitting position
- Be cautious in using alcohol, while standing for long periods or exercising, and during hot weather because of enhanced orthostatic hypotensive effects
- Regular monitoring of laboratory tests (potassium, serum creatinine) and blood pressure is necessary to ensure safe use of the drug and avoid adverse effects

Key Points
- Furosemide is commonly used to treat edema. It must be monitored closely to make sure electrolyte disturbances and hypotension do not occur
- Furosemide is more commonly used than bumetanide, but sometimes formulary or other concerns necessitate use of one drug in place of the other. A 40 mg dose of oral furosemide is roughly equivalent to a 1 mg dose of oral bumetanide. For IV administration, the ratio is 20:1 furosemide to bumetanide.

Drug Class: Nitrates

Introduction
The nitrates are used for the treatment of angina, both unstable and chronic stable types. They are available in several formulations and dosage forms that differ in their onset and duration of action.

Mechanism of Action for the Drug Class
Nitrates relax vascular smooth muscle by stimulating intracellular cyclic guanosine monophosphate production. They cause predominantly venous dilation with some dose-dependent arterial effects.

Usage for the Drug Class
- Angina*, heart failure, hypertension, pulmonary hypertension
- Noncardiovascular uses: Esophageal spastic disorders

Adverse Reactions for the Drug Class: Most Common
- Headache, hypotension, lightheadedness, syncope, weakness

Major Drug Interactions for the Drug Class
Drugs Affecting Nitrates
- Alcohol: Can cause severe hypotension and syncope
- Calcium channel blockers: May increase orthostatic hypotension
- Sildenafil, tadalafil, vardenafil: Increased hypotensive effects (avoid use within 24 hours of each other)

Nitrate Effects on Other Drugs
- Antihypertensive agents: Additive hypotension

Counseling Points for the Drug Class
- Extended-release tablets and capsules: Do not crush or chew. Administer doses so a 12-hour "nitrate-free interval" occurs.
- Sublingual tablets: Place under tongue or between cheek and gum. Rest during administration, preferably seated. Do not swallow tablets. Should feel a slight burning sensation under the tongue, which means the drug is working. Do not remove tablets from original glass container.
- Transdermal patch: Apply once daily to skin site free of hair and not subject to excessive movement. Avoid areas with cuts or irritations. Do not apply to distal parts of the extremities. Use caution when discarding so as to keep out of the reach of children or pets. Remove at night for a 12-hour "nitrate-free interval."
- Headaches may occur and are a sign that the medication is working. Do not alter dosage schedule; aspirin or acetaminophen may be used to relieve pain.

Key Point for the Drug Class
- Nitrates are the drug of choice for quick relief of angina symptoms. They are also used for long-term prevention of angina symptoms, although not recommended as first-line in patients with recent myocardial infarction when β-blockers are preferred.

Members of the Drug Class
In this section: Isosorbide mononitrate, nitroglycerin (sublingual)

Others: Isosorbide dinitrate, nitroglycerin (capsules, injection, topical ointment, transdermal patch, translingual spray)

■ Isosorbide Mononitrate
Brand Names
Imdur, Ismo, Monoket

Generic Name
Isosorbide mononitrate

Dosage Forms
Tablets, extended-release tablets

Dosing
30–240 mg daily (divided doses if not the extended-release formulation)

Key Point
Used for long-term treatment of chronic angina

■ Nitroglycerin
Brand Name
Nitrostat

Generic Name
Nitroglycerin (sublingual)

Dosage Forms
Sublingual tablets

Dosing
- Dosing (sublingual tablets): 0.3–0.6 mg repeated at 5-minute intervals up to 3 doses as needed for relief of anginal attack. If pain continues after 1 tablet, notify physician immediately. May use prophylactically 5-10 minutes before activities that precipitate an attack.

Key Points
- Sublingual tablets are used for the relief of angina attacks only, not for long-term treatment of angina
- Sublingual tablets must be stored in original containers away from humidity and moisture
- Patients should not crush sublingual tablets; they should just place under tongue and allow to dissolve

Drug Class: Potassium-Sparing Diuretic, Aldosterone Antagonist

Introduction

The aldosterone antagonists can be used as diuretics; however, they are more commonly used as adjunctive therapy to prevent morbidity and mortality in patients with stage C or D heart failure.

Mechanism of Action for the Drug Class

Competitively inhibit aldosterone, which binds to aldosterone receptors of the distal tubules in the kidney. This action increases sodium chloride and water excretion but not potassium and hydrogen ions. Spironolactone may also block the effect of aldosterone on arteriolar smooth muscle.

Members of the Drug Class

In this section: Spironolactone
   Other: Eplerenone

■ Spironolactone

Brand Name
Aldactone

Generic Name
Spironolactone

Dosage Forms
Tablets

Usage
- Edema or ascites in patients with cirrhosis of the liver*, heart failure*, hyperaldosteronism, hypertension, hypokalemia, acne in women, hirsutism

Dosing
- 12.5–200 mg daily

- Renal dosage adjustment:
  ○ CrCl 10–50 ml/minute: Administer every 12–24 hours
  ○ CrCl <10 ml/minute: Avoid use

Adverse Reactions: Most Common
- Hyperkalemia, cramping, diarrhea

Adverse Reactions: Rare/Severe/Important
- Gynecomastia, renal dysfunction (increased SCr: avoid if SCr >2 mg/dl)

Major Drug Interactions
Drugs Affecting Spironolactone
- Potassium supplements: Increased risk of hyperkalemia

Spironolactone's Effect on Other Drugs
- ACE Inhibitors, ARBs, trimethoprim: Increased risk of hyperkalemia

Counseling Point
- Avoid ingestion of food high in potassium or use of salt substitutes or other potassium supplements without the advice of your healthcare professional

Key Points
- Spironolactone is used as a diuretic in patients with cirrhosis of the liver. Use in these patients requires much higher dosing (up to 200 mg daily) than what is recommended in patients with heart failure (maximum 50 mg daily). The main role of spironolactone in patients with heart failure is to reduce morbidity and mortality.
- Patients must be monitored closely for hyperkalemia and renal dysfunction because these could result in potentially fatal adverse effects (hyperkalemia-induced arrhythmias).

Drug Class: Thiazide Diuretics

Introduction

The thiazide diuretics are recommended for first-line therapy in the treatment of hypertension. They can also be used in patients with edema, often in combination with a loop diuretic for synergistic effects.

Mechanism of Action for the Drug Class

Inhibit reabsorption of sodium and chloride in the distal tubules resulting in increased urinary excretion of sodium and chloride.

Members of the Drug Class

In this section: Hydrochlorothiazide
   Others: Bendroflumethiazide, chlorothiazide, chlorthalidone, methyclothiazide

■ Hydrochlorothiazide

Brand Name
Microzide

Generic Name
Hydrochlorothiazide

Dosage Forms
Tablets, capsules

Usage
- Hypertension*, edema
- Noncardiovascular use: Treatment of lithium-induced diabetes insipidus

Dosing
- 12.5–50 mg daily
- Renal dosage adjustment:
  - Ineffective if CrCl <30 ml/minute (except in combination with loop diuretics)

Adverse Reactions: Most Common
- Hypokalemia, orthostatic hypotension, stomach upset

Adverse Reactions: Rare/Severe/Important
- Hypochloremic alkalosis, photosensitivity

Major Drug Interactions
Drugs Affecting Hydrochlorothiazide
- Loop diuretics: Enhanced diuresis
- NSAIDs: May decrease efficacy of thiazides

Hydrochlorothiazide's Effect on Other Drugs
- Digoxin: Thiazide-induced hypokalemia may precipitate digitalis-induced arrhythmias
- Dofetilide: Increased levels, leading to ventricular arrhythmias (contraindicated)
- Lithium: Increased levels

Counseling Points
- Take in the morning to avoid increased urination at night
- Antihypertensive effects may take several days

Key Points
- The thiazide diuretics can be used in the treatment of mild hypertension. They can also be used for edema; however, they often only work for mild edema, and a loop diuretic is often required for more severe edema associated with heart failure.
- The 50-mg dose of hydrochlorothiazide has increased adverse effects without added efficacy and should generally be avoided

---

Drug Class: Vasodilator–Hydralazine

Introduction
Hydralazine is used for the treatment of refractory hypertension and heart failure. It is often not used first-line because of its inconvenient dosing schedule. It is sometimes used in heart failure in combination with nitrates in patients who do not respond to or are intolerant of ACE inhibitors or ARBs.

Mechanism of Action for the Drug Class
Hydralazine directly relaxes vascular smooth muscle resulting in peripheral vasodilation.

■ Hydralazine

Brand Name
Apresoline

Generic Name
Hydralazine

Dosage Forms
Tablets, injection

Usage
- Hypertension*, heart failure* (in combination with nitrate therapy)

Dosing
- Initial dose:
  - 10 mg four times daily
- Dosing adjustments:
  - Up to 300 mg/day in 3–4 divided doses
- Renal dosage adjustment:
  - CrCl 10–50 ml/minute: Administer every 8 hours

Adverse Reactions: Most Common
- Angina, headache, nausea/vomiting, tachycardia

Adverse Reactions: Rare/Severe/Important
- Drug-induced lupus-like syndrome (with higher doses)

Major Drug Interactions
None significant

Counseling Points

- Hydralazine must be taken 3–4 times daily
- Let your healthcare provider know if any lupus-like symptoms develop (fever, arthralgia, myalgia, malaise, pleuritic chest pain, edema, maculopapular facial rash)

Key Points

- Hydralazine is effective in the treatment of hypertension. It is also used for the treatment of heart failure in combination with nitrate therapy.

- Patient compliance may be an issue because it must be taken multiple times a day
- Hydralazine is a classic example of a drug that causes lupus-like syndrome. This adverse effect abates with discontinuation.

Combination Drug Therapies

Introduction

The use of antihypertensive agents in combination is common. To decrease the pill burden and improve compliance, combination antihypertensive therapies combine two active drugs into one pill. These formulations should not be used as initial therapy because they are not easy to titrate and should therefore only be used once it is known what doses of medication a patient requires. Most combinations include a thiazide diuretic. Available combination products are summarized in Table 5–1.

TABLE 5–1
Combination Antihypertensive Agents

Drug Class	Brand Name(s)	Generic Names	Other Similar Drugs
ACE inhibitors in combination with HCTZ	Zestoretic, Prinzide	Lisinopril/HCTZ	Benazepril/HCTZ, captopril/HCTZ, enalapril/HCTZ, fosinopril/HCTZ, moexipril/HCTZ, quinapril/HCTZ
Angiotensin receptor blockers in combination with HCTZ	Hyzaar	Losartan/HCTZ	Candesartan/HCTZ, eprosartan/HCTZ, irbesartan/HCTZ, olmesartan/HCTZ, telmisartan/HCTZ, valsartan/HCTZ
Dihydropyridine calcium channel blocker in combination with ACE inhibitor	Lotrel	Amlodipine/benazepril	None
β-Blockers in combination with thiazide diuretics	Ziac	Bisoprolol/HCTZ	Atenolol/chlorthalidone, metoprolol/HCTZ, propranolol/HCTZ
Thiazide diuretics in combination with potassium-sparing diuretics	Dyazide, Maxzide, Maxzide-25	Triamterene/HCTZ	None

1. Which of the following requires dosage adjustments in patients with renal dysfunction?
   A. Betapace
   B. Cartia XT
   C. Cordarone
   D. Lopressor

2. All of the following are potential adverse effects of amiodarone except
   A. Corneal microdeposits
   B. Bradycardia
   C. Hypothyroidism
   D. Renal failure

3. Which of the following is an appropriate indication for the use of amlodipine?
   A. Acute myocardial infarction
   B. Atrial fibrillation
   C. Chronic stable angina
   D. Heart failure

4. Which of the following is a common adverse effect of terazosin?
   A. Edema
   B. Orthostatic hypotension
   C. Skin hypersensitivity
   D. Torsades de pointes

5. Catapres-TTS-2 should be changed
   A. Every 12 hours
   B. Daily
   C. Every other day
   D. Every 7 days

6. Abrupt discontinuation of which of the following can cause rebound hypertension?
   A. Amiodarone
   B. Clonidine
   C. Furosemide
   D. Ramipril

7. All of the following can increase digoxin levels except
   A. Amiodarone
   B. Cyclosporine
   C. Diltiazem
   D. Furosemide

8. Which of the following would be an appropriate digoxin maintenance dose?
   A. 0.125 mg every 8 hours
   B. 0.25 g daily
   C. 125 mg daily
   D. 250 µg daily

9. Which of the following is most likely to cause peripheral edema as a side effect?
   A. Atenolol
   B. Furosemide
   C. Nifedipine
   D. Nitroglycerin

10. All of the following have the potential to cause hyperkalemia except
    A. Aldactone
    B. Avapro
    C. Benazepril
    D. Furosemide

11. The maximum dose recommendation for spironolactone in patients with heart failure is
    A. 10 mg daily
    B. 50 mg daily
    C. 200 mg daily
    D. 400 mg daily

12. The most common adverse effect of verapamil is
    A. Constipation
    B. Corneal microdeposits
    C. Renal dysfunction
    D. Thyroid disorders

13. All of the following have the potential to cause hypokalemia except
    A. Hydrochlorothiazide
    B. Lasix
    C. Lotrel
    D. Ziac

14. Hydralazine is used for which of the following indications?
    A. Edema
    B. Hypertension
    C. Lupus
    D. Myocardial infarction

15. Which of the following products contain an ACE inhibitor?
    A. Dyazide
    B. Hyzaar
    C. Zestoretic
    D. Ziac

Central Nervous System Agents

Christine Fitzgerald, PharmD, BCPS
Susan Kent, PharmD, CGP
Joel Shuster, PharmD, BCPP

Drug Class: 5-HT Receptor Antagonists

Introduction

Sumatriptan is a selective agonist of vascular serotonin type 1-like receptors for the acute management of migraine headaches. It is highly effective in many patients but must be avoided in those with concurrent cardiovascular disease.

Mechanism of Action for the Drug Class

$5HT_1$ receptor agonist at extracerebral and intracranial blood vessels, likely resulting in vasoconstriction and decreased trigeminal nerve transmission.

Members of the Drug Class

In this section: Sumatriptan
    Others: Almotriptan, eletriptan, frovatriptan, naratriptan, rizatriptan, zolmitriptan

■ Sumatriptan

Brand Name

Imitrex

Generic Name

Sumatriptan

Dosage Forms

Tablets, injection, nasal spray

Usage

- Acute treatment of migraine in adults with or without aura*, acute treatment of cluster headache episodes

Dosing

- Oral: 25–200 mg
- Injectable: 6–12 mg SUB-Q injection
- Nasal spray: 5–20 mg as 1 spray in 1 nostril (10 mg given as one 5-mg spray in *each* nostril) up to 40 mg/day
- Renal dosage adjustment:
  ○ No formal recommendations. Use caution in hemodialysis patients.
- Hepatic dosage adjustment:
  ○ Bioavailability of oral sumatriptan is increased with liver disease. If treatment is needed, do not exceed single doses of 50 mg.
  ○ Use of all dosage forms is contraindicated with severe hepatic impairment

Adverse Reactions: Most Common

- Paresthesias, hot/cold skin sensations, flushing, fatigue, somnolence, nausea, vomiting, unpleasant taste in mouth, dry mouth, headache, photosensitivity
- Injectable: local injection site reactions

Adverse Reactions: Rare/Severe/Important

- Chest, jaw, neck tightness, coronary vasospasm, MI, arrhythmia, seizure

Major Drug Interactions

Drugs Affecting Sumatriptan

- Sibutramine, MAOIs, ergotamines: Increased risk of serotonin syndrome

Contraindications

- Ischemic heart disease (angina, MI, CVA, TIA), peripheral vascular syndromes, uncontrolled hypertension, ischemic bowel disease, severe hepatic impairment (Child Pugh C), hemiplegic or basilar migraine, hypersensitivity, use of an ergotamine derivative (dihydroergotamine, methysergide) within 24 hours, use of another $5HT_1$ agonist within 24 hours, use of an MAOI within 2 weeks of sumatriptan therapy

Counseling Points

- Take at first sign of migraine attack. This is used to reduce migraine, not to prevent or reduce the number of attacks.
- Follow exact instructions for use. Do not re-dose if no response is achieved.
- Do not take sumatriptan within 24 hours of using an ergot medication or another serotonin agonist. Do not take sumatriptan with recent use of an MAOI (2 weeks).

- Wear sunscreen and proper clothing when in the sun
- Report any risk factors for heart disease or any unusual side effects immediately (chest tightness or pain, acute abdominal pain, excessive drowsiness)

Key Points
- Complete history/physical and medication history are imperative prior to initiating sumatriptan
- Demonstrate proper SUB-Q injection technique
- Sumatriptan is used to reduce migraine attack, not to prevent or reduce the number of attacks

---

Drug Class: Anorexiant

Introduction
Obesity is increasing in prevalence worldwide. To be successful in weight loss, it has been suggested a goal weight should be predefined and a weight loss program should include diet, exercise, and behavior modification, and possibly a pharmacologic agent. Debate continues on the appropriateness of weight loss medications due to the controversy surrounding the deaths and medical complications caused by the combination product Fen-Phen (fenfluramine and phentermine). Phentermine is still available.

Mechanism of Action for the Drug Class
Phentermine is a sympathomimetic amine that stimulates the CNS. The mechanism of action in treating obesity is unknown.

Members of the Drug Class
In this section: Phentermine
   Others: Benzphetamine, diethylpropion, phendimetrazine, sibutramine

■ Phentermine

Brand Names
Adipex-P, Ionamin, Fastin

Generic Name
Phentermine

Dosage Forms
Tablets, capsules

Usage
- Obesity* (short-term use)

Dosing
- 37.5 mg daily (as hydrochloride) or 15–30 mg in 1–2 divided doses (as resin complex)

Adverse Reactions: Most Common
- Increased blood pressure, palpitations, arrhythmias, GI discomfort, insomnia, nervousness

Adverse Reactions: Rare/Severe/Important
- Primary pulmonary hypertension, valvular heart disease, psychiatric reactions

Major Drug Interactions
Drugs Affecting Phentermine
- MAOIs: Contraindicated due to the risk of severe, possibly fatal adverse reactions

Counseling Points
- Take hydrochloride formulation at breakfast or 1–2 hours after breakfast
- Avoid late night dosing. Resin complex formulation administer before breakfast or at least 10–14 hours before retiring.

Key Points
- Schedule IV medication. Contraindicated in patients with a history of drug abuse.
- Use for patients with a BMI ≥ 30 kg/m^2 or with patients with a BMI ≥ 27 kg/m^2 in the presence of other risk factors (hypertension, DM, dyslipidemia)
- Should be used in conjunction with a weight management program
- Use with caution in diabetics. Glucose requirements may change.
- Structurally similar to amphetamines but has less severe CNS stimulation and a lower abuse potential
- Additional contraindications include advanced arteriosclerosis, cardiovascular disease, moderate to severe hypertension, pulmonary hypertension, hyperthyroidism, glaucoma, and agitated psychological states

---

Drug Class: Antianxiety Agents, Benzodiazepines

Introduction
Benzodiazepines (BZDs) are utilized in a broad spectrum of CNS disorders, though primarily as antianxiety, anticonvulsant, or hypnotic agents. The agents within the class have many similarities, and the differences between them are mostly pharmacokinetic.

Mechanisms of Action for the Drug Class

Benzodiazepines facilitate the activity of the inhibitory neurotransmitter GABA (gamma-aminobutyric acid) and other inhibitory transmitters by binding to specific benzodiazepine receptors.

Adverse Reactions for the Drug Class: Most Common

- Sedation, somnolence, memory impairment, coordination problems, dizziness, and dysarthria

Adverse Reactions for the Drug Class: Rare/Severe/Important

- Withdrawal syndrome and respiratory depression (particularly with other CNS depressants)

Counseling Points for the Drug Class

- Avoid alcohol while on BZD therapy because it can lead to possibly fatal respiratory depression
- Avoid activities that require mental alertness (e.g., driving) until the effects of the medication are known and comfortable. Follow this advice whenever the dose is increased also.
- Do not abruptly discontinue BZD therapy because withdrawal effects are likely

Key Points for the Drug Class

- The BZDs are Schedule IV medications that may be habit forming. Be cautious using BZDs in patients with a history of substance abuse.
- Patients who receive chronic BZDs will need to be tapered off of the medication gradually
- Contraindicated in narrow-angle glaucoma and pregnancy

Members of the Drug Class

In this section: Alprazolam, clonazepam, diazepam, lorazepam

Others: Chlordiazepoxide, clorazepate, midazolam, oxazepam

■ Alprazolam

Brand Names

Xanax, Xanax XR, Alprazolam Intensol, Niravam

Generic Name

Alprazolam

Dosage Forms

Tablets, extended-release tablets, oral disintegrating tablets (ODTs), solution

Usage

- Anxiety disorders*, panic disorders, alcohol withdrawal

Dosing

- 0.25–0.5 mg three times daily; titrate to a maximum dose of 10 mg/day

Dosing in Hepatic Impairment

- Reduce dosing by 50–60% or avoid use

Major Drug Interactions

Drugs Affecting Alprazolam

- CNS depressants and alcohol: Increase CNS depression
- Cimetidine, oral contraceptives, fluoxetine, valproic acid, azole antifungals: Increase serum concentrations (contraindicated with ketoconazole and itraconazole)

Counseling Points

- Do not push ODTs through the blister pack foil. Peel back foil, remove tablet with dry finger, and place the tablet on tongue. Medication does not require water.
- Do not chew, crush, or break extended-release tablets

Key Points

- Abuse potential may be higher with this agent compared to other BZDs due to its rapid action
- Withdrawal symptoms are more likely with a short-acting BZD, such as alprazolam. Discontinue medication slowly especially when used for >3 months.

■ Clonazepam

Brand Names

Klonopin, Klonopin Wafers

Generic Name

Clonazepam

Dosage Forms

Tablets, ODTs

Uses

- Panic disorder*, seizures (Lennox–Gastaut, akinetic, myoclonic, absence)*, restless legs syndrome, social phobia, acute mania associated with bipolar, multifocal tic disorders \Tourette's

Dosing

- 0.25–0.5 mg twice or three times daily, to a maximum dose of 20 mg/day

Dosing in Hepatic Impairment

- Contraindicated in severe hepatic disease

Major Drug Interactions

Drugs Affecting Clonazepam

- Phenytoin, carbamazepine, and phenobarbital: Decrease serum concentrations
- Azole antifungals: Increase serum concentrations
- CNS depressants and alcohol: Increase CNS depression

Counseling Point

- Do not push ODTs through the blister pack foil. Peel back foil, remove tablet with dry finger, and place the tablet on tongue. Medication does not require water.

Key Points

- Some clinicians use once-daily bedtime dosing due to the drug's long half-life
- Often used as an aid in the withdrawal of patients addicted to other BZDs

■ Diazepam

Brand Names
Valium, Diastat, Diazepam Intensol, Diastat AcuDial

Generic Name
Diazepam

Dosage Forms
Tablets, solution, injection, rectal gel

Usage
- Anxiety disorders*, acute alcohol withdrawal, seizures (adjunctive therapy, status epilepticus)*, skeletal muscle relaxant, preoperative and procedural sedation and amnesia

Dosing
- Anxiety disorders and muscle relaxant:
  - Initial dose: 2–10 mg/day in 2–4 divided doses
- Acute alcohol withdrawal:
  - Initial dose: 30–40 mg/day in 3–4 divided doses
- Status epilepticus:
  - Initial dose: 5–10 mg IV every 5–10 minutes; maximum dose 30 mg
- Dosing in hepatic impairment:
  - Contraindicated in severe hepatic disease

Major Drug Interactions
Drugs Affecting Diazepam
- CNS depressants and alcohol: Increase CNS depression
- Cimetidine, oral contraceptives, fluoxetine, valproic acid, azole antifungals: Increase serum concentrations (contraindicated with ketoconazole and itraconazole)
- Ranitidine and antacids: Decrease serum concentrations

Key Points
- Diazepam is also contraindicated with myasthenia gravis, severe respiratory insufficiency, and sleep apnea
- Use with caution or not at all in the elderly due to long half-life

■ Lorazepam

Brand Names
Ativan, Lorazepam Intensol

Generic Name
Lorazepam

Dosage Forms
Tablets, solution, injection

Usage
- Anxiety disorders*, seizures (status epilepticus)*, insomnia, acute alcohol withdrawal, sedation*, agitation*, antiemetic

Dosing
- Anxiety disorders:
  - Initial dose: 2–3 mg/day given in 2–3 divided doses
- Status epilepticus:
  - Initial dose: 4 mg IV in 10–15 minutes; maximum dose 8 mg
- Agitation:
  - Initial dose: 1–2 mg
- Sedation in ICU setting:
  - Initial dose: Intermittent 0.02 mg–0.06 mg/kg IV; continuous infusion 0.01–0.1 mg/kg per hour IV

Major Drug Interactions
Drugs Affecting Lorazepam
- Valproic acid and probenecid: Increase serum levels (reduce lorazepam dose by 50%)

Key Points
- There is a risk of propylene glycol toxicity when using the parental formulation. Monitor with prolonged use or higher doses.
- Although specific dose recommendations are not available, use with caution in patients with renal or hepatic impairment

---

Drug Class: Antianxiety Agent, Nonbenzodiazepine

Introduction

Buspirone is the only drug within this class. Although used for anxiety disorders, it is not a benzodiazepine (BZD) and is chemically unrelated to other CNS agents. Unlike BZDs, it lacks anticonvulsant and sedative properties and therefore has less overall clinical utility. However, buspirone lacks issues that can be problematic with BZD use. Buspirone is less sedating, has less CNS side effects, and a higher threshold of interaction with other CNS depressants and alcohol. Physical dependency and with-drawal symptoms have not been seen with buspirone. Buspirone can be a good antianxiety agent to use in patients who are unable to tolerate BZDs due to undesirable side effects and interactions, patients with a history of drug or alcohol abuse, and the elderly.

Mechanism of Action for the Drug Class

Buspirone's mechanism of action is primarily unknown. The drug has a high affinity for serotonin receptors and a moderate affinity for dopamine type-2 receptors.

■ Buspirone

Brand Name
BuSpar

Generic Name
Buspirone

Dosage Forms
Tablets

Usage
- Anxiety disorders*, aggression, depression, premenstrual syndrome, nicotine dependence

Dosing
- Initial dose: 15 mg/day in 2 divided doses. Titrate to a maximum dose of 60 mg/day.

Adverse Reactions: Most Common
- Dizziness, lightheadedness, headache, nausea, nervousness, excitement

Adverse Reactions: Rare/Severe/Important
- Extrapyramidal symptoms, restless legs syndrome

Major Drug Interactions
Drugs Affecting Buspirone
- Erythromycin, cimetidine, ketoconazole, itraconazole, clarithromycin, diltiazem, verapamil: Increase serum levels
- Rifampin, phenytoin, phenobarbital, carbamazepine, fluoxetine: Decrease serum levels, compromising efficacy

Buspirone's Effect on Other Drugs
- MAOIs: Warning of concomitant use due to risk of hypertensive crisis
- Haloperidol: Increases serum levels

Counseling Points
- Antianxiety effects may not be seen for at least a week or more
- Should not be stopped abruptly
- Use with caution in patients with renal and hepatic impairment

Key Points
- Abuse potential is low compared to BZDs
- Buspirone will not treat BZD withdrawal symptoms

Drug Class: Anticonvulsants

Introduction

Anticonvulsants are used for a broad spectrum of CNS on-label and off-label indications including seizure disorders, trigeminal and postherpetic neuralgias, bipolar disorders, neuropathic pain, migraine, mood disorders, and many others. The treatment goal in epilepsy is seizure-free control on as few antiepileptic drugs (AEDs) as possible with little to no side effects. But achieving a balance between superior efficacy and side effects is not easily obtainable for many patients. There are many adverse reactions to these medications, and the FDA has issued a special drug class warning of increased suicide behavior or ideation for all AEDs. Patients and family members should be made aware of the increased risk of suicidal thoughts and behavior. With any AED, patients should check with their physician before discontinuing medication. A gradual taper in dose may be required to prevent seizures and status epilepticus. Many AEDs are a substrate to or strongly inhibit/induce the CYP enzyme system, resulting in multiple drug interactions. In addition, pregnant patients who remain on AEDs should be encouraged to enroll in the North American Antiepileptic Drug Pregnancy Registry.

Mechanisms of Action for the Drug Class

Multiple mechanisms of action are used within this drug class and in many cases are unknown. Generally, when used for seizure disorders, control is achieved through alteration of sodium and/or calcium ion channels and/or neurotransmitters including γ-aminobutyric acid (GABA) and glutamate.

Members of the Drug Class

In this section: Carbamazepine, gabapentin, lamotrigine, levetiracetam, oxcarbazepine, phenobarbital, phenytoin, pregabalin, topiramate, valproate/divalproex

Others: Ethosuximide, felbamate, fosphenytoin, lincosamide, pentobarbital, primidone, tiagabine, vigabatrin, zonisamide

■ Carbamazepine

Brand Names
Carbatrol, Epitol, Equetro, Tegretol, Tegretol XR

Generic Name
Carbamazepine

Dosage Forms
Tablets, extended-release tablets, chewable tablets, extended-release capsules, suspension

Usage
- Seizures (partial, generalized tonic-clonic seizures, and mixed types), trigeminal neuralgia, acute manic and mixed episodes associated with bipolar 1 disorder (Equetro only)*, psychiatric disorders (unipolar depression, schizoaffective disorder, resistant schizophrenia, posttraumatic stress disorder), withdrawal from alcohol, cocaine, or benzodiazepines, restless legs syndrome, and many others

Dosing

- Seizure disorders:
  - Initial dose: Adults and children >12 years of age: 200 mg twice a day (tablets or capsules) or 400 mg four times a day (suspension). Increase at weekly intervals by <200 mg/day using a twice-daily regimen of formulations or three to four times/day divided dosing schedule IR and suspension formulations until optimal control is attained. Usual maintenance dose is 800–1200 mg/day.
- Trigeminal neuralgia:
  - Initial dose: 100 mg twice daily on the first day (50 mg four times a day with suspension). Increase by up to 200 mg/day using 100-mg increments every 12 hours (50 mg four times daily of suspension) as needed. Do not exceed 1200 mg/day.
- Acute mania and mixed episodes with bipolar 1 disorder (Equetro only):
  - Initial dose: 200 mg twice a day. Increase daily dose in increments of 200 mg/day until optimal response is achieved.
- Pharmacokinetic monitoring:
  - Target serum concentrations: 4–12 µg/ml

Adverse Reactions: Most Common

- Dizziness, drowsiness, ataxia, nausea, vomiting, diplopia, headache

Adverse Reactions: Rare/Severe/Important

- Hematologic (aplastic anemia, leukopenia, agranulocytosis, eosinophilia, thrombocytopenia), hepatic dysfunction, dermatologic reactions (toxic epidermal necrolysis, Stevens–Johnson syndrome), SIADH, cardiac conduction disturbances, hyponatremia

Major Drug Interactions

Drugs Affecting Carbamazepine

- Carbamazepine induces its own metabolism
- Cimetidine, erythromycin, clarithromycin, fluoxetine, valproic acid, protease inhibitors, azole antifungals, isoniazid, propoxyphene, diltiazem, and others: Increase carbamazepine serum concentrations
- Phenobarbital, primidone, rifampin, and phenytoin: Decrease serum concentrations of carbamazepine

Carbamazepine's Effect on Other Drugs

- Induces the metabolism of felbamate, lamotrigine, 10-monohydroxy metabolite (active metabolite of oxcarbazepine), phenytoin, protease inhibitors, clozapine, cyclosporine, olanzapine, risperidone, tiagabine, topiramate, valproic acid, zonisamide, doxycycline, oral contraceptives, theophylline, warfarin, and others, which leads to decreased serum concentration and possible therapeutic failure
- Concomitant use with MAOIs is contraindicated

Counseling Points

- Do not crush or chew extended-release tablets or capsules. Extended-release tablet coating is not absorbed and is excreted in the feces. Tablet coatings may be noticeable in the stool. Capsules may be opened and sprinkled over applesauce.
- Notify your healthcare provider if any of the following symptoms occur: unusual bleeding, bruising, fever, sore throat, rash or ulcer in the mouth
- If using oral contraceptives, consider an additional or alternative method of birth control
- May cause drowsiness, dizziness, or blurred vision. Observe caution when driving or performing tasks requiring alertness, coordination, or physical dexterity until the effects of the medication are familiar.

Key Points

- There is a U.S. **black box warning** for development of toxic epidermal necrolysis (TEN) or Stevens–Johnson syndrome (SJS) with an increased incidence in patients of Asian descent with the HLA-B*1502 allele. These patients should be screened for the presence of the HLA-B*1502 allele. If positive, carbamazepine should not be started.
- There is a **black box warning** for the development of aplastic anemia and agranulocytosis
- Carbamazepine is metabolized through CYP-450 3A4 to an active metabolite, 10, 11-epoxide. The active metabolite is metabolized through epoxide hydrolase. Carbamazepine is a strong inducer of CYP-450 enzymes. Be alert to any new medications added or discontinued from a patient's drug regimen because this could affect medication blood levels.
- Because of autoinduction, the half-life of the drug and its serum levels may change over the first few weeks of therapy. Patients must be observed closely and dosing must be individualized.

■ Gabapentin

Brand Name
Neurontin

Generic Name
Gabapentin

Dosage Forms
Tablets, capsules, suspension

Usage

- Seizures (adjunctive therapy in the treatment of partial seizures with and without secondary generalization)*, postherpetic neuralgia, pain (neuropathic, chronic, and postoperative pain), diabetic peripheral neuropathy*, vasomotor symptoms associated with menopause, fibromyalgia, social phobia, and many others

Dosing

- Adjunctive therapy for partial seizures and diabetic peripheral neuropathy
  - Initial dose: Initiate therapy with a dose of 300 mg three times daily. Increase at weekly intervals to 1.8 g daily. Maximum dose up to 3.6 g daily.
- Postherpetic neuralgia:
  - Initial dose: Initiate therapy with 300 mg on day 1, 300 mg twice a day on day 2, and 300 mg

three times a day on day 3. Titrate dose as needed for pain relief up to a daily dose of 1.8 g.

- Renal impairment adjustment:
  - Dose adjustments need to be made for renal impairment when CrCl <60 mL/minute

Adverse Reactions: Most Common
- Fatigue, somnolence, dizziness, peripheral edema, nystagmus, ataxia

Adverse Reactions: Rare/Severe/Important
- Aggressive behavior in children

Major Drug Interactions
Drugs Affecting Gabapentin
- Aluminum-containing antacids (decrease bioavailability by 20%)

■ Lamotrigine
Brand Names
Lamictal, Lamictal XR, Lamictal CD, Lamictal ODT

Generic Name
Lamotrigine

Dosage Forms
Tablets, chewable dispersible tablets. Starter kits are available for initial dosing titration when patients are already receiving valproic acid (blue kit), or carbamazepine, phenytoin, phenobarbital, primidone, or rifampin (green kit). The orange starter kit is used when titration is not affected by another concomitant medication.

Usage
- Seizures adjunctive therapy (generalized seizures of Lennox–Gastaut syndrome, partial seizures, and primary generalized tonic-clonic seizures)*, seizures conversion to monotherapy (partial seizures in patients who are currently taking valproic acid, carbamazepine, phenobarbital, phenytoin, or primidone as the single AED)*, maintenance treatment of bipolar 1 disorder

Dosing
- Seizure disorders (adjunctive therapy) and bipolar disorder:
  - Initial dose: Initial dosing and titration schedules depend on concomitant medications. Initiating at a higher dose or titrating at an accelerated rate increases the incidence of lamotrigine-associated rash. The initial dose of lamotrigine is 25 mg every other day for 1–2 weeks for patients currently on valproic acid. The initial dose of lamotrigine is 50 mg a day for 1–2 weeks for patients currently on carbamazepine, phenobarbital, phenytoin, primidone, or rifampin. If a patient is on any other AED, the initial dose is 25 mg/day for 1–2 weeks. Follow specific dosing guidelines for titration beyond weeks 1–2.

- Seizure disorders: Conversion to monotherapy:
  - Initial dose: Follow specific guidelines to appropriately titrate lower doses of valproic acid, carbamazepine, phenobarbital, phenytoin, and primidone while increasing doses of lamotrigine
- Dosing in hepatic impairment:
  - Reduce dosing by 25–50% and titrate to clinical effectiveness in moderate to severe hepatic impairment

Adverse Reactions: Most Common
- Headache, dizziness, rash, diplopia, nausea, somnolence, ataxia, rhinitis

Adverse Reactions: Rare/Severe/Important
- Dermatologic reactions (TEN, SJS), hypersensitivity reactions (multiorgan failure/dysfunction, blood dyscrasias)

Major Drug Interactions
Drugs Affecting Lamotrigine
- Valproic acid: Increases lamotrigine concentrations and effects
- Oral contraceptives, rifampin, carbamazepine, phenytoin, primidone, oxcarbazepine, and phenobarbital may decrease lamotrigine concentrations

Counseling Points
- Women should alert their physician if they plan on starting or stopping oral contraceptives
- It is very important to slowly increase daily dosage as directed. Use a calendar to assist in this process.
- Notify your healthcare provider immediately if you develop a rash

Key Points
- There is a **black box warning** for risk of life-threatening serious rashes, including TEN or SJS and/or rash-related deaths. The risk of rash is increased in the pediatric population, with concomitant use with valproic acid, with doses greater than the recommended initial dose, and when upward dose titration occurs too quickly. Patients should always be monitored for rash when starting therapy with this agent.
- Do not rechallenge a patient with lamotrigine if a rash has occurred with prior use
- This medication has been confused with the antifungal medication Lamisil

■ Levetiracetam
Brand Names
Keppra, Keppra XR

Generic Name
Levetiracetam

Dosage Forms
Tablets, solution, injection

Usage
- Seizures (adjunctive therapy for partial, myoclonic, and primary generalized tonic-clonic)*, manic bipolar 1 disorder, migraine prophylaxis

Dosing

- 500 mg twice a day, titrated every 2 weeks up to 3000 mg twice a day
- Renal dosing adjustments:
  - Required when CrCl <80 mL/minute

Adverse Reactions: Most Common

- Asthenia, somnolence, dizziness, vomiting, anorexia, infection

Adverse Reactions: Rare/Severe/Important

- Thrombocytopenia, coordination difficulties, behavior abnormalities (depression, nervousness, mood swings, irritability, agitation)

Counseling Point

- May cause drowsiness, dizziness, or blurred vision. Observe caution when driving or performing tasks requiring alertness, coordination, or physical dexterity.

■ Oxcarbazepine

Brand Name
Trileptal

Generic Name
Oxcarbazepine

Dosage Forms
Tablets, suspension

Usage

- Seizures (monotherapy and adjunctive therapy in partial seizures)*, bipolar disorders, neuropathic pain

Dosing

- Initial dose: 300 mg twice a day
- Dose adjustments need to be made for renal impairment when CrCl <30 mL/minute

Adverse Reactions: Most Common

- Dizziness, somnolence, diplopia, fatigue, nausea, vomiting, ataxia, abnormal vision, abdominal pain, tremor, abnormal gait

Adverse Reactions: Rare/Severe/Important

- Hyponatremia (monitoring serum levels should be considered during maintenance treatment), anaphylactic reactions and angioedema, multiorgan hypersensitivity reactions, dermatological reactions (TEN and/or SJS), psychomotor slowing, hematologic (agranulocytosis, aplastic anemia, pancytopenia)

Major Drug Interactions

Drugs Affecting Oxcarbazepine

- Phenobarbital, carbamazepine, valproic acid, phenytoin, and verapamil: Decrease serum concentrations of MHD (active metabolite), compromising effectiveness

Oxcarbazepine's Effect on Other Drugs

- Decreases serum concentrations of oral contraceptives, felodipine, and lamotrigine
- Increases serum concentrations of phenytoin and phenobarbital

Counseling Points

- If using oral contraceptives, consider an additional or alternative method of birth control
- May cause drowsiness, dizziness, or blurred vision. Observe caution when driving or performing tasks requiring alertness, coordination, or physical dexterity.
- Notify physician if any of the following symptoms occur: Unusual bleeding, bruising, fever, sore throat, rash or ulcer in the mouth

Key Points

- Oxcarbazepine has an active metabolite, 10-monohydroxy metabolite (MHD)
- Of patients with a history of a hypersensitivity reaction to carbamazepine, approximately 25–30% experience a hypersensitivity reaction to oxcarbazepine
- Has not been shown to cause autoinduction
- Due to oxcarbazepine's influence on the CYP-450 enzymatic system, be alert to any new medications added or discontinued from a patient's drug regimen because it could affect medication blood levels

■ Phenobarbital

Brand Name
Luminal

Generic Name
Phenobarbital

Dosage Forms
Tablets, capsules, elixir, injection

Usage

- Sedative/hypnotic*, seizure disorders* (partial and generalized tonic-clonic seizures, status epilepticus)

Dosing

- Seizure disorders:
  - Initial dose: Loading dose: 10–20 mg/kg, initial dose: 1–3 mg/kg per day
- Sedation:
  - Initial dose: 30–120 mg/day in divided doses; use with caution in patients with renal or hepatic impairment
- Pharmacokinetic monitoring:
  - Target serum concentration: 10–40 µg/ml

Adverse Reactions: Most Common

- Fatigue, drowsiness, decreased cognitive function, hyperactivity in children

Adverse Reactions: Rare/Severe/Important

- Respiratory depression (contraindication in severe respiratory disorders), hepatotoxicity (contraindicated in severe liver dysfunction), rash (including SJS), osteomalacia (chronic administration), acute intermittent porphyria (contraindicated in porphyria), hematologic disorders

Major Drug Interactions

Drugs Affecting Phenobarbital

- Cimetidine, felbamate, valproic acid: Increase serum concentrations

Phenobarbital's Effect on Other Drugs

- Decreases serum concentrations: Carbamazepine, lamotrigine, 10-monohydroxy metabolite of oxcarbazepine, doxycycline, theophylline, verapamil, valproic acid, warfarin, zonisamide
- Decreased efficacy of oral contraceptives and metronidazole

Counseling Points

- Avoid use with other CNS depressants including alcohol to prevent excessive sedation
- May cause drowsiness. Observe caution when driving or performing tasks requiring alertness, coordination, or physical dexterity.
- If using oral contraceptives, consider an additional or alternative method of birth control
- Alert your pharmacist or physician of any additional or discontinued medications

Key Points

- Schedule IV medication. Addiction is rare in patients taking phenobarbital for epilepsy, but this drug is contraindicated in patients with previous addiction to sedative/hypnotics.
- Due to phenobarbital's influence on the CYP-450 enzymatic system, be alert to any new medications added or discontinued from a patient's drug regimen because it could affect medication concentrations
- The half-life of this drug is approximately 80 hours

■ Phenytoin

Brand Names

Dilantin, Phenytek

Generic Name

Phenytoin

Dosage Forms

Capsules, chewable tablets, suspension, injection

Usages

- Seizures* (generalized tonic-clonic and complex partial seizures and prevention and treatment of seizures occurring during or following head trauma/neurosurgery, status epilepticus)

Dosing

- Status epilepticus:
  - Initial dose: Loading dose 15–20 mg/kg, maximum rate 50 mg/minute
- Seizure disorders:
  - Initial dose: 100 mg three times a day, titrated to target serum concentrations
- Pharmacokinetic monitoring:
  - Target serum concentration: 10–20 µg/ml total phenytoin, or free phenytoin serum concentrations of 1–2 µg/ml

- Free fraction of phenytoin increases in low albumin states

Adverse Reactions: Most Common

- Lethargy, fatigue, dizziness, blurred vision, nystagmus (an initial symptom of toxicity), cognitive impairment, gingival hyperplasia, acne, hirsutism, coarsening of facial features

Adverse Reactions: Rare/Severe/Important

- Rash (SJS and TEN), osteomalacia, folate deficiency, blood dyscrasias, hepatitis, lupus-like reactions, lymphadenopathy, porphyria, arrhythmias following rapid IV administration, seizures and coma at toxic levels, teratogenic (fetal hydantoin syndrome)

Major Drug Interactions

Drugs Affecting Phenytoin

- Antacids: Decrease bioavailability
- Carbamazepine, chronic alcohol ingestion, folic acid, and valproic acid: Decrease serum concentration
- Cimetidine, acute alcohol ingestion, fluconazole, isoniazid, and warfarin: Increase serum concentration

Phenytoin's Effect on Other Drugs

- Decreased serum concentrations: Carbamazepine, felbamate, lamotrigine, 10 monohydroxy metabolite of oxcarbazepine, tiagabine, topiramate, valproic acid, zonisamide, folic acid, and vitamin D
- Increases lithium toxicity
- Decreased efficacy: Oral contraceptives

Counseling Points

- Avoid alcoholic beverages
- If using oral contraceptives, consider an additional or alternative method of birth control

Key Points

- There is a black box warning for the development of TEN and/or SJS with an increased incidence in patients of Asian descent with the HLA-B*1502 allele
- Due to phenytoin's influence on the CYP-450 and UGT enzymatic system, be alert to any new medications added or discontinued from a patient's drug regimen because it could affect medication blood levels
- Drug interactions are complicated. Phenytoin is highly protein bound; thus drugs that displace phenytoin from protein-binding sites increase free phenytoin levels. Monitoring serum concentrations or free phenytoin levels if displacement from protein-binding sites is suspected and clinical response is important.
- The suspension formulation of this drug interacts with tube feedings. If a patient requires tube feedings, separate dosing of the suspension formulation at least 2 hours before and 2 hours after tube feeding. Consider switching to the injection formulation if interruption of tube feeding is not feasible.
- This drug is metabolized by Michaelis–Menten pharmacokinetics. Saturation of metabolism can occur at

doses used clinically resulting in a disproportionally large increase in the serum concentration compared to a small dosage increase
- Serum concentration levels need to be corrected for significant renal dysfunction and/or hypoalbuminemia. Alternatively, obtain a free phenytoin level.

■ Pregabalin

Brand Name
Lyrica

Generic Name
Pregabalin

Dosage Forms
Capsules

Usage
- Seizures (adjunctive therapy for partial onset)*, diabetic peripheral neuropathy*, postherpetic neuralgia, fibromyalgia*, general anxiety disorder, central pain

Dosing
- Initial dose: 50 mg three times a day or 75 mg two times a day. Dose can be increased to a maximum of 300 mg/day within 1 week.
- Dose adjustments need to be made for renal impairment when CrCl <60 mL/minute

Adverse Reactions: Most Common
- Peripheral edema, increased appetite, weight gain, constipation, dry mouth, ataxia, dizziness, somnolence, euphoria, difficulty with concentrating and attention, blurred vision, diplopia

Adverse Reactions: Rare/Severe/Important
- Angioedema, hypersensitivity reaction, creatine kinase elevations, thrombocytopenia, P-R interval prolongation

Counseling Points
- Let your healthcare practitioner know about any muscle pain or tenderness, swelling of face or mouth, or swelling of hands, legs, or feet
- May cause drowsiness. Observe caution when driving or performing tasks requiring alertness, coordination, or physical dexterity

Key Point
- Schedule V medication

■ Topiramate

Brand Name
Topamax

Generic Name
Topiramate

Dosage Forms
Tablets, capsules

Usage
- Seizures (monotherapy or adjunctive therapy for partial onset seizures and primary generalized tonic-clonic seizures, adjunctive treatment of seizures associated with Lennox–Gastaut syndrome)*, prophylaxis of migraine headache*, cluster headache, neuropathic pain, bipolar disorder, withdrawal from alcohol, weight loss

Dosing
- Seizure disorders:
  - Initial dose: 25–50 mg daily and increased weekly by 25–50 mg until an effective dose of 200–400 mg/day is reached in two divided doses
- Migraine prophylaxis:
  - Initial dose: 25 mg daily and increased weekly by 25 mg until an effective dose is reached at 50 mg twice a day
- Renal impairment:
  - CrCl <70 mL/minute: Start at 50% the usual adult dose
- Use with caution in patients with hepatic impairment

Adverse Reactions: Most Common
- CNS (dizziness, ataxia, somnolence, psychomotor slowing, confusion, nervousness, memory impairment), loss of appetite, taste alteration, abnormal vision, fatigue, paresthesia

Adverse Reactions: Rare/Severe/Important
- Metabolic acidosis, precipitation of manic or hypomanic states in patients with bipolar disorder, oligohidrosis, hyperthermia, depression, kidney stones (concomitant use with carbonic anhydrase inhibitors should be avoided), hyperammonemia (concomitant use with valproic acid), myopia

Major Drug Interactions
Drugs Affecting Topiramate
- Phenytoin, carbamazepine, valproic acid, and pioglitazone: Decrease serum concentrations up to 40% or more
- Hydrochlorothiazide, lamotrigine, metformin: Increase serum concentrations

Topiramate's Effect on Other Drugs
- Phenytoin and metformin: Increase serum concentrations
- Pioglitazone, valproic acid, lithium, and risperidone: Decrease serum concentrations
- Decreases efficacy of oral contraceptives

Counseling Points
- Drink lots of fluid to prevent the formation of kidney stones
- Use caution with other CNS medications and alcohol due to increased risk of CNS side effects
- If using oral contraceptives, consider an additional or alternative method of birth control

■ Valproate/Devalproex

Brand Names

Depakene, Depacon, Depakote, Depakote ER, Depakote Sprinkle, Stavzor

Generic Names

Valproate sodium, valproic acid, and divalproex sodium (divalproex is converted to the active moiety, valproic acid, in the GI tract)

Dosage Forms

Tablets (immediate, delayed, and extended-release), capsules (immediate and delayed-release), syrup, injection

Usage

- Seizures (monotherapy and adjunctive therapy for simple and complex absence seizures, and complex partial seizures, adjunctive therapy for multiple seizure types)*, manic episodes associated with bipolar disorder*, prophylaxis for migraine headaches*, mood disorders

Dosing

- Seizure disorders:
  - Initial dose: 10–15 mg/kg per day. Titrate dose by 5–10 mg/kg per day weekly until a therapeutic response is observed or intolerable side effects. Maximum dose: 60 mg/kg per day.
- Mania:
  - Initial dose: 750 mg in divided doses. Titrate dose as rapidly as tolerated to control symptoms.
- Migraine prophylaxis:
  - Initial dose: 250 mg twice a day. Titrate up to 100 mg/day.
- Pharmacokinetic monitoring:
  - Target serum concentration is 50–100 µg/mL, although some patients may be well-controlled on higher or lower serum concentrations

Adverse Reactions: Most Common

- GI (nausea, vomiting, anorexia initially), weight gain with chronic use, drowsiness, ataxia, alopecia, blurred vision, asthenia

Adverse Reactions: Rare/Severe/Important

- Hepatotoxicity (can be fatal, usually occurs within the first 6 months of therapy), pancreatitis (can be fatal), teratogenic, hyperammonemia, thrombocytopenia, hypothermia, multiorgan hypersensitivity, contraindicated in patients with urea cycle disorder

Major Drug Interactions

Drugs Affecting Valproate/Divalproex

- Phenytoin, phenobarbital, primidone, carbamazepine, lamotrigine, rifampin, carbapenem antibiotics, and topiramate: Decrease serum concentration
- Cimetidine, aspirin, and felbamate: Increase serum concentration

Valproate/Divalproex's Effect on Other Drugs

- Increased serum concentrations: Benzodiazepines, zidovudine, tricyclic antidepressants, phenobarbital, 10, 11-carbamazepine epoxide (an active metabolite)

Counseling Point

- Contact healthcare provider if nausea, vomiting, anorexia, lethargy, or jaundice occur because these may be signs of liver problems

Key Points

- There are **black box warnings** for hepatotoxicity, pancreatitis, and teratogenicity
- GI side effects can be reduced by using the delayed release formulation
- Due to valproate/divalproex's influence on the CYP-450 enzymatic system, be alert to any new medications added or discontinued from a patient's drug regimen because it could affect medication concentrations

---

Drug Class: Antidepressants, Miscellaneous

Introduction

This group of antidepressants encompasses some first-line agents and drugs that may have less sexual side effects than the more commonly used SSRIs.

Mechanism of Action for the Drug Class

Block presynaptic reuptake of serotonin and/or norepinephrine, thereby increasing concentrations of these CNS neurotransmitters in the synapse. Bupropion is also a weak inhibitor of dopamine reuptake. Mirtazapine has central presynaptic alpha$_2$-adrenergic antagonism that leads to increased release of serotonin and norepinephrine.

Counseling Points for the Drug Class

- All antidepressants require several weeks of continuous use before symptoms improve. Patients should be cautioned that some side effects will probably occur before the therapeutic effect.
- The most important aspect of treating depression may be that therapy must continue for 6–9 months after improvement. Stopping the drug therapy too soon greatly increases the risk of depression returning.

Key Point for the Drug Class

- There is a **black box warning** for all antidepressants that these drugs increase the risk of suicidal thinking and behavior in children, adolescents, and young adults (18–24 years of age) with major depressive disorder (MDD) and other psychiatric disorders

Members of the Drug Class
In this section: Bupropion, mirtazapine, nefazodone, trazodone

■ Buproprion

Brand Names
Wellbutrin, Wellbutrin-SR, Wellbutrin XL, Zyban, Budeprion, Others

Generic Name
Bupropion

Dosage Forms
Oral tablets, sustained-release tablets

Usage
- Depression*, smoking cessation*

Dosing
- Depression:
  ○ Start with 100 mg twice daily of the immediate-release formulation or 150 mg in A.M. once daily with the sustained-release or extended-release forms. Increase to the 300-mg target dose by day 4.
- Smoking cessation:
  ○ Start with 150 mg/day for 3 days; then increase to 150 mg twice daily
- Renal/hepatic dosage adjustment:
  ○ Start with reduced dosage and monitor carefully

Adverse Reactions: Most Common
- Headache, insomnia, xerostomia, weight loss

dry mouth due to lack of saliva

Adverse Reactions: Rare/Severe/Important
- Seizures

Major Drug Interactions
- Do not use with MAOIs

Key Points
- Bupropion was removed from the market many years ago due to the risk of seizures at doses >450 mg/day. At that time, the recommended daily doses were higher.
- Bupropion is particularly useful for patients suffering sexual side effects or excessive sedation from other agents
- Start elderly patients at half the usual initial doses

■ Mirtazapine

Brand Names
Remeron, Remeron Sol Tabs

Generic Name
Mirtazapine

Dosage Forms
Oral tablets, ODTs

Usage
- Treatment of depression

Dosing
- 15 mg daily at bedtime is initial dose that is increased to 30–45 mg/day. Maximum dose: 45 mg/day.
- Renal/hepatic dosage adjustment:
  ○ Start with reduced dosage and monitor carefully

Adverse Reactions: Most Common
- Somnolence, xerostomia, increased appetite, constipation

Major Drug Interactions
- Do not use within 14 days of an MAOI or with sibutramine

Counseling Point
- Because sleepiness is common with mirtazapine, it is best to take before bedtime

Key Points
- Paradoxically, higher doses (30–45 mg) may be less sedating than initial 15-mg dose
- May cause less sexual side effects as compared with the SSRIs
- Start elderly patients at half the usual initial dose

■ Nefazodone

Brand Name
Serzone (now *removed* from market as a brand name)

Generic Name
Nefazodone

Dosage Forms
Oral tablets

Usage
- Treatment of depression

Dosing
- Initial dose is 100 mg twice daily, which is increased to target dose of 300–600 mg daily

Adverse Reactions: Most Common
- Sedation, headache, dizziness

Adverse Reactions: Rare/Severe/Important
- Liver failure (drug has a **black box warning** for hepatotoxicity)

Major Drug Interactions
Drugs Affecting Nefazodone
- CYP3A3 and 3A4 inhibitors like amiodarone, erythromycin, grapefruit juice, diltiazem, verapamil, and others: Increase nefazodone concentrations

Nefazodone's Effect on Other Drugs

- Increased concentrations: Triazolam (a contraindicated drug), other benzodiazepines, some antipsychotic agents, lovastatin, simvastatin, and many others

Key Points

- Nefazodone is chemically related to trazodone, which may cause priapism. Rare cases of priapism have been reported.
- Nefazodone can be fairly sedating. Give larger portion of daily dosage at bedtime, if possible.
- Check LFTs on a regular basis
- Low incidence of sexual dysfunction
- Medication errors possible because of the similar-sounding and similar available doses of Seroquel (an antipsychotic agent)
- Start elderly patients at half the usual initial doses

■ Desyrel

Brand Name

Desyrel

Generic Name

Trazodone

Dosage Forms

Oral tablets

Usage

- Depression, nighttime sedation*

Dosing

- 150 mg/day (divided in 2–3 doses) is starting dose that can be increased to 300–500 mg daily as a target dose for depression
- 50 mg: 150 mg is used for nighttime sedation

Adverse Reactions: Most Common

- Sedation, dizziness, headache

Adverse Reactions: Rare/Severe/Important

- Priapism

Major Drug Interactions

Drugs Affecting Trazodone

- CYP3A4 inhibitors (e.g., sibutramine, venlafaxine, protease inhibitors, some SSRIs): Increase trazodone's effects

Trazodone's Effect on Other Drugs

- Increases effect of alcohol and other CNS depressants

Key Points

- Often used as a hypnotic due to its sedative properties. Many authorities frown on such usage, especially when used with antipsychotic therapy.
- Anticholinergic effects may be seen with high doses
- Should be taken with food to cut down on peak concentrations that may lead to lightheadedness
- Start elderly patients at half the usual initial doses

Drug Class: Antidepressants: Serotonin-Norepinephrine Reuptake Inhibitors

Introduction

This small class of newer antidepressants has less sexual side effects and patient-friendly adverse effect profiles. They are used similarly to other antidepressants. Duloxetine is also used for the management of certain pain syndromes.

Mechanism of Action for the Drug Class

These medications block the neuronal reuptake of serotonin and norepinephrine.

Counseling Points for the Drug Class

- All antidepressants require several weeks of continuous use before symptoms improve. Patients should be cautioned that some side effects will probably occur before the therapeutic effect. "Be patient and don't give up on the drug too soon."
- The most important aspect of treating depression may be that therapy must continue for 6–9 months *after* the patient has shown improvement. Stopping the drug therapy too soon greatly increases the risk of relapse. "Keep taking the medication even after the symptoms improve."

Key Point for the Drug Class

- There is a **black box warning** for all antidepressants that they increase the risk of suicidal thinking and behavior in children, adolescents, and young adults (18–24 years of age) with MDD and other psychiatric disorders

Members of the Drug Class

In this section: Duloxetine, venlafaxine
Others: Desvenlafaxine, milnacipran

■ Duloxetine

Brand Name

Cymbalta

Generic Name

Duloxetine

Dosage Forms

Delayed-release capsules, enteric-coated pellets

Usage

- Treatment of depression*, generalized anxiety disorder, and the pain syndromes associated with diabetic neuropathy* and fibromyalgia

Dosing

- Initial dose: 40–60 mg daily in 1 or 2 doses, to a maximum of 120 mg daily
- Avoid in patients with hepatic impairment or renal dysfunction where CrCl <30 ml/minute

Adverse Reactions: Most Common

- Nausea, headache, somnolence, dry mouth, insomnia, other GI complaints

Adverse Reactions: Rare/Severe/Important

- Syndrome of inappropriate antidiuretic hormone

Major Drug Interactions

- Contraindicated with MAOIs and sibutramine

Drugs Affecting Duloxetine

- CYP2D6 and 1A2 inhibitors (paroxetine, fluvoxamine): Increased duloxetine effects

Duloxetine's Effect on Other Drugs

- Increases effect of alcohol and other CNS depressants, thioridazine, β agonists

Key Points

- May take 2–3 weeks for best effects to occur. Doses may need to be titrated upward.
- Drug should be tapered off over a 2-week period when discontinuing therapy
- May be confused with fluoxetine (Prozac)

■ Venlafaxine

Brand Names
Effexor, Effexor-XR

Generic Name
Venlafaxine

Dosage Forms
Oral tablets, extended-release capsules and tablets

Usage

- Depression*, GAD*, SAD, panic disorder, hot flashes, OCD, ADHD

Dosing

- Usual starting dose for most indications is 75 mg daily that should be increased to 150 mg by days 4–7
- Target dose range is 150–225 mg daily
- Maximum dose is 375 mg daily
- Renal dosage adjustment:
  - Reduce in patients with CrCl <70 ml/minute

Adverse Reactions: Most Common

- Headache, insomnia, nervousness, somnolence, GI complaints, increased diastolic blood pressure, dizziness

Adverse Reactions: Rare/Severe/Important

- SIADH

Major Drug Interactions

Drugs Affecting Venlafaxine

- CYP2D6 and 3A4 inhibitors: Increase venlafaxine effects

Venlafaxine's Effects on Other Drugs

- Increased effects: CNS depressants, trazodone

Key Points

- Because of the unusual side effect of hypertension, patients should have their blood pressure checked regularly, especially patients on higher doses
- Drug should be tapered off over a 2-week period when discontinuing therapy
- Not FDA approved for use in children
- Start elderly patients at half the usual initial dose

Drug Class: Antidepressants, Selective Serotonin Reuptake Inhibitors

Introduction

This class of agents seemed to replace the tricyclic antidepressants when they came to the market in the late 1980s. These agents are among the most widely prescribed medications in the United States. They are used for MDD and various anxiety disorders.

Mechanism of Action for the Drug Class

Block presynaptic reuptake of serotonin, thereby increasing the concentration of this CNS neurotransmitter in the synapse.

Counseling Points for the Drug Class

- All antidepressants require several weeks of continuous use before symptoms improve. Patients should be cautioned that some side effects will probably occur before the therapeutic effect.
- The most important aspect of treating depression may be that therapy must continue for 6–9 months after improvement. Stopping the drug therapy too soon greatly increases the risk of depression returning.
- All SSRIs may cause somnolence or insomnia. Each patient's response should determine if once-daily dosing is in the A.M. or P.M.

Key Point for the Drug Class

- There is a **black box warning** for all antidepressants that these drugs increase the risk of suicidal thinking and behavior in children, adolescents, and young adults (18–24 years of age) with MDD and other psychiatric disorders

Members of the Drug Class

In this section: Citalopram, escitalopram oxalate, fluoxetine, paroxetine, sertraline
  Other: Fluvoxamine

■ Citalopram

Brand Name
Celexa

Generic Name
Citalopram

Dosage Forms
Oral tablets, oral solution

Usage
- Depression*, OCD

Dosing
- Initial dose is 20 mg/day that can be increased in 1–2 weeks to 40 mg daily if little or no response; maximum dose is 60 mg/day
- Do not exceed 20 mg in patients with hepatic impairment

Adverse Effects: Most Common
- GI complaints: Nausea, loss of appetite; somnolence or insomnia, sexual dysfunction, headache

Adverse Effects: Rare/Severe/Important
- Hyponatremia, SIADH

Major Drug Interactions
- Contraindicated with MAOIs or sibutramine

Drugs Affecting Citalopram
- Strong CYP2D6, 2C19, 3A4 inhibitors including quinidine, some protease inhibitors, ticlopidine: Increased effects
- Carbamazepine: Decreases citalopram levels

Citalopram's Effect on Other Drugs
- Increases effect: CNS depressants, buspirone, clozapine
- Serotonin agonists (e.g., "triptans") may result in serotonin syndrome

Counseling Point
- Start elderly patients at half the usual initial doses

Key Point
- Drug should be tapered off over a 2-week period when discontinuing therapy

■ Escitalopram Oxalate

Brand Name
Lexapro

Generic Name
Escitalopram oxalate

Dosage Forms
Oral tablets, oral solution

Usage
- Depression*, GAD

Dosing
- Initial dose is 10 mg/day, which may be increased to 20 mg after 1–2 weeks
- Maximum dose is 20 mg/day

Adverse Reactions: Most Common
- Nausea, loss of appetite, somnolence or insomnia, headache, sexual dysfunction

Adverse Reactions: Rare/Severe/Important
- Hyponatremia, SIADH

Major Drug Interactions
- Contraindicated with MAOIs or sibutramine

Drugs Affecting Escitalopram
- Strong CYP2D6, 2C19, 3A4 inhibitors including quinidine, some protease inhibitors, ticlopidine: Increase effects of escitalopram
- Serotonin agonists (e.g., "triptans") may result in serotonin syndrome

Escitalopram's Effect on Other Drugs
- Increases effect of CNS depressants, buspirone, clozapine

Counseling Point
- Start elderly patients at half the usual initial doses

Key Points
- Drug should be tapered off over a 2-week period when discontinuing therapy
- This drug is simply the S-enantiomer of the generically available citalopram and may not have advantages over citalopram

■ Flouoxetine

Brand Names
Prozac, Prozac Weekly, Sarafem

Generic Name
Fluoxetine

Dosage Forms
Oral capsules; delayed-release capsules: 90 mg; oral tablets: 10 mg; oral solution

Usage
- Depression*, OCD, bulimia nervosa, premenstrual dysphoric disorder (PMDD)*, panic disorder, selective mutism

Dosing

- Usual initial dose 10–20 mg/day
- Dose adjustments may be made every 2 weeks to a maximum dose of 80 mg daily
- High end of dose range often required for OCD and bulimia nervosa
- Once-weekly dosing with 90-mg delayed-release capsule may replace 20 mg daily dosage (rarely used product)
- Use lower doses and monitor closely in patients with severe renal or hepatic disease

Adverse Reactions: Most Common

- Nausea, loss of appetite, insomnia, sexual dysfunction, headache, nervousness (CNS stimulation)

Adverse Reactions: Rare/Severe/Important

- Hyponatremia, SIADH

Major Drug Interactions

- Contraindicated with MAOIs, sibutramine, thioridazine, ziprasidone

Drugs Affecting Fluoxetine

- Carbamazepine: Decreases fluoxetine levels
- CYP2C9 and 2D6 inhibitors: Increase fluoxetine levels

Fluoxetine's Effect on Other Drugs

- Strong CYP2D6 and 2C9 inhibitor and moderate inhibitor of CYP 1A2 and 2C19; may increase levels of alcohol, phenytoin, clozapine, tramadol, others

Key Points

- Fluoxetine should always be given in the morning to avoid insomnia. It is the most stimulating agent of the SSRIs.
- Appetite suppression is common, and the drug is sometimes used for obesity
- The parent molecule and active metabolite, norfluoxetine, have a very long half-life. Therefore, steady-state concentrations may not be reached for weeks, and drug may remain in the body for weeks after discontinuation.
- Use cautiously and at reduced dosages in elderly (because of its long half-life), if at all

■ Paroxetine

Brand Names
Paxil, Paxil CR

Generic Name
Paroxetine

Dosage Forms
Oral tablets, controlled-release tablets, oral suspension

Usage

- Depression*, OCD*, panic disorder, SAD, GAD*, posttraumatic stress disorder*, PMDD

Dosing

- Initial dose is usually 10–20 mg/day. May increase by 10 mg every 1–2 weeks with a maximum dose of 60 mg/day.
- Higher doses necessary in the treatment of OCD and panic disorder
- Use lower doses and monitor closely in patients with severe renal or hepatic disease

Adverse Reactions: Most Common

- Nausea, loss of appetite, somnolence or insomnia, headache, sexual dysfunction

Adverse Reactions: Rare/Severe/Important

- Hyponatremia, SIADH

Major Drug Interactions

- Contraindicated with MAO inhibitors, sibutramine, tamoxifen, thioridazine

Drugs Affecting Paroxetine

- Buspirone, cimetidine, tramadol: Increase levels of paroxetine
- Carbamazepine: Decreases paroxetine levels

Paroxetine's Effect on Other Drugs

- Strong inhibitor of CYP2D6 and moderate inhibitor of CYP 2B6
- Increases levels of CNS depressants, β-blockers, carbamazepine, buspirone

Key Points

- May cause more sexual dysfunction than other SSRIs
- Paroxetine has the most drug interactions of all of the SSRIs
- Use cautiously and at reduced dosages in elderly (because of its long half-life)
- No real advantage to patented controlled-release form
- Pregnancy category D

■ Sertraline

Brand Name
Zoloft

Generic Name
Sertraline

Dosage Forms
Oral tablets, solution

Usage

- Depression*, OCD*, panic disorder*, PTSD*, eating disorders, SAD, GAD

Dosing

- Initial dose is 25–50 mg/day, which is usually increased to an effective range of 100–200 mg daily
- Use cautiously in patients with hepatic impairment due to extensive hepatic metabolism of this agent

Adverse Reactions: Most Common

- GI complaints: Nausea, loss of appetite, somnolence or insomnia, headache, sexual dysfunction

Adverse Reactions: Rare/Severe/Important

- Hyponatremia, SIADH

Major Drug Interactions

- Contraindicated with MAOIs, sibutramine, thioridazine

Drugs Affecting Sertraline

- Strong CYP2D6 inhibitors: Increase effects of sertraline

Sertraline's Effects on Other Drugs

- Moderate inhibitor of CYP2B6, 2C19, 2D6
- May increase effects of carbamazepine, phenytoin, CNS depressants, clozapine, risperidone

Key Points

- There are less clinically significant drug interactions with this agent compared to other SSRIs
- Initial doses usually must be increased for full therapeutic effect: Probably more so than with other SSRIs
- Start elderly patients at half the usual initial doses

Drug Class: Antidepressants, Tricyclics

Introduction

This is the oldest group of antidepressant agents. Because of many adverse effects, especially their anticholinergic and sedative properties, these medications are not used very often for depression anymore. The possibility of death upon overdose is another drawback with these agents. These drugs are more commonly used for the treatment of chronic nerve pain conditions at lower doses than those used to treat depression.

Mechanism of Action for the Drug Class

Block presynaptic reuptake of serotonin and/or norepinephrine, thereby increasing concentrations of these CNS neurotransmitters in the synapse.

Counseling Points for the Drug Class

- All antidepressants require several weeks of continuous use before symptoms improve. Patients should be cautioned that some side effects will probably occur before the therapeutic effect.
- The most important aspect of treating depression may be that therapy must continue for 6–9 months after improvement. Stopping the drug therapy too soon greatly increases the risk of depression returning.
- Orthostatic hypotension is possible with these agents. Advise patients to take a full minute at the side of the bed before getting up in the morning.
- Sedation may get less with continued treatment
- Recommend sugarless drinks, candies, and gum for dry mouth. More water is the easiest and most convenient "therapy" for dry mouth and to prevent constipation.

Key Point for the Drug Class

- There is a **black box warning** for all antidepressants that these drugs increase the risk of suicidal thinking and behavior in children, adolescents, and young adults (18–24 years of age) with MDD and other psychiatric disorders

Members of the Drug Class

In this section: Amitriptyline, doxepin, nortriptyline
   Others: Amoxapine, clomipramine, desipramine, imipramine, protriptyline, trimipramine

■ Amintriptyline

Brand Name
Elavil

Generic Name
Amitriptyline

Dosage Forms
Oral tablets, injection

Usage

- Depression, neuropathic pain syndromes*, migraine prophylaxis

Dosing

- Initial dose is usually 10–25 mg at bedtime. To prevent severe side effects, dose should be increased gradually. Adjustments should be made every 2–3 days at 10–25 mg increments.
- May take weeks to get response after leveling off dosage at approximately 150 mg daily. Dose may need to be increased gradually to 200 mg or more. Maximum dose is 300 mg daily.
- Pharmacokinetic monitoring:
  - One of a few tricyclic antidepressants where blood level data is sometimes used. Therapeutic levels of amitriptyline and its active metabolite, nortriptyline, should be in the range of 100–250 ng/ml.
  - Levels are rarely drawn

Adverse Reactions: Most Common
Pharmacokinetic monitoring:

- Anticholinergic effects (dry mouth, constipation, urinary hesitancy, blurred vision), orthostatic hypotension, sedation

Adverse Reactions: Rare/Severe/Important

- AV conduction changes, heart block, MI

Major Drug Interactions

- Contraindicated with MAOIs, sibutramine, thioridazine, ziprasidone

Drugs Affecting Amitriptyline

- CYP2D6 inhibitors (e.g., quinidine, protease inhibitors) may increase the effects of amitriptyline as will SSRIs, valproic acid, cimetidine, and tramadol
- Carbamazepine, barbiturates, rifamycins will decrease effects of amitriptyline

Amitriptyline's Effect on Other Drugs

- Amitriptyline increases effects of CNS depressants, anticholinergic drugs, α1-agonists, quinidine, tramadol, thioridazine, antiarrhythmics

Key Points

- Start elderly patients at half the usual initial doses
- Metabolized to the active nortriptyline metabolite

■ Doxepin

Brand Names
Sinequan, Prudoxin, Zonalon

Generic Name
Doxepin

Dosage Forms
Oral capsules, cream, oral solution

Usage
- Depression*, pruritic skin conditions

Dosing
- Initial dose is 25–50 mg at bedtime. May be increased very gradually to 150–300 mg over 2–3 weeks.
- Topical product is applied as a thin film four times daily

Adverse Reactions: Most Common (*Oral*)
- Anticholinergic effects (dry mouth, constipation, urinary hesitancy, blurred vision), orthostatic hypotension, sedation

Adverse Reactions: Rare/Severe/Important (*Oral*)
- AV conduction changes, heart block, MI

Major Drug Interactions
- Contraindicated with MAOIs, sibutramine, thioridazine, ziprasidone

Drugs Affecting Doxepin
- CYP2D6 inhibitors (e.g., quinidine, protease inhibitors) may increase the effects of doxepin as will SSRIs, valproic acid, and tramadol
- Carbamazepine will decrease effects of doxepin

Doxepin's Effect on Other Drugs
- Doxepin increases effects of CNS depressants, anticholinergic drugs, α1-agonists, quinidine, tramadol

Key Points

- Dosage should be limited to bedtime to make use of sedative effects. Elderly more prone to experience "hangover effect."
- Start elderly patients at half the usual initial dose

■ Nortriptyline

Brand Names
Pamelor, Aventyl

Generic Name
Nortriptyline

Dosage Forms
Oral capsules, solution

Usage
- Depression

Dosing
- Initial dose is 25–50 mg/day that may be increased slowly to a maximum dose of 150 mg/day
- Pharmacokinetic monitoring:
  - One of a few tricyclic antidepressants where blood level data is sometimes used. Therapeutic levels of nortriptyline should be in the range of 50–150 ng/ml.
  - Levels are *rarely* drawn

Adverse Reactions: Most Common
- Anticholinergic effects (dry mouth, constipation, urinary hesitancy, blurred vision), orthostatic hypotension, sedation
- These effects are less than that of the parent compound, amitriptyline

Adverse Reactions: Rare/Severe/Important
- AV conduction changes, heart block, MI

Major Drug Interactions
- Contraindicated with MAOIs, sibutramine, thioridazine, ziprasidone

Drugs Affecting Nortriptyline
- CYP2D6 inhibitors (e.g., quinidine, protease inhibitors) may increase the effects of nortriptyline as will SSRIs, valproic acid, and tramadol
- Carbamazepine will decrease effects of nortriptyline

Nortriptyline's Effect on Other Drugs
- Nortriptyline increases effects of CNS depressants, anticholinergic drugs, α1-agonists, quinidine, tramadol

Key Points
- Nortriptyline, a secondary amine tricyclic, is the active metabolite of amitriptyline
- Less sedating than amitriptyline
- Also used sometimes in chronic pain syndromes
- Start elderly patients at half the usual initial dose

Drug Class: Antimanic Agent (Mood Stabilizer)

Introduction

This class of psychiatric agents is essentially made up of lithium and valproic acid (and its congeners). Valproic acid is covered in the section on anticonvulsant agents. These drugs are mainstays in the acute and maintenance therapy of the bipolar disorders.

Mechanism of Action for Lithium

Multiple effects on CNS neurotransmitters via altered cation transport across cell membranes. May have some effect on uptake of serotonin and norepinephrine.

■ Lithium

Brand Names

Eskalith, Eskalith CR, Lithobid

Generic Names

Lithium carbonate, lithium citrate (liquid formulations)

Dosage Forms

Oral capsules and tablets, oral controlled- and sustained-release tablets, oral syrup

Usage

- Bipolar disorder*, augmenting agent for refractory depression

Dosing

- Initial dose is 600–1200 mg/day (in 2–3 divided doses)
- Dose adjustments made based on serum levels
- Renal dosage adjustment:
  ○ Should not be used with severe renal impairment
- Pharmacokinetic monitoring:
  ○ Drug levels should be drawn 10–12 hours after dose
  ○ Desired levels are 0.8–1.2 mEq/liter in acute mania
  ○ Maintenance levels are usually kept at 0.5–0.9 mEq/liter

Adverse Reactions: Most Common

- GI complaints, dizziness, polydipsia, tremor, sedation, leucocytosis

Adverse Reactions: Rare/Severe/Important

- Hypothyroidism, arrhythmias

Major Drug Interactions

Drugs Affecting Lithium

- Diuretics, NSAIDs, tetracyclines, angiotensin receptor antagonists: Decrease excretion of lithium, increasing lithium serum levels
- High sodium intake: Increases excretion of lithium, decreases lithium levels

Lithium's Effect on Other Drugs

- MAOIs: Possibility of severe CNS reactions
- CNS neurotoxicity has been rarely reported when lithium is added to some antipsychotic agents, SSRIs, TCAs, and phenytoin

Counseling Points

- Drug concentration monitoring is frequently performed
- Inform your healthcare practitioner before taking new medications including OTC products because many can interact with lithium

Key Points

- Contraindicated in severe renal or cardiac disease and in pregnancy
- After long-term use, hypothyroidism may develop in up to 10% of patients. Treat with levothyroxine.
- Drug is not metabolized, but is excreted through kidneys unchanged
- Lithium will be reabsorbed when extra sodium is excreted due to diuretic therapy, heavy perspiration, etc.
- Diuretics, ACE inhibitors, NSAIDs, increase lithium concentrations. Use with caution or decrease lithium dose and monitor concentrations.

Drug Class: Antipsychotic Agents, Atypical

Introduction

These agents are now recommended as first-line agents for the treatment of psychotic diagnoses. They have less movement side effects as compared to the older or conventional "typical" antipsychotic drugs like haloperidol and fluphenazine. The incidence of other adverse effects may also be somewhat lower.

Mechanism of Action for the Drug Class

These agents have effects on multiple CNS neurotransmitter systems. Dopamine inhibition (D_1, D_2, and D_4 receptors) and serotonin antagonism (5-HT_2), along with unknown effects on glutamate and GABA lead to the therapeutic effects in the treatment of schizophrenia and other psychotic states.

Counseling Points for the Drug Class

- Where appropriate, suggest to patients that they speak to their physician about receiving their entire daily dose at bedtime
- Patients must not use alcohol or other CNS depressants
- Patients should use caution in hot weather. May cause thermoregulatory changes.
- Patients must immediately report hyperpyrexia, especially when associated with muscle rigidity and altered mental status (signs of neuroleptic malignant syndrome [NMS])
- The risks of extrapyramidal reactions should be explained. Patients should be told to report abnormal involuntary body movements or abnormal muscle contractions. If there is an acute problem, they should contact their physician immediately or go to the emergency department of their local hospital.
- Patients should not double their dose if there is a missed dose. They should go back on their regular schedule.
- Where possible, explain that their illness is a biological problem. They have done nothing wrong to have their problems.
- Explain that drugs of abuse will make their symptoms worse.
- Patients should not stop their medication or stop regular visits to their healthcare practitioners

Key Points for the Drug Class

- **Black box warning:** Patients with dementia-related behavioral disorders treated with atypical antipsychotics are at an increased risk of death compared to placebo
- Glucose control must be monitored with all atypical antipsychotic agents

Members of the Drug Class

In this section: Aripiprazole, olanzapine, quetiapine, risperidone, ziprasidone

Others: Clozapine, paliperidone

◼ Aripiprazole

Brand Name
Abilify

Generic Name
Aripiprazole

Dosage Forms
Oral tablets, ODTs, oral solution, injection solution

Usage
- Schizophrenia*, bipolar disorder*, augmenting agent in treatment of MDD

Dosing
- Initial dose of 10–15 mg daily that may be increased over a few weeks to a maximum of 30 mg daily

- Higher doses may be used in acute treatment of bipolar disorder
- Lower doses used as adjunct to treatment of depression

Adverse Effects: Most Common
- Agitation, insomnia, headache, akathisia, and other extrapyramidal effects

Adverse Effects: Rare/Severe/Important
- NMS, hyperglycemia, drug-induced diabetes mellitus

Major Drug Interactions
- Major substrate of CYP2D6, 3A4

Drugs Affecting Aripiprazole
- Inhibitors of CYP450 such as fluoxetine, paroxetine, quinidine, azole antifungals, and clarithromycin increase aripiprazole effects

Aripiprazole's Effect on Other Drugs
- Inducers of CYP450 such as carbamazepine, phenobarbital, and phenytoin decrease aripiprazole effects

Key Points
- This drug is usually used as a long-term agent
- This agent may have a slightly different mechanism of action than the other atypical antipsychotic agents. It may have more and various effects on serotonin receptors than any other of the atypical agents.
- May not cause weight gain like other atypical agents and it is often used for this reason
- There have been medication errors because the drug's generic name has confused some healthcare professionals who believe that this drug is a proton pump inhibitor or an antifungal agent

◼ Olanzapine

Brand Names
Zyprexa, Zyprexa Zydis, Zyprexa Relprevv

Generic Name
Olanzapine

Dosage Forms
Oral tablets, ODTs, injection, long-acting injection

Usage
- Schizophrenia*, bipolar disorder*, psychosis/agitation associated with Alzheimer's disease

Dosing
- Initial dose is usually 5–10 mg/day, which may be increased over 1–2 weeks to 15–20 mg daily. Maximum daily dose of 20 mg daily is often exceeded up to 30 mg daily.

Adverse Effects: Most Common
- Somnolence, headache, weight gain, lipid abnormalities

Adverse Effects: Rare/Severe/Important
- NMS, hyperglycemia, drug-induced diabetes mellitus, extrapyramidal effects

Major Drug Interactions
Drugs Affecting Olanzapine
- CYP1A2 inhibitors (fluvoxamine, ketoconazole, others) will increase effects of olanzapine
- Rifampin, carbamazepine, and omeprazole decrease olanzapine levels

Olanzapine's Effect on Other Drugs
- Increases effect of CNS depressants

Counseling Point
- Olanzapine frequently causes drowsiness. Use caution when driving or performing activities that require mental alertness. These effects are more common at the beginning of therapy.

Key Points
- This drug is usually used as a long-term agent
- Weight gain is a significant adverse effect. It may lead to diabetes.

◼ Quetiapine
Brand Name
Seroquel

Generic Name
Quetiapine

Dosage Forms
Oral tablets, extended-release tablets

Usage
- Schizophrenia*, bipolar disorder*, bipolar depression

Dosing
- Initial dose is usually 25–50 once or twice daily, which may be increased every few days to usual target dose of 400–500 mg daily. Maximum dose of 800 mg daily.

Adverse Effects: Most Common
- Somnolence, headache, sedation, weight gain (due to effects on appetite center), lipid abnormalities

Adverse Effects: Rare/Severe/Important
- Neuroleptic malignant syndrome, hyperglycemia, drug-induced diabetes mellitus, extrapyramidal effects

Major Drug Interactions
Drugs Affecting Quetiapine
- Strong CYP3A4 inducers (e.g., carbamazepine, phenytoin, phenobarbital) will decrease effect of quetiapine
- CYP3A4 inhibitors like the azole antifungals and protease inhibitors will increase effects of quetiapine

Quetiapine's Effect on Other Drugs
- Increases effect of CNS depressants

Counseling Point
- Will cause drowsiness. Use caution when driving or performing activities that require mental alertness.

These effects are more common at the beginning of therapy.

Key Points
- This drug is usually used as a long-term agent
- This agent has been used in low doses (25–50 mg) as a hypnotic agent. This suboptimal practice should be discouraged.

◼ Risperidone
Brand Name
Risperdal, Risperdal-M

Generic Name
Risperidone

Dosage Forms
Oral tablets, oral solution, ODTs, extended-release injection

Usages
- Schizophrenia*, bipolar disorder*, autism, Tourette's syndrome

Dosing
- Initial dose is usually 1 mg twice daily that can be increased every 1–2 days to target dose of 4–6 mg daily. Maximum dose is 16 mg daily.
- Renal dosage adjustment:
  - Initial doses should be halved in patients with renal impairment
  - Careful monitoring is required for continued therapy

Adverse Effects: Most Common
- Somnolence, headache, sedation, weight gain, lipid abnormalities, extrapyramidal side effects

Adverse Effects: Rare/Severe/Important
- Neuroleptic malignant syndrome, hyperglycemia, drug-induced diabetes mellitus

Major Drug Interactions
Drugs Affecting Risperidone
- Carbamazepine will decrease levels of risperidone
- CYP2D6 inhibitors like paroxetine, quinidine, and some protease inhibitors will increase the effects of risperidone

Risperidone's Effect on Other Drugs
- Increases effect of CNS depressants

Counseling Point
- May cause drowsiness. Use caution when driving or performing activities that require mental alertness. These effects are more common at the beginning of therapy.

Key Points

- **Black box warning:** Patients with dementia-related behavioral disorders treated with atypical antipsychotics are at an increased risk of death compared to placebo
- This drug is usually used as a long-term agent
- May prolong QT interval
- The orthostatic hypotensive effects are due to α-adrenergic blockade and are most commonly seen at initiation of therapy
- Extrapyramidal symptoms are more common with this agent than with other atypical antipsychotics, especially at doses >4–5 mg daily

■ Ziprasidone

Brand Name
Geodon

Generic Name
Ziprasidone

Dosage Forms
Oral capsules, injection

Usage
- Schizophrenia*, bipolar disorder*, acute agitation in patients with schizophrenia (injection)*

Dosing
- Initial oral doses are 20–40 mg twice daily that can be rapidly increased to target dose of 80 mg twice daily. It should be given with morning and evening meals.
- IM dosing for acute agitation is 10–20 mg/dose up to 40 mg/day. Oral therapy should replace continual IM injections.

Adverse Effects: Most Common
- Headache, somnolence, extrapyramidal side effects

Adverse Effects: Rare/Severe/Important
- NMS, hyperglycemia, drug-induced diabetes mellitus

Major Drug Interactions
Drugs Affecting Ziprasidone
- Azole antifungals and ciprofloxacin may increase ziprasidone's effect

Ziprasidone's Effect on Other Drugs
- Increases effect of CNS depressants
- Use cautiously with drugs that prolong the QTc interval because additive prolongation can occur

Counseling Point
- May cause drowsiness. Use caution when driving or performing activities that require mental alertness. These effects are more common at the beginning of therapy.

Key Points
- This drug is usually used as a long-term agent
- May prolong QTc interval. Monitoring is important, particularly for patients on other QTc-prolonging agents.

Drug Class: Cholinesterase Inhibitors

Introduction
Donepezil, a piperidine derivative, is a centrally active, reversible inhibitor of acetylcholinesterase used in the treatment of dementia of the Alzheimer's type. The drug is structurally unrelated to other anticholinesterase agents.

Mechanism of Action for the Drug Class
Reversibly inhibits the enzyme acetylcholinesterase, thereby increasing acetylcholine concentrations.

Members of the Drug Class
In this section: Donepezil
Others: Galantamine, rivastigmine, tacrine

■ Donepezil

Brand Names
Aricept, Aricept ODT

Generic Name
Donepezil

Dosage Forms
Tablets

Usage
- Treatment of mild, moderate, or severe dementia of the Alzheimer's type*, ADHD, behavioral syndromes in dementia, mild–moderate dementia associated with Parkinson's disease, Lewy body dementia

Dosing
- Alzheimer's disease:
  - 5 mg/day at bedtime; may increase to 10 mg/day at bedtime after 4–6 weeks

Adverse Reactions: Most Common
- Nausea, vomiting, diarrhea, bradycardia, hypertension, dizziness, headache, insomnia, fatigue

Adverse Reactions: Rare/Severe/Important
- Atrioventricular block, torsades de pointes

Major Drug Interactions

Drugs Affecting Donepezil

- Cholinergic agents: Additive cholinergic side effects
- Decreased effectiveness: Anticholinergic agents, St. John's wort
- Increased adverse effects/toxicity: Gingko biloba

Donepezil's Effect on Other Drugs

- Nondepolarizing neuromuscular-blocking agents: exaggerated muscle relaxation

Counseling Points

- Administer at bedtime without regard to food
- Allow ODT tablet to dissolve completely on tongue and follow with water
- Donepezil is not a cure but may help reduce symptoms of Alzheimer's disease

- Improvement associated with donepezil therapy is not maintained following discontinuance of the drug. Contact prescriber before discontinuing medication.
- Report severe nausea, vomiting, diarrhea, anorexia, dehydration, or weight loss
- GI upset is usually transient and occurs at dose titration

Key Points

- Effects will vary from patient to patient but may be observed as subtle improvement in cognition, function, or behavior over time
- Benefits associated with donepezil therapy are not maintained following discontinuance of the drug, suggesting that the underlying disease process of dementia is not altered by this medication
- GI upset generally resolves in 1–3 weeks

Drug Class: Dopamine Agonists (Anti-Parkinson's Agent)

Introduction

These pharmacologically dissimilar agents both have an effect on dopamine receptors. Carbidopa/levodopa is a combination product used primarily for the treatment of Parkinson's disease (PD). Ropinirole hydrochloride is a non-ergoline dopamine agonist that has a higher specificity to D_3 subtypes of dopamine receptors. Normal motor function depends on the synthesis and release of dopamine by neurons projecting from the substantia nigra to the corpus striatum. The progressive degeneration of these neurons that occurs in PD disrupts this pathway and results in decreased levels of dopamine. Striatal dopamine levels in symptomatic PD are decreased by 60–80%.

Mechanism of Action for the Drug Class

Levodopa circulates in the plasma to the blood–brain barrier (BBB), where it crosses and is converted to dopamine; carbidopa inhibits peripheral decarboxylation of levodopa, decreasing the conversion to dopamine in peripheral tissues. This results in higher plasma levels of levodopa available at the BBB. The proposed mechanism of action of ropinirole is due to stimulation of postsynaptic dopamine D_2-type receptors within the caudate putamen in the brain. Ropinirole also has moderate in vitro affinity for opioid receptors.

Adverse Reactions for the Drug Class: Most Common

- Loss of appetite, nausea, vomiting, constipation, abdominal pain, dizziness, headache, fatigue

Adverse Reactions for the Drug Class: Rare/Severe/Important

- Heart disease, orthostatic hypotension, dose-related dyskinesia, somnolence, hallucinations, psychotic disorders

Counseling Points for the Drug Class

- Take exactly as directed; do not change dosage or discontinue without consulting prescriber. Do not crush sustained-release form.
- Take with meals if GI upset occurs, before meals if dry mouth occurs, after eating if drooling or nausea occur
- Do not use alcohol and prescription/OTC sedatives or CNS depressants without consulting prescriber. Urine or perspiration may appear darker.
- Use caution when driving, climbing stairs, or engaging in tasks requiring alertness
- Use caution when rising from sitting or lying position
- Report exacerbation of underlying depression or psychosis
- Report unresolved constipation or vomiting, CNS changes, increased muscle spasticity or rigidity, unusual skin changes, or significant worsening of condition

Members of the Drug Class

In this section: Carbidopa/levodopa, ropinirole

Others: Amantadine, bromocriptine, entacapone, pramipexole

■ Carbidopa/Levodopa

Brand Names
Sinemet, Sinemet CR, Parcopa

Generic Name
Carbidopa/Levodopa

Dosage Forms
Tablets: Immediate-release, sustained-release, orally disintegrating

Usage
- PD*, RLS, amblyopia (poor vision)

Dosing
- PD:
  - Immediate-release tablet:
    - Initial: Carbidopa 25 mg/levodopa 100 mg three times a day titrated to desired effects. Use of more than one dosage strength or dosing four times a day may be required. Maximum dose is 8 tablets of any strength per day or 200 mg carbidopa and 2000 mg levodopa.
  - Sustained-release tablet:
    - Initial: Carbidopa 50 mg/levodopa 200 mg two times a day, at intervals not <6 hours
    - Dosage adjustment: May adjust every 3 days; intervals should be between 4 and 8 hours during the waking day (maximum: 8 tablets per day)

Major Drug Interactions
Drugs Affecting Carbidopa/Levodopa
- Increased effect: MAOIs
- Decreased effect: Antipsychotics, iron salts, metoclopramide, phenytoin, pyridoxine
- Herbal considerations: Avoid kava kava

Key Points
- Therapeutic effects may take several weeks or months to achieve, and frequent monitoring may be needed during first weeks of therapy
- Use of MAOIs concurrently or within 2 weeks of carbidopa/levodopa is contraindicated
- Patients using concomitant antihypertensives may be at an increased risk for orthostatic hypotension
- Avoid high-protein diets and high doses (>200 mg/day) of vitamin B_6 (pyridoxine)
- False-positive or false-negative urinary glucose results may occur with certain testing agents; false-positive urine ketone results may occur with certain testing agents

■ Ropinirole

Brand Names
Requip, Requip XL

Generic Name
Ropinirole

Dosage Forms
Tablets: Immediate-release, extended-release

Usage
- PD, early PD not receiving concomitant levodopa therapy, advanced PD on concomitant levodopa therapy, moderate to severe primary RLS

Dosing
- PD (immediate-release): Titrate weekly to therapeutic response in an ascending dose schedule from an initial dose of 0.25 mg three times daily to a maximum dose of 24 mg/day in divided doses
- PD discontinuation taper: Ropinirole should be gradually tapered over 7 days
- PD (extended-release): Initial dose is 2 mg once daily orally, titrated at a weekly or longer interval to therapeutic response at 2 mg daily increments to a maximum dose of 24 mg/day. When discontinuing, gradually taper over 7 days.
- RLS: Begin with 0.25 mg once daily and titrate as needed to a maximum of 4 mg
  - All doses are once daily 1–3 hours before bedtime; doses should be titrated when appropriate, based on clinical response and efficacy
  - Doses up to 4 mg per day may be discontinued without tapering

Major Drug Interactions
Drugs Affecting Ropinirole
- Increased effect: Ciprofloxacin, CYP1A2 inhibitors, estrogen derivatives, MAOIs
- Decreased effect: Antipsychotics, CYP1A2 inducers, metoclopramide
- Herbal considerations: Avoid kava kava, gotu kola, valerian, St. John's wort

Key Points
- Titrate dosing to achieve desired clinical response
- If therapy with a potent inhibitor of CYP1A2 is stopped or started during treatment with ropinirole, adjustment of ropinirole dose may be required
- May switch directly from immediate-release ropinirole; start an extended-release dose that matches most closely with the total daily immediate-release dose

---

Drug Class: Sedative-Hypnotic Agent, Benzodiazepine

Introduction

A few benzodiazepines have a place in therapy for short-term treatment of insomnia. As with all sleep agents, caution needs to be exercised to prevent habitual use and disturbance of a patient's natural sleep pattern. In addition, use should be limited in duration (7–10 days) to prevent potential increased reliance on higher dosing at bedtime. Benzodiazepines are a Schedule IV medication and can be habit forming. As with use in other indications, if patients have used the benzodiazepine long-term, they should be counseled not to discontinue benzodiazepines abruptly. A gradual taper is required to avoid rebound, relapse, and withdrawal symptoms.

Mechanism of Action for the Drug Class

Benzodiazepines facilitate the activity of the inhibitory neurotransmitter GABA and other inhibitory transmitters by binding to specific benzodiazepine receptors

Members of the Drug Class

In this section: Temazepam
    Others: Estazolam, flurazepam, quazepam, triazolam

■ Temazepam

Brand Name
Restoril

Generic Name
Temazepam

Dosage Forms
Capsules

Usage
- Short-term treatment of insomnia*, anxiety, panic attacks

Dosing
- Insomnia:
  ○ 7.5–30 mg at bedtime

- Use with caution in patients with renal and hepatic impairment

Adverse Reactions: Most Common
- CNS-related (sedation, somnolence, memory impairment, coordination problems, dizziness), emergence of complex behavior ("sleep driving")

Adverse Reactions: Rare/Severe/Important
- Withdrawal syndromes and respiratory depression (especially additive with other CNS depressants or alcohol), anaphylaxis reactions (angioedema, dyspnea, throat closing, nausea, vomiting)

Major Drug Interactions
Drugs Affecting Temazepam
- Oral contraceptives decrease serum levels

Temazepam's Effect on Other Drugs
- CNS depressants: Additive CNS depression

Counseling Points
- Ingesting alcoholic beverages during benzodiazepine therapy is very dangerous and must be avoided
- Take just before going to sleep
- Only used when needed and for the short term (7–10 days) to prevent habit-forming use

Key Points
- As a drug class, all benzodiazepines are contraindicated in narrow-angle glaucoma and pregnancy (Class D)
- Elderly patients are the most susceptible to adverse effects and should be started with the 7.5-mg dose

---

Drug Class: Sedative-Hypnotic Agent, Nonbenzodiazepine

Introduction

A newer drug class of sedative-hypnotic medications has supplanted much of the use of benzodiazepines for treatment of insomnia. Although structurally, the nonbenzodiazepines do not resemble the benzodiazepines, they do function in a similar fashion and have very similar side-effect profiles and patient counseling points. As with all sleep agents, caution needs to be exercised to prevent habitual use and disturbance of a patient's natural sleep pattern. These agents are Schedule IV medications and may be habit-forming. Use should be limited in duration to prevent potential increased reliance on higher dosing at bedtime.

Mechanism of Action for the Drug Class

Although not benzodiazepines, they similarly facilitate the activity of the inhibitory neurotransmitter GABA.

Counseling Points for the Drug Class
- Alcohol use while taking these medications can be dangerous and should be avoided
- Do not abruptly discontinue these drugs. A gradual taper is required to avoid rebound, relapse, and withdrawal symptoms. Insomnia is common after abruptly stopping sleeping aids.
- Only use when needed and for short-term duration
- Take just before going to sleep

Members of the Drug Class
In this section: Zolpidem, eszopiclone
Others: Ramelteon, zaleplon

■ Zoplidem

Brand Names
Ambien, Ambien CR

Generic Name
Zolpidem

Dosage Forms
Tablets, sublingual tablets, spray

Usage
- Short-term and long-term treatment of insomnia

Dosing
- Initial dose: immediate-release, sublingual, and spray 10 mg at bedtime. Extended-release, 12.5 mg at bedtime (1 spray = 5 mg)
- Use with caution in patients with hepatic impairment

Adverse Reactions: Most Common
- CNS related (sedation, somnolence, dizziness), emergency of complex behavior ("sleep driving"), headache, diarrhea

Adverse Reactions: Rare/Severe/Important
- Withdrawal syndromes and respiratory depression (especially additive with other CNS depressants or alcohol; use with caution in patients with mild to moderate COPD or sleep apnea), CNS depression, depression, anaphylaxis reactions (angioedema)

Major Drug Interactions
Drugs Affecting Zolpidem
- Azole antifungal agents, ritonavir, and SSRIs increase serum concentrations
- Rifampin decreases serum concentrations

Zolpidem's Effect on Other Drugs
- CNS depressants (additive CNS depression)

Counseling Point
- Do not crush controlled-release tablets. Place sublingual tablets under the tongue and do not swallow or administer with water.

Key Points
- Reevaluate patient needs after 7–10 days of use. Zolpidem has been studied for use up to 35 days.
- Elderly patients are the most susceptible to side effects. Starting doses of the immediate-release, sublingual, and spray should be 5 mg at bedtime. The starting dose for the extended-release tablet should be 6.25 mg at bedtime.

- Use the immediate-release tablets for patients who require medication to initiate sleep. Use the extended-release tablets for patients who require medication to maintain sleep throughout the night.

■ Exzopiclone

Brand Name
Lunesta

Generic Name
Eszopiclone

Dosage Forms
Tablets

Usage
- Insomnia

Dosing
- Initial dose: 2 mg at bedtime
- Use with caution in patients with hepatic impairment

Adverse Reactions: Most Common
- CNS-related (sedation, somnolence, dizziness, abnormal dreams, memory impairment), emergency of complex behavior ("sleep driving"), decreased inhibition, dry mouth, impaired coordination, unpleasant taste

Adverse Reactions: Rare/Severe/Important
- Withdrawal syndromes and respiratory depression (especially additive with other CNS depressants or alcohol; use with caution in patients with compromised lung function), CNS depression, depression, anaphylaxis reactions (angioedema, throat closing, dyspnea), chest pain, peripheral edema

Major Drug Interactions
Drugs Affecting Eszopiclone
- Azole antifungal agents, clarithromycin, and ritonavir increase serum concentrations

Eszopiclone's Effect on Other Drugs
- CNS depressants (additive CNS depression)

Key Points
- Reevaluate patient needs after 7–10 days of use. Eszopiclone has been studied for use up to 6 months.
- Elderly patients are the most susceptible to side effects. The starting dose should be 1 mg at bedtime.

Drug Class: Skeletal Muscle Relaxants

Introduction
Centrally acting skeletal muscle relaxants are used for the short-term treatment of skeletal muscle pain and discomfort.

Mechanism of Action for the Drug Class
The exact mechanism of action is unclear, but the clinical effects of this class may be associated with general depression of the CNS. These agents typically have no direct

effect on skeletal muscle. Baclofen exerts its effects as an agonist at presynaptic GABA$_B$ receptors, acting mainly at the spinal cord level to inhibit the transmission of both monosynaptic and polysynaptic reflexes, with resultant relief of muscle spasticity. Cyclobenzaprine is structurally related to the TCAs. It acts primarily at the brainstem within the CNS. Carisoprodol is metabolized to meprobamate, which has anxiolytic and sedative effects. Tizanidine is an imidazole derivative chemically related to clonidine, exhibiting α2-adrenergic agonist properties.

Members of the Drug Class
In this section: Baclofen, carisoprodol, cyclobenzaprine, metaxalone, methocarbamol, tizanidine
Others: Chlorzoxazone, dantrolene, orphenadrine

■ Baclofen

Brand Name
Lioresal

Generic Name
Baclofen

Dosage Form
Injection, tablet

Usage
• Treatment of muscle spasm associated with acute painful musculoskeletal conditions*, treatment of reversible spasticity associated with multiple sclerosis or spinal cord lesions, intractable hiccups, intractable pain relief, bladder spasticity, trigeminal neuralgia, cerebral palsy, Huntington's chorea

Dosing
• Oral: 5 mg three times a day, may increase 5 mg/dose every 3 days to a maximum of 80 mg/day
• Intrathecal:
  ○ Test dose: 50–100 μg, doses >50 μg should be given in 25-μg increments, separated by 24 hours, until a 4- to 8-hour positive clinical response is seen. Patients not responding to screening dose of 100 μg should not be considered for chronic infusion/implanted pump.
  ○ Maintenance: After positive response to test dose, a maintenance intrathecal infusion can be administered via an implanted intrathecal pump. Initial pump dose: Infusion at a 24-hourly rate dosed at twice the test dose.
• Renal dosage adjustment: May be necessary to reduce dosage; no specific guidelines have been established

Adverse Reactions: Most Common
• Nausea, vomiting, drowsiness, dizziness, headache, poor muscle tone, weakness

Adverse Reactions: Rare/Severe/Important
• Constipation (significant with intrathecal use), withdrawal reactions with abrupt discontinuation (more severe with intrathecal use), coma, seizure

Major Drug Interactions
Baclofen's Effect on Other Drugs
• Increased effect of alcohol, CNS depressants
• Herbal considerations: Avoid valerian, St. John's wort, kava kava, gotu kola

Counseling Points
• Take as prescribed. Do not discontinue this medicine without consulting prescriber.
• Do not take any prescription or OTC sleep-inducing drugs, sedatives, or antispasmodics without consulting prescriber. Avoid alcohol use.
• Use caution when driving or engaging in tasks requiring alertness until response to drug is known
• Frequent small meals or lozenges may reduce GI upset

Key Points
• Avoid abrupt withdrawal of drug. Encourage consistent and early refills of medication to minimize the risk of significant sequelae of withdrawal.
• Avoid alcohol and other CNS depressants

■ Carisoprodol

Brand Name
Soma

Generic Name
Carisoprodol

Dosage Forms
Tablets

Usage
• Treatment of muscle spasm associated with acute painful musculoskeletal conditions*, pain associated with TMJ disorder

Dosing
• 250–350 mg three times daily and at bedtime
• Hepatic impairment: Use lower initial doses and increase gradually as needed and tolerated

Adverse Reactions: Most Common
• Dizziness, headache, somnolence

Adverse Reactions: Rare/Severe/Important
• Paradoxical CNS stimulation, seizure, drug abuse/dependence, withdrawal symptoms

Major Drug Interactions
Drugs Affecting Carisoprodol
  ○ CYP2C19 inhibitors (moderate and strong)

Carisoprodol's Effect on Other Drugs
  ○ Ethanol, CNS depressants: Additive CNS depression

Counseling Points
• Do not use alcohol, prescription/OTC sedatives, CNS depressants, or psychotropic agents without consulting prescriber

- Use caution when driving, climbing stairs, or engaging in tasks requiring alertness
- Use caution when rising from sitting or lying position
- Report syncope, tachyarrhythmia, or excessive somnolence
- Monitor for and report signs/symptoms of seizures when withdrawing from prolonged therapy
- Avoid meprobamate while on carisoprodol therapy
- If next dose is more than 1 hour late, skip the missed dose

Key Points

- Carisoprodol should only be used for short periods (2–3 weeks) due to lack of evidence of effectiveness with prolonged use
- Carisoprodol is metabolized to meprobamate, which has anxiolytic and sedative effects. Avoid concurrent use of these two agents.

■ Cyclobenzaprine

Brand Names
Amrix, Flexeril

Generic Name
Cyclobenzaprine

Dosage Forms
Capsules (extended-release), tablets

Usage

- Treatment of muscle spasm associated with acute painful musculoskeletal conditions

Dosing

- Capsule, extended-release:
  - 15 mg once daily; some patients may require up to 30 mg once daily
- Tablet, immediate-release:
  - 5 mg three times a day; may increase to 7.5–10 mg three times a day if needed
- Hepatic impairment:
  - Capsule, extended-release: Not recommended in mild to severe impairment
  - Tablet, immediate-release:
    - Mild impairment: Initial: 5 mg; use with caution; titrate slowly, and consider less frequent dosing
    - Moderate–severe impairment: Use not recommended

Adverse Reactions: Most Common

- Palpitations, nervousness, confusion, dizziness, headache, somnolence, bad taste in mouth, constipation, indigestion, nausea, dry mouth, blurred vision

Adverse Reactions: Rare/Severe/Important

- Cholestasis, hepatitis, jaundice, cardiac dysrhythmia, anaphylaxis, immune hypersensitivity reaction

Major Drug Interactions

- Consider all drug interactions with TCAs as possible interactions with cyclobenzaprine

Drugs Affecting Cyclobenzaprine
- Increased level/effect: CYP1A2 inhibitors, pramlintide
- Decreased level/effect: Acetylcholinesterase inhibitors, peginterferon α-2b

Cyclobenzaprine's Effect on Other Drugs
- Increased level/effect: Ethanol, anticholinergic drugs, CNS depressants, MAOIs
- Decreased level/effect: Acetylcholinesterase inhibitors

Counseling Points

- Avoid activities requiring mental alertness or coordination until drug effects are realized
- Watch for potential anticholinergic side effects
- Report signs/symptoms of decreased hepatic function, especially if you have preexisting hepatic disease
- Report lack of symptom improvement within 2–3 weeks of therapy
- Avoid alcohol and other CNS depressants while taking this drug
- Avoid concomitant use of TCAs or guanethidine during therapy with this drug

Key Points

- Not intended for long-term use. Do not use for >2–3 weeks.
- Use caution in patients with hepatic impairment
- Not effective for spasticity associated with cerebral palsy
- Given structural similarity to TCAs, advise patients of anticholinergic side effects and precautions. Avoid concomitant use with MAOIs.

■ Metaxalone

Brand Name
Skelaxin

Generic Name
Metaxalone

Dosage Forms
Tablets

Usage

- Treatment of muscle spasm associated with acute painful musculoskeletal conditions

Dosing

- 800 mg three to four times a day
- Renal impairment:
  - No specific dosage recommendations; use caution in mild–moderate impairment
  - Contraindicated in severe renal impairment
- Hepatic impairment:
  - No specific dosage recommendations; use caution in mild–moderate impairment
  - Contraindicated in severe hepatic impairment

Adverse Reactions: Most Common

- Drug-induced GI disturbances, nausea, vomiting, dizziness, headache, somnolence, nervousness

Adverse Reactions: Rare/Severe/Important

- Hemolytic anemia, leukopenia, jaundice, hypersensitivity

Major Drug Interactions

Effect of Metaxalone on Other Drugs

- Increased level/effect: ethanol, CNS depressants, psychotropics
- Herbal considerations: Avoid valerian, St. John's wort, kava kava, gotu kola

Counseling Points

- Avoid activities requiring mental alertness or coordination until drug effects are realized
- Inform diabetic patients that metaxalone may cause false-positive results for certain urine glucose tests
- Avoid alcohol and other CNS depressants while taking this drug
- If the next dose is >1 hour past regular dosing time, skip the missed dose
- Report signs/symptoms of decreased hepatic function, especially if you have preexisting hepatic disease

Key Points

- Use caution in patients with significant renal or hepatic impairment
- May cause leukopenia; use caution with clozapine and carbamazepine
- Monitor relevant laboratory values for renal and hepatic function

■ Methocarbamol

Brand Name

Robaxin

Generic Name

Methocarbamol

Dosage Forms

Injection, tablets

Usage

- Treatment of muscle spasm associated with acute painful musculoskeletal conditions*, supportive therapy in tetanus

Dosing

- Muscle spasm:
  - Oral: 1.5 g four times a day for 2–3 days (up to 8 g/day for severe conditions), then decrease to 4–4.5 g/day in 3–6 divided doses
  - IM, IV: 1 g every 8 hours if oral not possible; injection should not be used for >3 consecutive days. If condition persists, may repeat course of therapy after a drug-free interval of 48 hours.

- Tetanus:
  - IV: Initial dose: 1–3 g; may repeat dose every 6 hours until oral dosing is possible; injection should not be used for >3 consecutive days
- Renal impairment:
  - Do not administer injectable formulation to patients with renal dysfunction
  - Use lower initial oral doses and increase gradually as needed and tolerated
- Hepatic impairment:
  - Specific dosing guidelines are not available; plasma protein binding and clearance are decreased; half-life is increased
  - Use lower initial oral doses and increase gradually as needed and tolerated

Adverse Reactions: Most Common

- Flushing, pruritus, rash, urticaria, indigestion, nausea, vomiting, dizziness, headache, nystagmus, somnolence, vertigo, nervousness, blurred vision, conjunctivitis

Adverse Reactions: Rare/Severe/Important

- Bradyarrhythmia, hypotension, syncope, leukopenia, anaphylaxis, seizure (IV formulation)

Major Drug Interactions

Methocarbamol's Effect on Other Drugs

- Ethanol, CNS depressants, pyridostigmine
- Herbal considerations: Avoid valerian, St. John's wort, kava kava, gotu kola

Counseling Points

- Do not increase dose or discontinue without consulting prescriber. Take as directed.
- Avoid alcohol and other CNS depressants while taking this drug
- Avoid activities requiring mental alertness or coordination until drug effects are realized
- Drug may color urine brown, black, or green
- Report excessive drowsiness or mental agitation, chest pain, skin rash, swelling of mouth/face, difficulty speaking, or vision changes
- If the next oral dose is >1 hour late, skip the missed dose

Key Points

- Do not use the injection formulation for >3 consecutive days
- Use caution in patients with renal and hepatic impairment
- Injectable product is *not* recommended in patients with renal dysfunction

■ Tizanidine

Brand Name

Zanaflex

Generic Name

Tizanidine

Dosage Forms

Capsules, tablets

Usage

- Treatment of muscle spasm associated with acute painful musculoskeletal conditions*, tension headaches, low back pain*, trigeminal neuralgia

Dosing

- Usual initial dose: 4 mg, may increase by 2–4 mg as needed for satisfactory reduction of muscle tone every 6–8 hours to a maximum of 3 doses totaling 36 mg in any 24-hour period
- Renal impairment:
  - Reduce dose with a CrCl <25 ml/minute
- Hepatic impairment:
  - Avoid use if possible. If drug is necessary, use lowest possible doses while monitoring for hypotension.

Adverse Reactions: Most Common

- Hypotension, dry mouth, vomiting, constipation, abnormal LFTs, dizziness, somnolence, nervousness, muscle weakness, speech or vision disturbances

Adverse Reactions: Rare/Severe/Important

- Orthostatic hypotension, angina, heart failure, MI, syncope, leukopenia, thrombocytopenia, hepatitis

Major Drug Interactions

- Avoid concomitant use with ciprofloxacin or fluvoxamine

Drugs Affecting Tizanidine

- Increased effects are seen with β-blockers, ciprofloxacin, CYP1A2 inhibitors, herbal products with hypotensive properties, MAOIs, estrogens, phosphodiesterase 5 inhibitors, pentoxifylline
- Decreased effects occur with antidepressants (α2-antagonists), herbal products with hypertensive properties, methylphenidate, SSRIs/SNRIs, TCAs

Tizanidine's Effect on Other Drugs

- Increased effects: Ethanol, CNS depressants, antihypertensives
- Herbal considerations: Avoid valerian, St. John's wort, kava kava, gotu kola

Counseling Points

- Avoid activities requiring mental alertness until drug effects are realized
- Rise slowly from a lying/seated position because this drug may cause hypotension
- Although this drug may be taken with or without food, take the drug the same way every time. Inconsistent administration with regards to food may enhance or delay onset and change the adverse effect profile.
- Do not discontinue the drug suddenly
- Do not drink alcohol while taking this drug

Key Points

- Tizanidine is chemically related to clonidine and has α2-adrenergic agonist properties
- Use with caution in the elderly
- Discuss risks of sudden discontinuation of drug
- Follow maximum daily dosing guidelines

Drug Class: Smoking Cessation Aid, Partial Nicotinic Agonist

Introduction

Varenicline is the first drug in its pharmacologic class and is considered a second-line treatment option as a smoking cessation aid. As a partial agonist at the nicotinic acetylcholine receptor, varenicline produces the reward experience of smoking but at a significantly lower level than nicotine. In addition, it also helps alleviate the symptoms of nicotine withdrawal.

Mechanism of Action for the Drug Class

Partial neuronal α-4, β-2 receptor agonist within the mesolimbic dopamine system.

■ Varenicline

Brand Name

Chantix

Generic Name

Varenicline

Dosage Forms

Tablets

Usage

- Smoking cessation aid

Dosing

- Initial dose: Day 1–3: 0.5 mg daily; day 4–7: 0.5 mg twice a day; day 8 onward: 1 mg twice a day
- Renal impairment: Adjust dose for CrCl <30 ml/minute

Adverse Reactions: Most Common

- Nausea, somnolence, dizziness, insomnia, headache, abnormal dreams, GI discomfort

Adverse Reactions: Rare/Severe/Important

- Neuropsychiatric events (**black box warning**, depression, suicidal-related events, changes in behavior, aggression, hostility, agitation) angioedema, hypersensitivity reactions, rash (SJS, erythema multiforme), loss of consciousness, difficulty concentrating

Counseling Points

- The patient and family members need to be aware of potential mood changes and suicidal thoughts. Report any changes in behavior and mood to the prescriber.
- Instruct patient to start drug 1 week before target quit date
- If a patient cannot tolerate side effects, temporarily reduce the dose
- If patient has successfully quit by week 12, he or she may remain on the drug for an additional 12 weeks.

If the patient was not successful by week 12 and continues to smoke, stop the medication and do not continue for the additional 12 weeks.

- Take medication with a full glass of water
- May cause dizziness or loss of consciousness. Observe caution when driving or performing tasks requiring alertness, coordination, or physical dexterity
- Do not abruptly discontinue. Taper off.

Key Point

- The FDA has received an abundance of reported psychiatric side effects making varenicline one of the most reported prescription drugs at this time

---

Drug Class: Stimulants

Introduction

These CNS stimulants are primarily used for ADHD and narcolepsy or excessive daytime sleepiness (EDS). Stimulants increase alertness and prevent sleep, but their side-effect profile includes insomnia, heart palpitations, hypertension, and irritability. The goal of using these agents is to improve quality of life, but a balance needs to be found between benefit and risks.

Mechanism of Action for the Drug Class

Although the mechanism of action for modafinil is unknown, the other two drugs covered in this class are thought to mediate CNS stimulation through either the release of norepinephrine and dopamine (amphetamine/dextroamphetamine) or through blocking the reuptake of norepinephrine and dopamine (methylphenidate).

Members of the Drug Class

In this section: Amphetamine/dextroamphetamine, methylphenidate, modafinil

Others: Armodafinil, dextroamphetamine, lisdexamfetamine, methamphetamine

■ Amphetamine/Dextroamphetamine

Brand Names

Adderall, Adderall XR

Generic Name

Amphetamine/Dextroamphetamine

Dosage Forms

Immediate-release tablets, extended-release capsules

Usage

- ADHD*, narcolepsy*

Dosing

- ADHD:
  ○ Initial dose: Adults: IR 5 mg one to two times a day. Adults: ER 20 mg daily in the morning.
  ○ Initial dose: Children 3–5 years of age: IR 2.5 mg/day. Children >6 years of age: IR 5 mg/day one to two times a day. Extended-release: 5–10 mg daily.
  ○ Give the first dose on awakening.
- Narcolepsy:
  ○ Initial dose: Adults: IR 10 mg/day
  ○ Initial dose: Children 6–12 years of age: 5 mg/day. Children >12 years of age: Refer to adult dosing.

Adverse Reactions: Most Common

- Insomnia, headache, weight loss, loss of appetite, nervousness, abdominal pain

Adverse Reactions: Rare/Severe/Important

- Cardiac adverse effects including sudden death, drug abuse/dependency, sudden death in children (FDA special alert), suppression of growth may occur in children with long-term use, exacerbate preexisting or emergence of new psychiatric disorders, worsening of motor and vocal tics, aggression, seizures, visual disturbances, dependency

Major Drug Interactions

Drugs Affecting Amphetamine/Dextroamphetamine

- Antacids, acetazolamide, thiazides increase serum concentrations

Amphetamine/Dextroamphetamine's Effect on Other Drugs

- Concomitant use with MAOIs is contraindicated

Counseling Points

- Do not crush or chew sustained-release formulations. The contents of the capsules may be sprinkled on applesauce.
- Avoid evening doses to decrease risk of insomnia
- Consult physician before discontinuing drug

Key Points

- Amphetamine/dextroamphetamine has many contraindications. It is contraindicated in patients with cardiac structure abnormalities, advanced arteriosclerosis, symptomatic heart disease, and moderate–severe hypertension due to the possibility of sudden cardiac death. It is also contraindicated in patients with a history of drug dependence because it is a Schedule II controlled substance. It is further contraindicated in patients with hypersensitivity or idiosyncratic reactions to sympathomimetic amines, hyperthyroidism, glaucoma, and agitated states.
- Screen and monitor cardiovascular status of patients, blood pressure, heart rate, psychiatric history, growth and weight gain
- Drug holidays may be given to children being treated for ADHD to determine the need for continued treatment and allow "catch-up" growth

■ Methylphenidate

Brand Names
Ritalin, Ritalin SR, Ritalin LA, Concerta, Methylin, Methylin ER, Metadate ER, Metadate CD, Daytrana

Generic Name
Methylphenidate

Dosage Forms
Immediate-release and extended-release tablets, extended-release capsules, chewable tablets, transdermal system, solution

Usage

- ADHD*, narcolepsy*, depression, fatigue, traumatic brain injury

Dosing

- ADHD:
  - Initial dose: Adults: IR 10–60 mg/day in 2–3 divided doses. Adults: LA 20 mg daily in the morning.
  - Initial dose: Children >6 years of age: IR 5 mg twice a day
  - Sustained- and extended-release tablets have an 8-hour duration of action. Administer the 8-hour dose of the regular release tablets.
  - Initial dose Concerta: 18–36 mg once a day
  - Initial dose Metadate CD: 20 mg once a day
  - Initial dose Daytrana: 10-mg patch. Apply to hip 2 hours before effect is needed; remove 9 hours after application.

- Narcolepsy:
  - Initial dose: IR 10 mg two to three times a day

Adverse Reactions: Most Common

- Insomnia, headache, anorexia, loss of appetite, nervousness, dizziness, hyperhidrosis, nausea

Adverse Reactions: Rare/Severe/Important

- Cardiac-adverse events, dependency, contraindicated in patients with a history of alcohol or drug abuse, sudden death in children (FDA special alert), suppression of growth may occur in children with long-term use, exacerbate preexisting or emergence of new psychiatric disorders, worsening of motor and vocal tics, aggression, seizures, visual disturbances, contact dermatitis with transdermal application

Major Drug Interactions

Methylphenidate's Effect on Other Drugs

- Concomitant use with MAOIs or halogenated anesthetics is contraindicated
- Increased serum concentrations of SSRIs and warfarin

Counseling Points

- Do not crush or chew sustained-release or extended-release formulations. The contents of the capsules may be sprinkled on applesauce.
- Take IR, chewable tablets, and solution 30–45 minutes before meals
- Avoid evening doses to decrease risk of insomnia
- Drink at least 8 ounces of water with chewable tablets to avoid choking
- Consult physician before discontinuing drug

Key Points

- Methylphenidate has many contraindications. It is contraindicated in patients with structure cardiac abnormalities, advanced arteriosclerosis, symptomatic heart disease, and moderate to serve hypertension due to the possibility of sudden cardiac death. It is also contraindicated in patients with a history of drug dependence because it is a Schedule II controlled substance. It is further contraindicated in patients with hypersensitivity or idiosyncratic reactions to sympathomimetic amines, hyperthyroidism, glaucoma, agitated states, motor tics, and a family history of Tourette's syndrome.
- Screen and monitor cardiovascular status of patients, blood pressure, heart rate, psychiatric history, growth and weight gain
- Drug holidays may be given to children being treated for ADHD to determine the need for continued treatment and allow "catch-up" growth

■ Modafinil

Brand Name
Provigil

Generic Name
Modafinil

Dosage Forms

Tablets

Usage

- Improve wakefulness in patients with EDS associated with narcolepsy or shift-work sleep disorder*, adjunctive therapy for obstructive sleep apnea/hypopnea syndrome*, ADHD*, fatigue

Dosing

- ADHD:
  - Initial dose: 100–300 mg
- Narcolepsy and obstructive sleep apnea/hypopnea syndrome:
  - Initial dose: 200 mg daily taken in the morning
- Shift-work sleep disorder:
  - Initial dose: 200 mg daily taken 1 hour prior to shift work
  - Reduce dose by 50% in patients with severe hepatic impairment.

Adverse Reactions: Most Common

- Insomnia, headache, nervousness, dizziness, nausea, anxiety

Adverse Reactions: Rare/Severe/Important

- Hypertension, rash, SJS, multiorgan hypersensitivity reaction, angioedema, anaphylaxis, psychiatric symptoms

Major Drug Interactions

Modafinil's Effect on Other Drugs

- Decreases serum concentration of oral contraceptives

Counseling Points

- Avoid use with alcohol
- If using oral contraceptives, consider an additional or alternative method of birth control

Key Point

- Schedule IV medication that can produce psychoactive and euphoric effects. The abuse potential is similar to other CNS stimulant agents.

Review Questions

1. Which of the following benzodiazepines would *not* be given for seizure control?
   - A. Alprazolam
   - B. Clonazepam
   - C. Diazepam
   - D. Lorazepam

2. Which antiepileptic drug is available in an injectable formulation?
   - A. Lamotrigine
   - B. Levetiracetam
   - C. Oxcarbazepine
   - D. Topiramate

3. The target serum concentration for phenytoin is
   - A. 4–12 µg/ml
   - B. 10–20 µg/ml
   - C. 10–40 µg/ml
   - D. 50–100 µg/ml

4. Which medication can suppress growth in children with long-term use?
   - A. Adderall
   - B. Ambien
   - C. Lunesta
   - D. Provigil

5. The correct dosing regimen for the first 7 days of Chantix therapy is
   - A. Day 1–7: 0.5 mg daily
   - B. Day 1–3: 0.5 mg daily, then day 4–7: 0.5 mg twice a day
   - C. Day 1–3: 0.5 mg twice a day, then day 4–7: 1 mg twice a day
   - D. Day 1–7: 1 mg twice a day

6. Which of the following is *least* likely to cause withdrawal symptoms with abrupt discontinuation?
   - A. Ativan
   - B. BuSpar
   - C. Klonopin
   - D. Xanax

7. Which drug induces its own metabolism?
   - A. Keppra
   - B. Lamictal
   - C. Tegretol
   - D. Trileptal

8. Which of the following *pairs* of atypical antipsychotic agents cause the most extrapyramidal effects?
   - A. Quetiapine and ziprasidone
   - B. Ziprasidone and olanzapine
   - C. Ziprasidone and risperidone
   - D. Olanzapine and clozapine
   - E. Olanzapine and quetiapine

9. The most common side effects seen with the tricyclic antidepressants (TCAs) are
   A. Sedation and anticholinergic effects
   B. CNS stimulation and increased appetite
   C. Arrhythmias and hypertension
   D. Serotonin syndrome and/or akathisia
   E. Hiccups and fainting spells

10. Mirtazapine causes a fair amount of sedation at the recommended starting dose. It should always be given at bedtime. As the dose is increased, there seems to be less sedation.
    A. True
    B. False

11. Which common over-the-counter medication may cause a severe rise in lithium levels when administered concomitantly with normal lithium therapy?
    A. Loperamide (Imodium)
    B. Pseudoephedrine (Sudafed)
    C. Bismuth subsalicylate suspension (Kaopectate)
    D. Docusate sodium (Colace)
    E. Ibuprofen (Motrin-IB)

12. Which of the following *oral* psychiatric agents is available as a once-weekly dosage form?
    A. Mirtazapine
    B. Citalopram
    C. Haloperidol
    D. Fluoxetine
    E. Fluphenazine

13. The maximum daily dose for sumatriptan nasal spray is
    A. 40 mg
    B. 12 mg
    C. 100 mg
    D. 200 mg

14. One of your nursing home patients is started on Aricept. Which of the following counseling points is correct?
    A. GI upset usually resolves in 1–3 months
    B. Concomitant use of gingko biloba may lead to an increased risk of adverse effects or toxicity
    C. Aricept represents a cure for Alzheimer's disease
    D. Dose titration should occur after 7 days on 5 mg orally every day at bedtime

15. Which of the following skeletal muscle relaxants is structurally related to the tricyclic antidepressants (TCAs)?
    A. Zanaflex
    B. Skelaxin
    C. Amrix
    D. Soma

chapter 7

Endocrine Agents

Mirza Perez, PharmD, BCPS

Drug Class: Antiestrogens

Introduction

Tamoxifen is a selective estrogen receptor modulator (SERM) commonly used for the prevention and treatment of breast cancer.

Mechanism of Action for the Drug Class

Competes with estrogen for binding sites in target tissues such as breast, decreasing the effects of estrogen in those tissues.

Members of the Drug Class

In this section: Tamoxifen

 Tamoxifen

Brand Name
Nolvadex

Generic Name
Tamoxifen

Dosage Forms
Tablets

Usage
Breast cancer; reduction in breast cancer incidence in high-risk women*, treatment of ductal carcinoma in situ

Dosing
- Treatment of metastatic breast cancer:
  - 20–40 mg daily
- Adjuvant treatment for breast cancer, ductal carcinoma in situ, and reduction of breast cancer risk:
  - 20 mg daily for 5 years

Adverse Reactions: Most Common
- Hot flashes, mood changes, vaginal discharge or bleeding, menstrual irregularities

Adverse Reactions: Rare/Severe/Important
- Blood clots, hair loss, bone pain, endometrial hyperplasia

Major Drug Interactions
Drugs Affecting Tamoxifen
- Strong inhibitors or inducers of CYP2C9, CYP2D6, and CYP3A4: Increase or decrease efficacy (may increase risk of breast cancer)

Tamoxifen's Effect on Other Drugs
- Warfarin: Increases anticoagulant effects

Contraindications
- Women who require concomitant anticoagulant therapy
- Women with a history of deep vein thrombosis or pulmonary embolus
- Pregnancy

Counseling Point
- Take steps to avoid pregnancy when taking tamoxifen and during the 2 months after discontinuation

Key Points
- The benefits of tamoxifen as a treatment for breast cancer are firmly established and far outweigh the potential risks for most women
- Tamoxifen helps decrease bone loss in postmenopausal women

Drug Class: Bisphosphonates

Introduction

Bisphosphonates are used in the treatment and prevention of osteoporosis. There are specific dosing instructions that are important to prevent the common gastrointestinal side effects from these medications. Many of them have multiple dosing options, often for the same indications such as osteoporosis.

Mechanism of Action for the Drug Class

Inhibits osteoclastic-mediated bone resorption, preventing bone destruction.

Usage for the Drug Class

- Osteoporosis*, Paget's disease

Adverse Reactions for the Drug Class: Most Common

- Abdominal pain, dyspepsia, nausea, hypocalcemia

Adverse Reactions for the Drug Class: Rare/Severe/Important

- Bone/muscle pain, esophagitis, gastritis, esophageal ulcers, osteonecrosis of the jaw

Major Drug Interactions for the Drug Class

Drugs Affecting Bisphosphonates

- Aspirin: Increased risk of gastrointestinal-adverse events
- Nonsteroidal anti-inflammatory drugs (NSAIDs): Increased risk of gastrointestinal irritation
- Antacids: Decreased absorption of bisphosphonates

Contraindications for the Drug Class

- Patients with abnormalities of the esophagus such as strictures or achalasia
- Inability to sit upright or stand for at least 30 minutes

Counseling Points for the Drug Class

- Take bisphosphonates at least 30 minutes before the first food or beverage of the day with 6–8 oz of plain water only, first thing in the morning
- Do not lie down for 30 minutes after taking the medication and until after the first food of the day
- Do *not* chew or crush on tablets
- Notify your physician if new symptoms of heartburn, difficulty or pain on swallowing develop
- Take supplemental calcium and vitamin D if dietary intake is inadequate

Key Points for the Drug Class

- Hypocalcemia must be corrected before therapy is initiated
- Osteonecrosis of the jaw, usually related to tooth extraction and/or local infection with delayed healing, has been observed with the use of bisphosphonates. Bisphosphonate-associated osteonecrosis has been reported primarily in cancer patients receiving intravenous bisphosphonates. However, some cases have also been reported in patients receiving treatment for postmenopausal osteoporosis. The known risk factors for osteonecrosis include a cancer diagnosis, poor oral hygiene, concomitant therapies (i.e., radiotherapy, chemotherapy, or corticosteroids), and comorbid diseases (i.e., preexisting dental disease, anemia, infection, or coagulopathy). Patients who develop osteonecrosis of the jaw should be referred to an oral surgeon for care.

Members of the Drug Class

In this section: Alendronate, risedronate, ibandronate
    Others: Etidronate, pamidronate, zoledronic acid

■ Alendronate

Brand Names

Fosamax, Fosamax Plus D

Generic Name

Alendronate

Dosage Forms

Tablets, solution

Dosing

- Treatment of osteoporosis in men and postmenopausal women:
    - 70 mg once a week or 10 mg daily
- Prevention of postmenopausal osteoporosis:
    - 35 mg once a week or 5 mg daily
- Treatment of glucocorticoid-induced osteoporosis:
    - 5 mg daily (10 mg daily in postmenopausal women not on hormone replacement therapy)
- Treatment of Paget's disease:
    - 40 mg daily for 6 months
- Renal dosage adjustment:
    - Not recommended in patients with creatinine clearance (CrCl) <35 ml/minute

■ Risedronate

Brand Name

Actonel

Generic Name

Risedronate

Dosage Forms

Tablets

Dosing

- Treatment and prevention of osteoporosis in postmenopausal women:
    - 5 mg daily or 35 mg once weekly
- Treatment and prevention of glucocorticoid-induced osteoporosis:
    - 5 mg once daily

- Treatment of Paget's disease:
  - 30 mg once daily for 2 months. Retreatment may be necessary after 2 months of observation.
- Renal dosage adjustment:
  - Not recommended in patients with CrCl <30 ml/min

Ibandronate

Brand Name
Boniva

Generic Name
Ibandronate

Dosage Forms
Tablets, injection

Usage
- Uses of Injection
  - Treatment and prevention of osteoporosis*, hypercalcemia of malignancy*, metastatic bone disease*

Dosing
- Treatment of postmenopausal osteoporosis:
  - Oral: 2.5 mg once daily or 150 mg once a month
  - IV: 3 mg every 3 months
- Prevention of postmenopausal osteoporosis:
  - Oral: 2.5 mg once daily or 150 mg once a month
- Hypercalcemia of malignancy (unlabeled use):
  - IV: 2–4 mg over 2 hours
- Metastatic bone disease:
  - Oral: 50 mg once daily
  - IV: 6 mg over 1 hour every 3–4 weeks
- Renal dosage adjustments:
  - Avoid in CrCl <30 ml/minute

Drug Class: Calcitonin-Salmon

Introduction
Calcitonin-salmon is a synthetic version of the hormone calcitonin found in salmon, which is more active in humans than human calcitonin. Calcitonin is used for treating postmenopausal osteoporosis, Paget's disease, and hypercalcemia. It is most commonly given intranasally.

Mechanism of Action for the Drug Class
Directly inhibits osteoclastic bone resorption; promotes the renal excretion of calcium, phosphate, sodium, magnesium, and potassium by decreasing tubular reabsorption; increases the jejunal secretion of water, sodium, potassium, and chloride.

Members of the Drug Class
In this section: Calcitonin

Calcitonin

Brand Names
Miacalcin, Fortical

Generic Name
Calcitonin-salmon

Dosage Forms
Solution (intranasal spray), injection

Usage
- Osteoporosis*, treatment of Paget's disease, hypercalcemia

Dosing
- Use one spray per day intranasally in one nostril; alternate nostrils daily

Adverse Reactions: Most Common
- Allergic reactions, nasal mucosal alterations, rhinitis

Adverse Reactions: Rare/Severe/Important
- Epistaxis, sinusitis

Counseling Points
- Before priming the pump and using a new bottle, allow it to reach room temperature
- To prime (activate) the pump, the bottle should be held upright and the two white side arms of the pump depressed toward the bottle until a full spray is produced
- To administer the medication, the nozzle should be carefully placed into the nostril with the head in the upright position
- The pump should *not* be primed before each daily dose
- Take supplemental calcium and vitamin D if dietary intake is inadequate
- Store new unassembled bottles in the refrigerator
- Once the pump has been activated, store bottle in use at room temperature in an upright position for up to 35 days

Key Point
- Usually used when bisphosphonates are not tolerated

Drug Class: Sex Hormones—Estrogens, Progestins, Estrogen and Progestin Combinations, Estrogen and Androgen Combinations

Introduction

These medications are used mainly for the treatment of vasomotor symptoms associated with menopause and the prevention of osteoporosis. However, their use has decreased since the Women's Health Initiative (WHI) trial in 2002. This trial was terminated prematurely because of an increased risk of coronary heart disease and thromboembolic events in patients receiving the estrogen/progesterone combination. The interpretation of this study has been controversial based on the risk profile of the women included in the study.

Mechanism of Action for the Drug Class

Estrogens (estradiol, conjugated estrogen, esterified estrogen) are important in developing and maintaining the female reproductive system and secondary sex characteristics, promoting growth and development of the vagina, uterus, fallopian tubes, and breasts. Estrogens are also involved in shaping the skeleton and inhibiting bone resorption. Progestins (medroxyprogesterone) inhibit the secretion of gonadotropins, which in turn prevent follicular maturation and ovulation and results in endometrial thinning.

Adverse Reactions for the Drug Class: Most Common for Estrogen-Containing Products

- Vaginal bleeding, breast tenderness, nausea and vomiting

Adverse Reactions for the Drug Class: Most Common for Progestin-Containing Products

- Breakthrough bleeding, nausea

Adverse Reactions for the Drug Class: Rare/Severe/Important for Estrogen-Containing Products

- Weight gain, edema, headache, migraines

Adverse Reactions for the Drug Class: Rare/Severe/Important for Progestin-Containing Products

- Insomnia, somnolence

Major Drug Interactions for the Drug Class

Drugs Affecting Estrogen

- Barbiturates, rifampin, phenytoin, carbamazepine, and other agents that induce hepatic microsomal enzymes (CYP450 3A4): May lower estrogen levels

Estrogen's Effect on Other Drugs

- Corticosteroids: May increase the pharmacologic and toxicologic effects

Contraindications for the Drug Class

- Known or suspected pregnancy
- Undiagnosed abnormal vaginal bleeding
- Known or suspected breast cancer except for selected patients treated for metastatic disease
- Active thromboembolic disorders
- Severe liver disease

Counseling Points for the Drug Class (Estrogen)

- Estrogens have been reported to increase the risk of endometrial carcinoma in postmenopausal women
- Do not use estrogens with or without progestins to prevent heart disease, heart attacks, or strokes
- Do not use estrogens and progestins during pregnancy
- Notify a healthcare practitioner if any of the following occur: pain in the groin or calves, sharp chest pain or sudden shortness of breath, abnormal vaginal bleeding, missed menstrual period, lumps in the breast, sudden severe headache, vision or speech disturbance, weakness or numbness in an arm or leg, severe abdominal pain, yellowing of the skin or eyes, or severe depression
- Women with an intact uterus should also receive monthly progestins not estrogen-only products
- While you are on estrogens, you should visit your doctor at least once a year for appropriate follow-up

Members of the Drug Class (Estrogens)

In this section: Estradiol, estradiol transdermal system, conjugated estrogen
   Others: Esterified estrogens, estrone, estropipate

Members of the Drug Class (Progestins)

In this section: Medroxyprogesterone
   Others: Hydroxyprogesterone, norethindrone acetate, progesterone

■ Estradiol

Brand Name
Estrace

Generic Name
Estradiol

Dosage Forms
Tablets

Usage
Treatment of moderate to severe vasomotor symptoms*, vulvar and vaginal atrophy associated with menopause, female hypoestrogenism, breast cancer (palliation only), androgen-dependent carcinoma of the prostate, prevention of osteoporosis*, abnormal uterine bleeding due to hormonal imbalance

Dosing
- Treatment of moderate to severe vasomotor symptoms, vulvar and vaginal atrophy associated with menopause:
  - Initial dose: 1–2 mg daily adjusted to control symptoms. Administration should be cyclic, 3 weeks on,

1 week off. Attempts to discontinue or taper should be considered at 3- to 6-month intervals.

- Treatment of "female hypoestrogenism":
  - Initial dose: 1–2 mg daily adjusted to control symptoms
- Treatment of breast cancer for palliation only:
  - Initial dose: 10 mg three times daily for a period of at least 3 months
- Treatment of advanced androgen-dependent carcinoma of the prostate:
  - Initial dose: 1–2 mg three times daily adjusted to control symptoms
- Prevention of osteoporosis:
  - Initial dose: 0.5 mg administered cyclically (23 days on and 5 days off), dose adjusted to control menopausal symptoms

■ Estradiol Transdermal System

Brand Names
Climara, Vivelle, Estraderm

Generic Name
Estradiol transdermal system

Dosage Forms
Patch

Usage
Treatment of moderate to severe vasomotor symptoms and vulvar and vaginal atrophy; prevention of postmenopausal osteoporosis

Dosing
- Climara: 0.025–0.05 mg/day applied to the skin once weekly, adjusted based on symptoms
- Vivelle: 0.025–0.0375 mg/day applied to the skin twice weekly, adjusted based on symptoms
- Estraderm: 0.05 mg/day applied to the skin twice weekly, adjusted based on symptoms

Counseling Points
Guidelines for applying the transdermal system:
- Place the adhesive side on a clean, dry area of the lower abdomen or the upper quadrant of the buttock
- Do not apply the transdermal system to the breasts
- Rotate the sites of application, allowing an interval of at least 1 week between application to a particular site
- The area selected should not be oily, damaged, or irritated
- Apply the system immediately after opening the pouch and removing the protective lining
- Press the system firmly in place using the fingers for at least 10 seconds
- If a system falls off, apply a new one for the remainder of the 7-day dosing interval
- Only *one* system should be worn at any one time during the 7-day dosing interval
- Swimming, bathing, or using a sauna may decrease the adhesion of the system

Key Points
- In women who are taking oral estrogens, the transdermal system can be initiated 1 week after withdrawal of oral therapy
- Therapy may be given continuously in women who do not have an intact uterus. In patients with an intact uterus, therapy may be given on a cyclic schedule (3 weeks on, 1 week off)
- Climara is a continuous transdermal system for once-weekly administration; Vivelle and Estraderm are continuous-transdermal systems for twice-weekly administration

■ Conjugated Estrogen

Brand Name
Premarin

Generic Name
Conjugated estrogen

Dosage Forms
Tablets

Usage
Treatment of moderate to severe vasomotor symptoms*, vulvar and vaginal atrophy, female hypoestrogenism, prevention of osteoporosis*

Dosing
- 0.3–1.25 mg daily

Key Points
- Conjugated estrogens may be given continuously with no interruption in therapy or in cyclic regimens (regimens such as 25 days on drug followed by 5 days off)
- Attempts to discontinue or taper medication should be made at 3- to 6-month intervals

■ Medroxyprogesterone

Brand Names
Cycrin, Provera, Depo-Provera, Depo-Sub-Q Provera 104

Generic Name
Medroxyprogesterone

Dosage Forms
Tablets, injectable suspension

Usage
- Management of endometriosis-associated pain (Depo-Sub-Q Provera only), secondary amenorrhea, abnormal uterine bleeding due to hormonal imbalance, reduction of endometrial hyperplasia in postmenopausal women receiving estrogens, prevention of pregnancy*

Dosing
- Management of endometriosis-associated pain:
  - SUB-Q injection: 104 mg SUB-Q every 3 months (13 weeks)

- Secondary amenorrhea:
  - Tablets: 5 or 10 mg daily for 5–10 days
- Abnormal uterine bleeding due to hormonal imbalance:
  - Tablets: 5 or 10 mg daily for 5–10 days beginning on day 16 or day 21 of the menstrual cycle
- Reduction of endometrial hyperplasia in postmenopausal women receiving 0.625 mg of conjugated estrogens:
  - Tablets: 5 or 10 mg daily for 12–14 consecutive days per month, either beginning on the day 1 of the menstrual cycle or day 16 of the menstrual cycle
- Prevention of pregnancy:
  - IM Injection: 150 mg IM every 3 months (13 weeks)
  - SUB-Q Injection: 104 mg SUB-Q every 3 months (13 weeks)

Counseling Points

- Advise patients that at the beginning of Depo-Provera therapy their menstrual cycle may be disrupted and irregular and unpredictable bleeding or spotting may occur
- Progestin withdrawal bleeding usually occurs within 3–7 days after discontinuing oral therapy
- Depo-Sub-Q Provera should be given by SUB-Q injection into the anterior thigh or abdomen

Key Point

- Women who use Depo-Provera Contraceptive Injection (IM or SUB-Q) may lose significant bone mineral density. Bone loss is greater with increasing duration of use and may not be completely reversible. Depo-Provera Contraceptive Injection should be used as a long-term birth control method (e.g., >2 years) only if other birth control methods are inadequate.

■ Conjugated Estrogen/ Medroxyprogesterone Acetate

Brand Names
Prempro, Premphase

Generic Name
Conjugated estrogen/medroxyprogesterone acetate

Dosage Forms
Tablets

Usage

- Treatment of moderate to severe vasomotor symptoms*, vulvar and vaginal atrophy, prevention of postmenopausal osteoporosis*

Dosing

- Prempro: Start with 0.3 mg/1.5 mg with subsequent dosage adjustments based on patient response and symptoms. Patients should be treated with the lowest effective dose.
- Premphase: 0.625 mg tablet daily on days 1–14 and 0.625 mg/5 mg daily on days 15–28

Counseling Point

- Take as directed by prescriber

Key Point

- This medication is the drug of choice in women with an intact uterus

■ Esterified Estrogens and Methyltestosterone

Brand Names
Estratest, Estratest HS

Generic Name
Esterified estrogens and methyltestosterone

Dosage Forms
Tablets

Usage

- Treatment of moderate–severe vasomotor symptoms associated with menopause

Dosing

- 1 tablet daily (3 weeks on and 1 week off)

Counseling Points

- Take as directed by prescriber

Drug Class: Combined Oral Contraceptives (Monophasic)

Introduction

The administration of combined oral contraceptives is a contraceptive method that includes a combination of an estrogen and a progestin. When taken daily they inhibit ovulation. They are currently the most common form of pharmacologic birth control. Table 7–1 at the end of this section summarizes the available monophasic combined oral contraceptives.

Mechanism of Action for the Drug Class

The agents deliver a fixed dosage of estrogen and progestin throughout the cycle that inhibits ovulation by suppressing the gonadotropins, follicle-stimulating hormone (FSH), and luteinizing hormone (LH). Additionally, alterations in the genital tract, including cervical mucus (that inhibits sperm penetration) and the endometrium (that reduces the likelihood of implantation), may contribute to contraceptive effectiveness.

Members of the Drug Class

In this section: Combinations of ethinyl estradiol and levonorgestrel/norethindrone/desogestrel/drospirenone/norgestimate

Others: Combinations of ethinyl estradiol and ethynodiol, mestranol or norethindrone

Dosage Forms for the Drug Class

Tablets

Usage for the Drug Class

- Prevention of pregnancy in women, treatment of menorrhagia, pain associated with endometriosis, dysmenorrhea

Dosing for the Drug Class

- 21-day regimen: Day 1 of cycle is the first day of menstrual bleeding. Take 1 tablet daily for 21 days, beginning on day 5 of cycle. No tablets are taken for 7 days; whether bleeding has stopped or not, start a new course of 21 days.
- 24-day regimen: Take 24 days of active pills and 4 days of inert or iron tablets on the last 4 days of cycle
- 28-day regimen: To eliminate the need to count the days between cycles, some products contain 7 inert or iron-containing tablets to permit continuous daily dosage during the entire 28-day cycle. Take 7 inert or iron tablets on the last 7 days of cycle.

Adverse Reactions for the Drug Class: Most Common

- Nausea, vomiting, bloating, migraine headaches, edema, breast tenderness, breakthrough bleeding (most often in first few cycles of pills), change in menstrual flow, weight gain, tiredness, fatigue, depression

Adverse Reactions for the Drug Class: Rare/Severe/Important

- Myocardial infarction, thromboembolism, cerebral hemorrhage, hypertension, gallbladder disease

Major Drug Interactions for the Drug Class

Drugs Affecting Combined Oral Contraceptives

- Antibiotics: Menstrual irregularities and possible contraceptive failure
- Barbiturates, carbamazepine, griseofulvin, phenytoin, rifampin, protease inhibitors: Decreased efficacy via metabolic induction

Combined Oral Contraceptive Effects on Other Drugs

- Tricyclic antidepressants, β-blockers, theophylline, benzodiazepines: Increase effect via decreased metabolism

Contraindications for the Drug Class

- History of myocardial infarction, coronary artery disease, known or suspected breast carcinoma or estrogen-dependent neoplasm, hepatic adenomas/carcinomas, undiagnosed abnormal genital bleeding, thromboembolic disorder, pregnancy, acute liver disease

Counseling Points for the Drug Class

- Take oral contraceptive pills at exactly the same time every day for maximum effectiveness and do not exceed dosing intervals >24 hours
- Missing pills may reduce the effectiveness of the birth control and cause spotting or light bleeding
- Continue to take pills throughout all bleeding episodes
- Use an additional method of birth control for the first week of pills during the initial cycle of oral contraceptive pills
- Spotting or breakthrough bleeding may occur during the first few months of therapy. If bleeding lasts more than a few days and occurs in more than one cycle, consult your healthcare provider.
- Notify your healthcare provider if pregnancy is suspected or if any of the following occur: Sudden severe headache, visual disturbances, numbness in an arm or leg, severe abdominal pain, prolonged episodes of bleeding, or amenorrhea
- Appropriate action if one or more pills are missed:
  - If 1 pill is missed anytime in the cycle, take the pill as soon as you remember and the next pill at its regular time
  - If 2 pills are missed during the first 2 weeks of the cycle, take 2 pills daily for 2 days; then resume taking pills on their regular schedule. Use additional contraception (condom, etc.) for the remainder of the cycle.
  - If 2 pills are missed during the third week of the cycle and you are a day 1 starter, throw out the rest of the pack and start a new pack that same day. If you are a Sunday starter, keep taking 1 pill every day until Sunday. On Sunday throw out the rest of the pack and start a new pack that same day. Use additional contraception until the new pack of pills is started and for the first 7 days of the new cycle.
  - If 3 or more pills are missed and you are a day 1 starter, throw out the rest of the pack and start a new pack that same day. If you are a Sunday starter, keep taking 1 pill every day until Sunday. On Sunday throw out the rest of the pack and start a new pack that same day. Use additional contraception until the new pack of pills is started and for the first 7 days of the new cycle.

Key Points for the Drug Class

- Combined oral contraceptives should be prescribed with caution if ever, to smokers, >35 years of age
- Smokers <30 years of age who are otherwise healthy generally can use combined oral contraceptives
- Seasonale is a new combined oral contraceptive that provides continued estrogen and progesterone for 3 months

TABLE 7–1

Combined Oral Contraceptives (Monophasic)

Brand Name	Generic Name and Dosage
Alesse	Levonorgestrel: 0.1 mg
	Ethinyl estradiol: 20 µg for 21 days
Desogen	Desogestrel: 0.15 mg
	Ethinyl estradiol: 30 µg for 21 days
Loestrin FE 1/20	Norethindrone acetate: 1 mg
	Ethinyl estradiol: 20 µg for 21 days
	Ferrous fumarate: 75 mg for 7 days
Lo-Ovral	Norgestrel: 0.3 mg
	Ethinyl estradiol: 30 µg for 21 days
Ortho-Cyclen	Norgestimate: 0.25 mg
	Ethinyl estradiol: 35 µg for 21 days
Yasmin	Drospirenone: 3 mg
	Ethinyl estradiol: 30 µg for 21 days
Seasonale	Levonorgestrel: 0.15 mg
	Ethinyl estradiol: 30 µg for 84 days

Drug Class: Combined Oral Contraceptives (Biphasic)

Mechanism of Action for the Drug Class

These drugs inhibit ovulation (as explained in the monophasic drug class section). In this drug class, the amount of estrogen remains the same for the first 21 days of the cycle and decreases at the end of the cycle.

Members of the Drug Class

In this section: Combinations of ethinyl estradiol and desogestrel

Others: Combinations of ethinyl estradiol and norethindrone

■ Desogestrel/Ethinyl Estradiol

Brand Name

Mircette

Generic Name

Desogestrel/Ethinyl Estradiol

Dosage Forms

Tablets

Usage

- Prevention of pregnancy in women

Dosing

- Desogestrel 0.15 mg/Ethinyl Estradiol 20 µg for 21 days
- Placebo for 2 days
- Ethinyl estradiol 10 µg for 5 days

Drug Class: Combined Oral Contraceptives (Triphasic)

Mechanism of Action for the Drug Class

This drug inhibits ovulation (as explained in the monophasic drug class section). In this drug class, the estrogen amount remains the same or varies throughout the cycle; the progestin amount varies. Table 7–2 summarizes the available triphasic combined oral contraceptives.

Members of the Drug Class

In this section: Combinations of ethinyl estradiol and levonorgestrel/norethindrone/desogestrel/norgestimate

Dosage Forms

Tablets

Usage

- Prevention of pregnancy in women, treatment of moderate acne vulgaris in women ≥15 years of age

TABLE 7–2

Combined Oral Contraceptives (Triphasic)

Brand Name	Generic Name and Dosage
Ortho-Novum 7/7/7	Norethindrone: 0.5 mg/Ethinyl estradiol: 35 µg for 7 days Norethindrone: 0.75 mg/Ethinyl estradiol: 35 µg for 7 days Norethindrone: 1 mg/Ethinyl estradiol: 35 µg for 7 days
Ortho Tri-Cyclen	Norgestimate: 0.18 mg/Ethinyl estradiol: 35 µg for 7 days Norgestimate: 0.215 mg/Ethinyl estradiol: 35 µg for 7 days Norgestimate: 0.25 mg/Ethinyl estradiol: 35 µg for 7 days
Triphasil, Trivora	Levonorgestrel: 0.050 mg/Ethinyl estradiol: 30 µg for 6 days Levonorgestrel: 0.075 mg/Ethinyl estradiol: 40 µg for 5 days Levonorgestrel: 0.125 mg/Ethinyl estradiol: 30 µg for 10 days

Drug Class: Progestin-Only Oral Contraceptives

Mechanism of Action for the Drug Class

Progestins prevent conception by suppressing ovulation in approximately 50% of users: Thickening the cervical mucus to inhibit sperm penetration, lowering the midcycle LH and FSH peaks, slowing the movement of the ovum through the fallopian tubes, and altering the endometrium.

Members of the Drug Class

In this section: Norethindrone
   Others: Norgestrel

■ Norethindrone

Brand Name

Micronor

Generic Name

Norethindrone

Counseling Points

- Effectiveness may be dramatically reduced when progestin-only pills are taken >3 hours late; use a back-up non-pharmacologic method of contraception (such as condoms) for the next 48 hours whenever pills are taken ≥3 hours late
- Appropriate action if one or more progestin-only pills are missed:
  - If the pill is taken ≥3 hours late, take the pill as soon as remembered and use additional contraception for 48 hours
  - If 1 or more pills are missed, take it as soon as remembered. Take today's pill at its regular time, even if that means taking 2 pills in 1 day. Use additional contraception for 48 hours.

Drug Class: Selective Estrogen Receptor Modulators

Introduction

Raloxifene is one of the medications in the family of SERMs. It is more selective in its action than tamoxifen and is used in the treatment of osteoporosis and in the prevention of breast cancer in high-risk women.

Mechanism of Action for the Drug Class

Inhibits bone resorption and reduces biochemical markers of bone turnover.

Members of the Drug Class

In this section: Raloxifene

■ Raloxifene

Brand Name

Evista

Generic Name

Raloxifene

Dosage Forms

Tablets

Usage

- Prevention and treatment of postmenopausal osteoporosis*, risk reduction for invasive breast cancer in postmenopausal women with osteoporosis and in postmenopausal women with high risk for invasive breast cancer

Dosing

- 60 mg daily

Adverse Reactions: Most Common

- Hot flashes, nausea

Adverse Reactions: Rare/Severe/Important

- Muscle aches, vaginal bleeding, abdominal pain, thromboembolism

Major Drug Interactions

Drugs Affecting Raloxifene

- Cholestyramine: Reduced raloxifene absorption

Raloxifene's Effect on Other Drugs

- Levothyroxine: Decreased absorption
- Warfarin: May decrease prothrombin time by 10%

Contraindications

- Women who are or may become pregnant; history of venous thromboembolic events

Counseling Points

- Discontinue raloxifene at least 72 hours prior to and during prolonged immobilization to prevent clot formations
- Avoid prolonged restrictions of movement during travel because of the increased risk of blood clots
- Take supplemental calcium and vitamin D if daily intake is inadequate

Key Point

- Avoid in patients with a history of thromboembolic disorders

---

Drug Class: Glucocorticoids

Introduction

Glucocorticoids are anti-inflammatory, immunosuppressant agents used in the treatment of a variety of diseases including those of allergic, dermatologic, endocrine, hematologic, inflammatory, neoplastic, nervous system, renal, respiratory, rheumatic, and autoimmune origin. They may be used in the management of cerebral edema, chronic swelling, as a diagnostic agent, diagnosis of Cushing's syndrome, antiemetic, and many other uses. They have significant adverse effects that can be dose- and duration-limiting. Converting from one glucocorticoid to another is a common practice. Approximate conversions are listed in Table 7–3.

Mechanism of Action for the Drug Class

The exact mechanism of glucocorticoids' effect is unknown. They inhibit interleukin-1 and various other cytokines that mediate inflammatory responses. They also decrease inflammation by suppression of migration of polymorphonuclear leukocytes and decreasing capillary permeability.

Members of the Drug Class

In this section: Methylprednisolone and prednisone, dexamethasone

Others: Betamethasone, cortisone, hydrocortisone, prednisolone, triamcinolone (these are other systemic glucocorticoids)

Usage for the Drug Class

- Treatment of multiple inflammatory conditions*, acute asthma, rheumatoid arthritis, dermatologic lesions such as keloids, autoimmune disorders such as multiple sclerosis, adrenogenital syndrome, adjunctive therapy of *Pneumocystis jiroveci* pneumonia (PCP)

Adverse Reactions for the Drug Class: Most Common

- Gastrointestinal irritation, increased appetite, nervousness/restlessness, weight gain, acne, glucose intolerance (transient), lipid abnormalities (transient)

Adverse Reactions for the Drug Class: Rare/Severe/Important

- Lower resistance to infections, adrenal suppression, rounding out of the face, hirsutism, glaucoma, osteoporosis, peptic ulceration

Major Drug Interactions for the Drug Class

Drugs Affecting Glucocorticoids

- Alcohol/NSAIDs: Increase risk of gastric ulceration
- Estrogens: May increase toxicity

Glucocorticoid Effects on Other Drugs

- Insulin/oral hypoglycemic agents: Increase glucose levels

Contraindications for the Drug Class

- Systemic fungal infections
- Administration of live vaccines concomitantly

Counseling Points for the Drug Class

- Take oral tablets with food
- Take oral tablets preferably in the morning

Key Points for the Drug Class

- Too rapid withdrawal of therapy, especially after prolonged use, may cause acute, possibly life-threatening adrenal insufficiency

TABLE 7–3

Glucocorticoid Conversion

Glucocorticoid	Equivalent Anti-Inflammatory Dose
Cortisone	25 mg
Hydrocortisone	20 mg
Prednisone	5 mg
Prednisolone	5 mg
Methylprednisolone	4 mg
Triamcinolone	4 mg
Betamethasone	0.75 mg
Dexamethasone	0.75 mg

- The prescribed dosages of glucocorticoids vary depending on the compound used and the nature of the patient's condition. Depending on these factors, the dose may be taken once a day, over the course of several doses spaced evenly throughout the day, or even every other day.

Methylprednisolone and Prednisone

Brand Names
Medrol and Medrol Dosepak, Depo-Medrol, Solu-Medrol

Generic Name
Methylprednisolone

Dosage Forms
Tablets, injection

Brand Names
Deltasone, Orasone

Generic Name
Prednisone

Dosage Forms
Tablets, oral solution

Dosing
Treatment of acute asthma, including status asthmaticus and allergic rhinitis:
- Oral: 4–48 mg/day (methylprednisolone) or 5–60 mg/day (prednisone); individualize dose based on response
- Alternate-day oral therapy: Twice the daily dose may be administered every other day. If course of therapy is >10–14 days, therapy must be tapered when discontinuing.
- Dosepak: Taper each day according to manufacturer's instructions (6-day therapy starting with 24 mg day 1; decrease by 4 mg every day and finish with 4 mg on day 6)

- IV (sodium succinate): Loading dose: 2 mg/kg/dose then 0.5: 1 mg/kg/dose every 6 hours for 5 days

Treatment of rheumatoid arthritis:
- Intra-articular (acetate): Large joints (such as knees and ankles) 20–80 mg; medium joints (such as elbows and wrists) 10–40 mg; small joints (such as metacarpophalangeal) 4–10 mg

Dermatologic lesions:
- IM (acetate): 40–120 mg IM weekly for 1–4 weeks

Anti-inflammatory or immunosuppression:
- Oral, IV (sodium succinate): 0.5–2 mg/kg per day in divided doses every 6–12 hours
- Pulse therapy (IV): 250–1000 mg daily for 3 days

Acute exacerbation of multiple sclerosis:
- Oral: 200 mg (prednisone) daily for 1 week then 80 mg every other day for 1 month

Treatment of adrenogenital syndrome:
- IM (acetate): 40 mg every 2 weeks

Dexamethasone

Brand Names
Decadron, DexPak

Generic Name
Dexamethasone

Dosage Forms
Tablets, solution, injection

Usage
Treatment of a variety of diseases including those of allergic, dermatologic, endocrine, hematologic, inflammatory, neoplastic, nervous system, renal, respiratory, rheumatic, and autoimmune origin; may be used in the management of cerebral edema, chronic swelling, as a diagnostic agent, diagnosis of Cushing's syndrome, antiemetic

Dosing
- Anti-inflammatory:
  - Oral, IM, IV: 0.75–9 mg/day in divided doses every 6–12 hours
  - Intra-articular, intralesional, or soft tissue: 0.4–6 mg/day

- Cerebral edema:
  - IV: 10 mg stat, 4 mg IM/IV (should be given as sodium phosphate) every 6 hours until response is maximized

Key Point
- Dexamethasone is commonly used for the reduction of nerve swelling following nerve damage or neurosurgery. Dosage depends on the specific treatment.

Drug Class: Thyroid Hormones

Introduction
Thyroid hormones are chemical compounds that are essential for the function of every cell in the body. They help regulate growth and the body's metabolism. The two most important thyroid hormones are thyroxine (T4) and triiodothyronine (T3).

Mechanism of Action for the Drug Class
The effect of thyroid hormones is believed to be exerted through control of DNA transcription and protein synthesis. Their principal effect is to increase the metabolic rate of body tissues noted by increased respiratory rate, cardiac output, heart rate, protein, fat, and carbohydrate metabolism. They exert a profound effect on every organ system, particularly CNS development. Levothyroxine is a synthetic form of T4.

Members of the Drug Class
In this section: Levothyroxine sodium
  Others: Liothyronine, liotrix, thyroid (desiccated)

■ Levothyroxine Sodium

Brand Names
Levothroid, Levoxyl, Synthroid

Generic Name
Levothyroxine sodium

Dosage Forms
Tablets, injection

Usage
- Hypothyroidism*, myxedema coma

Dosing
Hypothyroidism:
- Oral: 100–125 µg/day. In patients >50 years of age or with underlying cardiac disease, the initial starting dose is 25–50 µg/day.
- Maximum dose: 300 µg/day

Myxedema coma:
- Initial dose: 300–500 µg IV
- Maintenance dose: 75–100 µg IV daily until stable

Adverse Reactions: Most Common
- Fatigue, increased appetite, weight loss, heat intolerance, hyperhidrosis

Adverse Reactions: Rare/Severe/Important
- Hair loss, menstrual irregularities, nervousness, irritability, insomnia

Major Drug Interactions
Drugs Affecting Levothyroxine
- Cholestyramine: Impairs absorption
- Estrogens: Increase serum thyroxine binding globulin thus decreasing free thyroxine concentrations
- Iron and calcium: Decrease absorption (separate administration)
- Raloxifene: Decreases absorption

Levothyroxine's Effect on Other Drugs
- Warfarin: Increased prothrombin time/international normalized ratio

Contraindications
- Untreated thyrotoxicosis, uncorrected adrenal insufficiency

Counseling Points
- Report any signs and symptoms of thyroid hormone toxicity such as chest pain, increased pulse rate, palpitations, excessive sweating, heat intolerance, and nervousness
- Take oral tablets first thing in the morning on an empty stomach at least ½ hour before any other food
- If you are receiving concomitant therapy with cholestyramine and levothyroxine, separate doses at least 4–5 hours apart

Key Points
- Thyroid-stimulating hormone T3, and T4 blood concentrations should be obtained every 6–8 weeks initially, then every 6–12 months until stable and annually thereafter and dose adjustments made accordingly
- Doses should be adjusted in 12.5- to 25-µg increments

Review Questions

1. Which of the following is a common adverse reaction of Nolvadex?
   A. Bone pain
   B. Dyspepsia
   C. Gastric ulcers
   D. Hot flashes

2. All of the following are important counseling points about bisphosphonates except
   A. Do not lie down for 30 minutes after taking bisphosphonates
   B. Most common adverse reaction is dizziness
   C. Take supplemental calcium and vitamin D
   D. Take 30 minutes before eating in the morning

3. Which of the following statements about Miacalcin is false?
   A. It has no major drug interactions
   B. Normal dose is 1 tablet by mouth twice daily
   C. Rhinitis is a common adverse reaction
   D. It is used for the treatment of osteoporosis

4. Which of the following is (are) common adverse reactions of combined oral contraceptives?
   A. Breakthrough bleeding
   B. Breast tenderness
   C. Nausea and vomiting
   D. All of the above are common adverse reactions

5. All of the following are contraindications for the use of combined oral contraceptives except
   A. Active thromboembolic disorders
   B. Gastric ulcer
   C. Pregnancy
   D. Severe liver disease

6. All of the following medications interact with combined oral contraceptives except
   A. Antacids
   B. Antibiotics
   C. Phenytoin
   D. Protease inhibitors

7. Which of the following combined oral contraceptives is indicated to be used for 84 consecutive days?
   A. Loestrin FE
   B. Mircette
   C. Ortho-Tri-Cyclen
   D. Seasonale

8. All of the following statements about Climara are true except
   A. Available as a transdermal patch
   B. Contains estrogen and progesterone
   C. Used for the treatment of vasomotor symptoms
   D. Used for the prevention of osteoporosis

9. All of the following statements about Evista are true except
   A. Contraindicated in patients with a history of venous thromboembolism
   B. Contraindicated in patients at risk for breast cancer
   C. Most common adverse reaction is hot flashes
   D. Used for the prevention and treatment of osteoporosis

10. Which of the following is (are) indications for the use of methylprednisolone?
    A. Acute asthma
    B. Hirsutism
    C. Rheumatoid arthritis
    D. A and C are correct

11. All of the following statements about levothyroxine are true except
    A. Increased appetite is a common adverse reaction.
    B. It comes as a tablet and injection.
    C. Lower doses are used in the elderly.
    D. Used for the treatment of hyperthyroidism.

12. Which of the following agents is a monophasic combined oral contraceptive?
    A. Desogen
    B. Mircette
    C. Prempro
    D. Triphasil

13. Which of the following is (are) important counseling point(s) about progestin-only contraceptives?
    A. Effectiveness may be dramatically reduced when pills are taken >3 hours late.
    B. Use a backup method of contraception (such as condoms) for the next 48 hours whenever pills are taken ≥3 hours late.
    C. If ≥1 pills are missed, take it as soon as possible. Take today's pill at its regular time, even if that means taking 2 pills in 1 day. Use additional contraception for 48 hours.
    D. All of the above are important counseling points.

14. Which of the following bisphosphonates can be dosed once every month?
    A. Actonel
    B. Boniva
    C. Fosamax
    D. All of the above can be dosed once monthly

15. All of the following statements about tamoxifen are true except
    A. Competes with estrogen for binding sites in target tissues such as breast
    B. Used in the treatment of breast cancer
    C. Increase anticoagulants effects of warfarin
    D. Contraindicated in patients with a history of colon cancer

CHAPTER 8

Gastrointestinal Agents

Jamila Stanton, PharmD, BCPS

Drug Class: 5-HT₃ Receptor Antagonists

Introduction

Serotonin subtype-3 (5-HT$_3$) receptor antagonists are most effective when used to prevent nausea and vomiting associated with moderate to highly emetogenic chemotherapeutic regimens, radiation therapy, and postoperative nausea and vomiting. With the exception of palonosetron, which differs from the other drugs in this class by having a longer half-life and stronger receptor affinity, these agents have not been consistently effective in preventing delayed chemotherapy-induced nausea and vomiting. Of note, alosetron, a 5-HT$_3$ antagonist approved in 2000, is only indicated in the treatment of severe diarrhea-predominant irritable bowel syndrome in women; this agent should not be used for antiemetic purposes.

Mechanism of Action for the Drug Class

Selective antagonist of serotonin subtype-3 (5-HT$_3$) receptors. 5-HT$_3$ receptors are present peripherally on vagal nerve terminals and centrally in the chemoreceptor trigger zone of the brain; these receptors are stimulated by serotonin release following cytotoxic drug administration and radiation therapy. Drugs in this class bind to the 5-HT$_3$ receptors located on the vagal neurons in the lining of the GI tract, blocking the signal to the vomiting center in the brain, thus preventing nausea and vomiting.

Members of the Drug Class

In this section: Ondansetron
    Others: Alosetron, dolasetron, granisetron, palonosetron

■ Ondansetron

Brand Name

Zofran

Generic Name

Ondansetron

Dosage Forms

Injection, oral solution, oral tablets, orally disintegrating tablets

Usage

- Prevention of chemotherapy-induced nausea and vomiting*, prevention of radiation-induced nausea and vomiting*, prevention and treatment of postoperative nausea and vomiting, hyperemesis gravidum*

Dosing

- Prevention of chemotherapy-induced nausea and vomiting:
  - Intravenous: 32 mg once daily given prior to chemotherapy
  - Oral: 24 mg given 30 minutes prior to chemotherapy or 8 mg 30 minutes prior to chemotherapy and repeat in 8 hours, then 8 mg every 12 hours for 1–2 days post chemotherapy (dosing regimen dependent on chemotherapy emetogenicity potential)
- Prevention of radiation-induced nausea and vomiting:
  - Oral: 8 mg 1–2 hours prior to radiotherapy, may repeat every 8 hours after radiotherapy
- Prevention of postoperative nausea and vomiting:
  - IV, IM: 4 mg as a single dose immediately before the induction of anesthesia; may be more effective if given at the end of surgery, immediately after anesthesia
  - Oral: 16 mg given 1 hour before induction of anesthesia
- Hyperemesis gravidum:
  - Oral: 8 mg every 12 hours
  - IV: 8 mg administered over 15 minutes every 12 hours or 1 mg/hour infused continuously for up to 24 hours
- Hepatic dosage adjustment:
  - Maximum daily dose of 8 mg in patients with severe liver disease (Child-Pugh Score ≥10)

Adverse Reactions: Most Common

- Headache, dizziness, constipation, malaise/fatigue, drowsiness

Adverse Reactions: Rare/Severe/Important
- Anaphylaxis/angioedema, elevated LFTs, EKG changes (especially with dolasetron)

Major Drug Interactions
Drugs Affecting Ondansetron
- Cytochrome P450 inducers (rifampin, rifabutin, phenytoin, carbamazepine): increase metabolism and clearance of ondansetron

Ondansetron's Effect on Other Drugs
- Apomorphine: Enhanced hypotensive effect of apomorphine

Contraindications
- Hypersensitivity to 5-HT$_3$ receptor antagonist or any component of the formulation

- Markedly prolonged QT interval or atrioventricular block II or III (dolasetron); patients receiving class I or III antiarrhythmic agents (dolasetron)

Counseling Point
- Do not remove the orally disintegrating tablets from blister pack until you are ready to take the medication; peel the backing off, do not push through the backing. Use dry hands, place the tablet on the tongue and swallow with saliva

Key Points
- The medication should be taken on a scheduled basis and not as needed. It is more effective in prevention of nausea and vomiting rather than treatment
- Use caution, especially with dolasetron, in patients with QT prolongation or on medications known to prolong the QT interval

---

Drug Class: Antacids

Introduction
The class of antacid agents encompasses a variety of aluminum, magnesium, and calcium products generally used to neutralize gastric acidity. Drugs in this class are available as single and combination therapy preparations in multiple dosage forms, including liquids, gelcaps, tablets, and chewable tablets. Most of these preparations are available over the counter (OTC); therefore healthcare providers should pay particular attention to the use of these products in patients with renal dysfunction, duration of use >2 weeks, and those taking prescription drugs known to interact with antacid compounds.

Mechanism of Action for the Drug Class
Neutralize gastric acid, inactivate pepsin, and bind bile salts.

Members of the Drug Class
In this section: Magnesium hydroxide/aluminum hydroxide (Maalox), calcium carbonate (Tums)

Others: Numerous preparations of single-ingredient or combinations of aluminum hydroxide, magnesium hydroxide, calcium carbonate ± simethicone are available

■ Magnesium Hydroxide/Aluminum Hydroxide

Brand Names
Maalox, Alamag Plus, Mintox Plus, Mi-Acid, Almacone

Generic Name
Magnesium hydroxide/aluminum hydroxide ± simethicone; chewable products may also contain calcium carbonate

Dosage Forms
Oral suspension, tablets, chewable tablets

Usage
- Acid indigestion*, heartburn*, short-term treatment of hyperphosphatemia in renal failure; aluminum hydroxide may also be used for prevention of GI bleeding and as an adjunctive agent in peptic ulcer disease

Dosing
- Liquid: 10–20 ml every 4–6 hours as needed before meals and at bedtime (see product-specific dosing)
- Tablets/chewable tablets: 2–4 tablets every 4–6 hours as needed before meals and at bedtime (see product-specific dosing)
- Renal dosage adjustment:
  - Use caution; aluminum and magnesium may accumulate (no specific dosing requirements)

Adverse Reactions: Most Common
- Constipation, diarrhea, chalky taste, abdominal cramps, nausea, vomiting

Adverse Reactions: Rare/Severe/Important
- Hypermagnesemia, aluminum-intoxication, hypophosphatemia, metabolic alkalosis, intestinal obstruction, dehydration

Major Drug Interactions
Magnesium Hydroxide/Aluminum Hydroxide's Effect on Other Drugs
- Antacid preparations have been reported to decrease the pharmacologic effect/exposure of many drugs when concomitantly administered. Good evidence supports a significant interaction with iron salts, tetracyclines, digoxin, dasatinib, isoniazid, itraconazole, ketoconazole, fluoroquinolones, mycophenolate, and thyroid hormones.

- Antacid preparations have been reported to increase the pharmacologic effect/exposure of the following drugs: Quinidine, sulfonylureas

Counseling Points

- Separate administration of antacid medications by at least 2 hours from other medications
- Use with caution if you have renal insufficiency. Contact a physician immediately if irregular heartbeat, severe stomach pain, or excessive weakness or tiredness occurs.
- Antacids should not be taken for longer than 2 weeks. Contact a physician if symptoms are not relieved promptly or symptoms return often

Key Points

- With easy OTC access to these agents, assess patients for potential drug interactions and renal impairment that may result in toxicity
- Symptoms that recur and persist beyond 2 weeks may be a sign of more serious disease; these patients should be referred to a physician

■ Calcium Carbonate

Brand Names
Tums, Maalox Regular Chewable, Calci-Chew, Rolaids, Chooz, Alka-Mints

Generic Name
Calcium carbonate

Dosage Forms
Chewable tablets, gum tablets, lozenges, liquid

Usage
Acid indigestion*, heartburn*, treatment/prevention of calcium deficiency*, hypophosphatemia in renal failure

Dosing

- Acid indigestion, heartburn:
  - 5–10 ml every 2 hours; maximum: 7000 mg calcium carbonate/24 hours (see product-specific dosing)
  - Tablets/chewable tablets: 1–4 tablets every 2 hours; maximum: 7000 mg calcium carbonate/24 hours (see product-specific dosing because tablet strengths vary)

- Treatment/Prevention of Calcium Deficiency:
  - 1–2 g of elemental calcium/day in 2–3 divided doses with meals (variable based on serum calcium and clinical condition)

Adverse Reactions: Most Common

- Constipation, bloating, gas, nausea, vomiting, abdominal pain, xerostomia

Adverse Reactions: Rare/Severe/Important

- Hypercalcemia, hypophosphatemia, milk-alkali syndrome

Major Drug Interactions
Calcium Carbonate's Effect on Other Drugs

- Calcium carbonate antacid preparations have been reported to decrease the pharmacologic effect/exposure of many drugs when concomitantly administered. Good evidence supports a significant interaction with iron salts, tetracyclines, fluoroquinolones, ketoconazole, itraconazole, salicylates, and thyroid hormones.
- Calcium carbonate antacid preparations have been reported to increase the pharmacologic effect/exposure of quinidine

Counseling Points

- Separate administration of antacid medications by at least 2 hours from other medications
- Chew tablets completely before swallowing; do not swallow whole
- For self-treatment antacids should not be taken for >2 weeks. Contact a physician if symptoms are not relieved promptly or symptoms return often.

Key Points

- With easy OTC access to these agents it is important to assess patients for potential drug interactions and more serious symptoms that require a physician's care
- Symptoms that recur and persist beyond 2 weeks may be a sign of more serious disease; these patients should be referred to a physician

---

Drug Class: Antidiarrheal/Antisecretory Agents

Introduction

Bismuth subsalicylate possesses antisecretory, anti-inflammatory, and antibacterial effects. Available OTC, it is used for a variety of indications including indigestion, upset stomach, and diarrhea. It is important to remember that an active component of this agent is salicylate, an aspirin derivative that may lead to toxicities in excessive doses or an inappropriate patient population.

Mechanism of Action for the Drug Class

The exact mechanism of action has not been determined. The salicylate moiety provides an antisecretory effect, and bismuth moiety exhibits antimicrobial activity directly against bacterial and viral GI pathogens; bismuth also has some antacid properties.

Members of the Drug Class

In this section: Bismuth subsalicylate/bismuth subgallate
  Others: None

Bismuth Subsalicylate/ Bismuth Subgallate

Brand Names
Pepto-Bismol, Kaopectate, Maalox Total Stomach Relief, Bismatrol

Generic Names
Bismuth subsalicylate, bismuth subgallate

Dosage Forms
Oral suspension, oral and chewable tablets

Usage
Indigestion*, diarrhea*, abdominal cramps, prevention and treatment of traveler's diarrhea, treatment of *Helicobacter pylori*–associated gastritis/ulcer (in combination only)

Dosing
- 2 tablets or 30 ml orally every 30–60 minutes as needed; maximum of 8 doses/24 hours

Adverse Reactions: Most Common
- Constipation, diarrhea, nausea, grayish-black tongue discoloration, grayish-black vomiting, grayish-black discoloration of stool

Adverse Reactions: Rare/Severe/Important
- Persistent tinnitus, hearing loss, nausea, vomiting, neurotoxicity with excessive doses (confusion, slurred speech, severe headache, muscle weakness, seizure)

Major Drug Interactions
Bismuth Subsalicylate/Bismuth Subgallate's Effect on Other Drugs
- Tetracycline, doxycycline: Decreased absorption and effectiveness

- Aspirin/anticoagulants: Use of multiple salicylates may lead to toxicity and increased risk of bleeding

Contraindications
- Children or teenagers with influenza or chicken pox due to the risk of Reye's syndrome, hypersensitivity to salicylates (including aspirin), coagulopathy, severe GI bleeding; not recommended for use in pregnancy: Pregnancy category C/D (third trimester)

Counseling Points
- Medication may temporarily darken the tongue and/or stools (nonharmful)
- Chew tablet well or shake suspension well before use
- Report any changes in hearing or ringing in your ears
- If diarrhea is accompanied by high fever, blood/mucus in the stool, or continues for >2 days, consult a physician

Key Points
- Bismuth subsalicylate is commonly used OTC drug for a variety of GI indications
- This medication may be harmful in large doses; neurotoxicity has been reported; any symptoms of encephalopathy should be reported to a physician
- Bismuth subsalicylate should be avoided in children and teenagers with viral symptoms or chicken pox

---

Drug Class: Antidiarrheals

Introduction
Antidiarrheals are widely available OTC and commonly used in the symptomatic treatment of diarrhea. Concurrent fluid and electrolyte replacement is often necessary in all age groups depending on the severity of diarrhea. Importantly, patients with bacterial enteritis should not use these agents; similarly, they should not be used if diarrhea is accompanied by high fever or blood in stool.

Mechanism of Action for the Drug Class
Acts peripherally on intestinal opioid receptors, to inhibit peristalsis and prolong transit time; reduces fecal volume, increases viscosity, and diminishes fluid and electrolyte loss; demonstrates antisecretory activity.

Members of the Drug Class
In this section: Loperamide, bismuth subsalicylate (see above)
Others: Diphenoxylate/atropine, multiple formulations of kaolin pectin ± activated attapulgite ± bismuth salts

Loperamide
Brand Names
Imodium, Imodium AD, K-Pek II

Generic Name
Loperamide

Dosage Forms
Caplets, capsules, tablets, oral liquid

Usage

- Symptomatic relief and control of acute nonspecific diarrhea (including traveler's diarrhea)*, treatment of chronic diarrhea associated with inflammatory bowel disease*, antineoplastic agents, and bowel resection

Dosing

- 4 mg orally, followed by 2 mg orally after each loose stool, up to 16 mg/day
- Dosing in hepatic impairment:
  - Caution in patients with hepatic impairment due to reduced first-pass metabolism; no specific dosing recommendations available

Adverse Reactions: Most Common

- Abdominal pain, constipation, dizziness, drowsiness, dry mouth

Adverse Reactions: Rare/Severe/Important

- Toxic megacolon, ileus, necrotizing enterocolitis

Major Drug Interactions

Drugs Affecting Loperamide

- Gemfibrozil and ketoconazole: Increased exposure to loperamide

Loperamide's Effect on Other Drugs

- Potentiate the adverse effects of CNS depressants, phenothiazines, and tricyclic antidepressants
- Saquinavir: Decreased plasma concentrations of saquinavir

Counseling Points

- May cause drowsiness or dizziness; exercise caution while driving or performing hazardous tasks
- Consult physician if acute diarrhea lasts >48 hours or is accompanied by severe abdominal pain, distention, or fever
- Maintain adequate hydration during treatment

Key Points

- Do not use in acute diarrhea associated with bacterial enteritis or *Clostridium difficile,* or for diarrhea associated with high fever or bloody stool
- Use with caution in treatment of AIDS patients; stop therapy at the sign of abdominal distention; cases of toxic megacolon have occurred in AIDS patients with infectious colitis

Drug Class: Antiflatulents

Introduction

Simethicone has been used as an adjunct in the treatment of various clinical conditions in which gas retention may be a problem including postoperative gaseous distention, air swallowing, dyspepsia, infant colic, peptic ulcer, spastic or irritable colon, and diverticulitis.

Mechanism of Action for the Drug Class

Decreases the surface tension of gas bubbles and thereby disperses and prevents gas pockets in the GI system.

Members of the Drug Class

In this section: Simethicone
Others: Charcoal, combination product charcoal/simethicone

■ Simethicone

Brand Names
Gas-X, Mylanta Gas, Mylicon, Phazyme

Generic Name
Simethicone

Dosage Forms
Softgels, chewable tablets, oral suspension (drops), oral strips

Usage

Relief of bloating*, pressure, and discomfort of gas; adjunctively in upper abdominal ultrasound to enhance delineation by reducing gas shadowing

Dosing

- 40–125 mg orally four times daily after meals and at bedtime

Adverse Reactions: Most Common

- Diarrhea, nausea, regurgitation, vomiting

Contraindications

- Known or suspected intestinal perforation and obstruction

Counseling Points

- This medication works best when taken after meals and at bedtime
- Avoid drinking carbonated beverages or eating foods that may cause an increase in stomach gas

Key Point

- Simethicone is a frequently used OTC medication for people of various ages, ranging from infants to adults. It may be used as needed for gas pain and discomfort, and it works optimally when taken after meals.

Drug Class: Bulk-Forming Laxatives

Introduction

Treatment and prevention of constipation should consist of bulk-forming agents in addition to dietary modifications that increase fiber intake. Bulk-forming laxatives usually have an effect within 12–24 hours and reach a maximum effect after several days. This class of medications includes several fiber products, including methylcellulose, polycarbophil, and psyllium, mostly available OTC.

Mechanism of Action for the Drug Class

Bulk-forming laxatives cause retention of fluid and an increase in fecal mass, resulting in stimulation of peristalsis.

Members of the Drug Class

In this section: Psyllium
   Others: Methylcellulose, polycarbophil, wheat dextrin

■ Psyllium

Brand Names

Fiberall, Genfiber, Konsyl, Metamucil, Reguloid

Generic Name

Psyllium

Dosage Forms

Capsules, powder, wafers

Usage

Dietary fiber supplement*, treatment of occasional and chronic constipation, irritable bowel syndrome, inflammatory bowel disease, diverticular disease, adjunctive agent for cholesterol lowering

Dosing

- Daily fiber recommended intake: Adults 19–50 years: Male: 38 g/day; female: 25 g/day
- 2.5–30 g orally daily in 1–3 divided doses

Adverse Reactions: Most Common

- Abdominal pain and cramping, constipation, diarrhea, flatulence

Adverse Reactions: Rare/Severe/Important

- Bronchospasm, bowel obstruction/impaction, esophageal obstruction

Major Drug Interactions

Psyllium's Effect on Other Drugs

- Carbamazepine: May decrease absorption/effectiveness of carbamazepine
- Antidiabetic agents: Additive blood glucose lowering

Contraindications

- Presence of abdominal pain, nausea, vomiting, intestinal obstruction, or fecal impaction

Counseling Points

- Powder: Mix in large glass of water or juice (≥8 oz) and drink immediately. Maintain adequate hydration and fiber intake during therapy. Do not inhale powder.
- Capsules and wafers: Take each dose with ≥8 oz of water
- Separate this medication from other medications by at least 1 hour
- Results may begin in 12 hours; full results may take 2–3 days
- Report persistent constipation; watery diarrhea; difficulty, pain, or choking with swallowing; do not use for >1 week without consulting a physician

Key Points

- Bulk-forming laxatives must be taken with plenty of fluids (8 oz per dose) to prevent bowel/esophageal obstruction and fecal impaction; elderly patients not receiving enough fluids may be at particularly high risk of these adverse effects
- Due to the potential adsorption of concomitantly administered medications, separate administration by at least 1 hour
- Specific formulations (sugar-free, sodium-free) are available for particular patient populations with dietary restrictions

Drug Class: Laxatives, Osmotic/Hyperosmolar

Introduction

Osmotic laxatives are commonly used in larger quantities prior to GI procedures to evacuate the bowel. In smaller quantities, they are generally used as an alternative to bulk-forming laxatives in the treatment of constipation, with safety and efficacy data extending through 6 months.

Mechanism of Action for the Drug Class

Polyethylene glycol is an osmotic agent that causes retention of water in the stool resulting in a softer stool and more frequent bowel movements.

Members of the Drug Class

In this section: Polyethylene glycol 3350
   Others: Glycerin, lactulose, sorbitol

Polyethylene Glycol 3350

Brand Name

MiraLAX

Generic Name

Polyethylene glycol 3350

Dosage Forms

Powder

Usage

Constipation (occasional and chronic)*

Dosing

- 17 g of powder (~1 heaping tablespoon) dissolved in 4–8 oz of water daily

Adverse Reactions: Most Common

- Nausea, abdominal fullness, diarrhea, flatulence, stomach cramps

Adverse Reactions: Rare/Severe/Important

- Dermatitis, rash, urticaria

Major Drug Interactions

- None reported

Contraindications

- Bowel obstruction, known or suspected

Counseling Points

- Mix 1 heaping tablespoon of powder in 8 oz of water and drink immediately. May take 2–4 days to produce bowel movement.
- Maintain adequate fluid intake throughout use
- Do not use this medicine for >2 weeks unless directed by your healthcare provider

Key Points

- MiraLAX may be better tolerated than other laxatives with regard to GI-adverse effects (gas and bloating); however, it can take up to 2–4 days to see results
- MiraLAX has been shown to be safe and effective for up to 6 months in trials treating chronic constipation; however, patients should consult their physician prior to use beyond 2 weeks

---

Drug Class: H₂ Receptor Antagonists

Introduction

H₂ receptor antagonists are used for the treatment of GI disorders where acid suppression is desired or for prevention of ulcers in critically ill patients. These agents are available as prescription products, as well as OTC formulations, making access to them widespread. They are commonly used for mild gastroesophageal reflux disease (GERD); however, they have been shown to be less effective than other acid-suppressive therapies in moderate–severe disease. In the treatment of peptic ulcer disease, H₂ receptor blockers may be used to heal ulcers or maintain ulcer healing; their efficacy in gastric ulcers induced by nonsteroidal anti-inflammatory drugs is variable and therefore not usually recommended.

Mechanism of Action for the Drug Class

Competitive inhibition of histamine at H₂ receptors of the gastric parietal cells, which inhibits gastric acid secretion; in addition, gastric volume and hydrogen ion concentration are also reduced.

Members of the Drug Class

In this section: Cimetidine, famotidine, ranitidine
   Others: Nizatidine

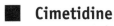 Cimetidine

Brand Name

Tagamet

Generic Name

Cimetidine

Dosage Forms

IV, tablets, oral solution

Usage

Treatment of GERD*, prevention or relief of heartburn*, acid indigestion, or sour stomach; prevention of upper GI bleeding in critically ill patients, short-term treatment and maintenance therapy of active duodenal ulcers, short-term treatment of gastric ulcers and gastric hypersecretory states, part of a multidrug regimen for *H. pylori* eradication

Dosing

- Oral: 300–800 mg one to four times daily (dose and frequency-dependent on indication)
- Oral (OTC): 200 mg twice daily
- IM/IV: 300 mg every 6–8 hours; infusion: 37.5–50 mg/hour (rate dependent on indication)
- Renal dose adjustment:
  - CrCl 10–50 ml/minute: Administer 50% of normal dose
  - CrCl <10 ml/minute: Administer 25% of normal dose
- Hepatic dose adjustment: Dosing adjustment in severe liver disease may be required; however, no specific recommendations are available

Adverse Reactions: Most Common

- Diarrhea, dizziness, headache, somnolence, gynecomastia

Adverse Reactions: Rare/Severe/Important

- Agranulocytosis, thrombocytopenia, confusion, necrotizing enterocolitis in fetus/newborn

Major Drug Interactions

Cimetidine's Effect on Other Drugs

- Increased effect/toxicity of dofetilide, lidocaine, phenytoin, procainamide, quinidine, theophylline, tricyclic antidepressants, calcium channel blockers, carbamazepine, warfarin, cyclosporine, SSRIs, sulfonylureas
- Decreased effect/absorption of iron salts, itraconazole, ketoconazole, atazanavir, dasatinib, fosamprenavir (theoretical), erlotinib

Counseling Points

- If you are using cimetidine to prevent heartburn, take oral formulations 30–60 minutes prior to meals
- If used for self-medication, do not use if you have difficulty swallowing, are vomiting blood, or have bloody or black stools; seek medical attention
- Heartburn or stomach pain that continues or worsens, or if use is required for >14 days, consult a physician

Key Points

- Cimetidine is an effective option for the treatment of multiple GI disorders requiring acid suppression
- Of the H_2 antagonists available, it has the most significant inhibition of multiple CYP enzymes, and therefore drug interactions
- Patients with renal and severe liver dysfunction should receive dosing adjustments to prevent adverse effects, such as confusion; this is particularly true for elderly patients
- Rapid IV administration has been associated with cardiac arrhythmias and hypotension, therefore intermittent or continuous infusions are preferred when IV administration is necessary

■ Famotidine

Brand Names
Pepcid, Pepcid AC

Generic Name
Famotidine

Dosage Forms
Oral suspension, tablets, chewable tablets, IV

Usage
Treatment of GERD*, relief of heartburn and acid indigestion*, stress ulcer prophylaxis in critically ill patients*, maintenance therapy and treatment of duodenal ulcer, acute treatment of gastric ulcer, pathologic hypersecretory conditions, part of a multidrug regimen for *H. pylori* eradication, symptomatic relief in gastritis

Dosing

- Oral/IV: 20–40 mg daily or twice daily (dose and frequency-dependent on indication; higher doses up to 160 mg every 6 hours have been used for hypersecretory conditions)
- Oral (OTC): 10–20 mg daily or twice daily
- Renal dose adjustment:
  - CrCl <50 ml/minute: Administer 50% of normal dose or increase dosing interval to every 36–48 hours

Adverse Reactions: Most Common

- Constipation, diarrhea

Adverse Reactions: Rare/Severe/Important

- Thrombocytopenia, confusion, necrotizing enterocolitis in fetus/newborn

Major Drug Interactions

Famotidine's Effect on Other Drugs

- Decreased effect/absorption of iron salts, itraconazole, ketoconazole, atazanavir, dasatinib, fosamprenavir (theoretical), erlotinib

Counseling Points

- If you are using famotidine to prevent heartburn, take oral formulations 15–60 minutes prior to meals
- If used for self-medication, do not use if you have difficulty swallowing, are vomiting blood, or have bloody or black stools; seek medical attention
- Heartburn or stomach pain that continues or worsens, or if use is required for >14 days, consult a physician

Key Points

- Famotidine is an effective option for the treatment of multiple GI disorders requiring acid suppression and is commonly used for stress ulcer prophylaxis in the ICU setting
- Unlike some other H_2 antagonists, it is not an inhibitor of the CYP enzyme system; therefore, drug interactions are limited to those drugs with decreased absorption in the altered gastric pH
- Patients with renal dysfunction should receive dosing adjustments to prevent adverse effects, such as confusion; this is particularly true for elderly patients

■ Ranitidine

Brand Name
Zantac

Generic Name
Ranitidine

Dosage Forms
Effervescent granules, IV, oral syrup, tablets, capsules

Usage
Treatment of GERD*, relief of heartburn*, indigestion, short-term and maintenance therapy of duodenal and gastric ulcers, erosive esophagitis, pathologic hypersecretory

conditions, part of a multidrug regimen for *H. pylori* eradication, prevention of stress-induced ulcers in critically ill patients

Dosing

- Oral: 150 mg one to four times daily (frequency-dependent on indication) or 300 mg daily (depending on indication)
- Oral (OTC): 75–150 mg twice daily
- IV: 50 mg every 6–8 hours; continuous infusion: 6.25 mg/hour
- Renal dose adjustment: CrCl <50 ml/minute: 150 mg orally every 24 hours or 50 mg IM/IV every 18–24 hours
- Hepatic dose adjustment: Minor changes in half-life, distribution, clearance, and bioavailability are possible; however, dosing adjustments are not necessary

Adverse Reactions: Most Common

- Abdominal pain, diarrhea, constipation, nausea, vomiting, dizziness, fatigue, agitation

Adverse Reactions: Rare/Severe/Important

- Anemia, thrombocytopenia, necrotizing enterocolitis in fetus or newborn, pancreatitis

Major Drug Interactions

Ranitidine's Effect on Other Drugs
- Increased effect/toxicity of glipizide, theophylline, procainamide (at doses >300 mg)

- Decreased effect/absorption of aspirin, atazanavir, dasatinib, erlotinib, gefitinib, fosamprenavir, itraconazole, ketoconazole, warfarin (variable)

Counseling Points

- If using ranitidine to prevent heartburn, take 30–60 minutes before having foods/drinks that cause heartburn
- If used for self-medication, do not use if you have difficulty swallowing, are vomiting blood, or have bloody or black stools; seek medical attention
- Heartburn or stomach pain that continues or worsens, or if use is required for >14 days, consult a physician
- Ranitidine effervescent granules should not be chewed, swallowed whole, or dissolved on tongue. Dissolve in at least 1 teaspoon of water; swallow when completely dissolved.

Key Points

- Ranitidine is a weak inhibitor of CYP 1A2 and 2D6, thus owing to its various drug interactions
- Ranitidine is generally well-tolerated and an effective treatment option for mild GERD symptoms and heartburn relief, especially in the outpatient setting
- Patients with renal dysfunction should receive dosing adjustments to prevent adverse effects, such as confusion; this is particularly true for elderly patients

---

Drug Class: Prokinetic Agents

Introduction

Metoclopramide is classified as both an antiemetic and prokinetic agent. It is frequently used in the treatment of gastroparesis and chemotherapy-induced nausea and vomiting. Although metoclopramide is generally well-tolerated, recent data have led to an FDA **black box warning** regarding chronic metoclopramide use and an increased risk of developing tardive dyskinesia.

Mechanism of Action for the Drug Class

Dual mechanism of action; blocks dopamine receptors in the chemoreceptor zone in the CNS and also enhances the response of acetylcholine in the upper GI tract causing enhanced motility and accelerated gastric emptying.

Members of the Drug Class

In this section: Metoclopramide
   Others: None

■ Metoclopramide

Brand Name
Reglan

Generic Name
Metoclopramide

Dosage Forms
IV, tablets, syrup

Usage

Diabetic gastroparesis*, prevention/treatment of nausea and vomiting associated with chemotherapy*, generalized nausea and vomiting*, gastroesophageal reflux, postpyloric placement of enteral feeding tubes

Dosing

- GERD, gastroparesis:
  - Oral/IV/IM: 10 mg four times daily, with meals and at bedtime
- Chemotherapy-induced nausea/vomiting:
  - IV: 1–2 mg/kg 30 minutes before chemotherapy, and repeated every 2 hours for two doses, then every 3 hours for three doses
  - Alternate dosing for low-risk chemotherapy: PO: 10–40 mg every 4–6 hours

- Renal dosage adjustment:
  - CrCl ≤40 ml/minute: Administer 50% of the normal dose

Adverse Reactions: Most Common
- Drowsiness, fatigue, restlessness, insomnia, extrapyramidal reactions (generally in the form of dystonic reactions or pseudoparkinsonism)

Adverse Reactions: Rare/Severe/Important
- Depression, NMS, tardive dyskinesia, tachyphylaxis

Major Drug Interactions
Drugs Affecting Metoclopramide
- Succinylcholine, anticholinergics (antagonize metoclopramide effects)

Metoclopramide's Effect on Other Drugs
- Anti-Parkinson's agents: Diminished therapeutic effect secondary to opposite mechanisms of action
- Antipsychotic agents: Increased risk of EPS
- Serotoninergic antidepressants: Increased risk of serotonin syndrome
- Cyclosporine: Increased absorption/effect

Contraindications
- GI obstruction, perforation or hemorrhage; pheochromocytoma; history of seizures or concomitant use of other agents likely to increase extrapyramidal reactions

Counseling Points
- If used for gastroparesis, take 30 minutes prior to meals
- Notify your physician if you experience any spastic or involuntary movements, altered mental status, or palpitations

Key Points
- Widespread use of metoclopramide is somewhat limited by its side effects. It has been associated with common side effects such as drowsiness, restlessness, and insomnia. Rare, but serious side effects include EPS, NMS, and the risk of serotonin syndrome with concomitant agents that effect serotonin. Depression, ranging from mild to severe, has also occurred in patients without a previous history of depression.
- Dystonic reactions are more common in elderly patients and young children/adults, and they occur more frequently with higher doses
- In 2009, the FDA issued a **black box warning** for the risk of tardive dyskinesia with high doses and prolonged use of metoclopramide

---

Drug Class: Proton Pump Inhibitors (PPIs)

Introduction
PPIs are well-tolerated and relatively safe options for the treatment of GI disorders requiring acid suppression therapy. They are considered first-line therapy in the treatment of moderate–severe GERD symptoms, erosive esophagitis, and treatment of NSAID-induced ulcers in the setting of continued NSAID use. A PPI-based multidrug regimen is also the first-line treatment for eradication of *H. pylori*–associated ulcers because they have been shown to be more effective than H₂ antagonist–based regimens. With such widespread use in recent years, data have emerged linking the long-term use of these agents to increased risk of pneumonia and *C. difficile*; however, a causative relationship has not been established.

Mechanism of Action of the Drug Class
PPI suppresses gastric acid secretion by inhibition of the H⁺/K⁺-ATPase in the gastric parietal cell.

Usage for the Drug Class
Acute treatment and maintenance therapy for erosive esophagitis*, treatment of GERD*, part of a multidrug regimen for *H. pylori* eradication*, prevention of gastric ulcers associated with continuous NSAID therapy*, long-term treatment of pathologic hypersecretory conditions including Zollinger–Ellison syndrome*, stress ulcer prophylaxis in critically ill patients*, relief of heartburn and indigestion*

Adverse Reactions for the Drug Class: Most Common
- Headache, dizziness, somnolence, diarrhea, constipation, nausea

Major Drug Interactions for the Drug Class
Proton Pump Inhibitor Effects on Other Drugs
- Decreased efficacy/absorption of itraconazole, ketoconazole, posaconazole, atazanavir, nelfinavir, delavirdine, dasatinib, erlotinib, clopidogrel (currently under investigation), mycophenolate mofetil
- Increased efficacy/toxicity of digoxin, benzodiazepines

Counseling Points for the Drug Class
- Take 1 hour before eating at the same time each day
- If used for self-medication, do not use if you have difficulty swallowing, are vomiting blood, or have bloody or black stools; seek medical attention

- Heartburn or stomach pain that continues or worsens, or if use is required for >14 days, consult a physician

Key Points for the Drug Class

- PPIs are generally considered interchangeable; selection of agent is usually based on cost and formulary considerations
- Multiple PPIs are available OTC; thus healthcare providers should assess patients for prolonged use, potential drug interactions, or symptoms of more serious disease that require a physician's attention
- Prolonged use of these agents has led to concern regarding the potential for adverse effects such as increased risk of pneumonia and *C. difficile* infections

Members of the Drug Class

In this section: Esomeprazole, lansoprazole, omeprazole, pantoprazole, rabeprazole

Others: Dexlansoprazole, omeprazole/sodium bicarbonate

▪ Esomeprazole

Brand Name

Nexium

Generic Name

Esomeprazole

Dosage Forms

Capsules, oral granules for suspension, IV

Dosing

- Oral/IV: 20–40 mg one to two times daily (dose- and frequency-dependent on indication)
- IV infusion: 80-mg bolus, followed by 8 mg/hour

Dosing in hepatic impairment:

- Severe hepatic impairment (Child-Pugh Class C): Maximum dose 20 mg/day

Administration:

- If using granules: Empty into container with 1 tablespoon of water and stir; leave 2–3 minutes to thicken. Stir and drink within 30 minutes.
- Esomeprazole capsule can be opened and contents mixed with 1 tablespoon of applesauce. Swallow immediately; mixture should not be chewed or warmed; IV esomeprazole is not more efficacious than oral therapy and is significantly more expensive.

▪ Lansoprazole

Brand Name

Prevacid

Generic Name

Lansoprazole

Dosage Forms

Capsules, disintegrating tablets

Dosing

- Oral: 15–30 mg one to three times daily (dose- and frequency-dependent on indication)
- Oral (OTC): 15 mg daily

Administration:

- If using orally disintegrating tablets: Do not swallow whole, do not chew. Place tablet on tongue; allow to dissolve (with or without water) until particles can be swallowed.
- Lansoprazole capsules may be opened and the intact granules sprinkled on 1 tablespoon of applesauce, pudding, cottage cheese, yogurt, or strained pears. The granules should then be swallowed immediately; capsules may be opened and emptied into about 60 ml orange juice, apple juice, or tomato juice; mix and swallow immediately.

▪ Omeprazole

Brand Name

Prilosec

Generic Name

Omeprazole

Dosage Forms

Capsules, tablets, granules for suspension

Dosing

- Oral: 20–40 mg one to two times daily (dose- and frequency-dependent on indication)
- Oral (OTC): 20 mg daily

Administration:

- Capsules may be opened and contents added to 1 tablespoon of applesauce, use immediately
- Granules for oral suspension: Empty the contents of the 2.5-mg packet into 5 ml of water (10-mg packet into 15 ml of water); stir. For NG tube administration, add 5 ml of water into a catheter-tipped syringe, and then add the contents of a 2.5-mg packet (15 ml water for the 10-mg packet); shake. Note: Regardless of the route of administration, the suspension should be left to thicken for 2–3 minutes prior to administration.

▪ Pantoprazole

Brand Name

Protonix

Generic Name

Pantoprazole

Dosage Forms

Tablets, IV, granules for suspension

Dosing

- Oral/IV push: 40–80 mg one to two times daily (dose- and frequency-dependent on indication)
- IV infusion: 80-mg bolus, followed by 8 mg/hour IV drip

Administration:
- Delayed-release oral suspension: Should only be administered in apple juice or applesauce and taken about 30 minutes before a meal. Do not administer with any other liquid or food.

■ Rabeprazole

Brand Name
AcipHex

Generic Name
Rabeprazole

Dosage Forms
Tablets

Dosing
- 20 mg one to two times daily; up to 60 mg twice daily (dose- and frequency-dependent on indication)

Drug Class: Anticholinergic/Antispasmodic Agents

Introduction
Anticholinergic agents such as dicyclomine are used in the treatment of GI motility disorders such as irritable bowel syndrome (IBS) and urinary incontinence. The use of anticholinergic agents is generally limited by their side effects, notable for dizziness, drowsiness, blurry vision, and dry mouth. There are limited data to support the efficacy of these agents, and many patients are unable to tolerate therapeutic doses; therefore, they are not considered first-line therapy for IBS or urinary incontinence.

Mechanism of Action for the Drug Class
Blocks the action of acetylcholine at parasympathetic sites in smooth muscle, secretory glands, and the CNS.

Members of the Drug Class
In this section: Dicyclomine

Others: GI anticholinergics: Hyoscyamine, scopolamine, belladonna, propantheline, atropine; urinary anticholinergics/antispasmodics: oxybutynin, tolterodine, trospium, solifenacin, darifenacin

■ Dicyclomine

Brand Name
Bentyl

Generic Name
Dicyclomine

Dosage Forms
Capsules, tablets, syrup, IV

Usage
Urinary incontinence*, IBS, infant colic, acute enterocolitis

Dosing
- Oral: 20–40 mg four times a day
- IM: 20 mg four times day; maximum of 1–2 days (do not administer IV)

Adverse Reactions: Most Common
- Dry mouth, dizziness, drowsiness, blurred vision, nausea, weakness, nervousness, light-headedness (parenteral dicyclomine), local irritation (parenteral dicyclomine)

Adverse Reactions: Rare/Severe/Important
- Decreased sweating, tachyarrhythmia, psychosis, difficulty breathing

Major Drug Interactions
Dicyclomine's Effect on Other Drugs
- Anticholinergic drugs: Belladonna/belladonna alkaloids may have additive anticholinergic effects/toxicities
- Acetylcholinesterase inhibitors: Theoretical interaction because they would likely antagonize the therapeutic effect of each other

Contraindications
- Obstructive diseases of the GI tract, severe ulcerative colitis, reflux esophagitis, unstable cardiovascular status in acute hemorrhage, obstructive uropathy, narrow-angle glaucoma, myasthenia gravis, infants <6 months of age

Counseling Points
- This drug may impair mental alertness; use caution when driving or engaging in tasks that require alertness
- Dicyclomine may cause constipation; increasing exercise, fluids, fruit, or fiber may help if patients experience this side effect

Key Point
- Dicyclomine is not considered a first-line therapy for urinary incontinence or IBS due to a lack of data supporting its efficacy over alternative agents and high incidence of side effects. Such side effects are notable for dizziness, drowsiness, dry mouth, blurry vision, nausea, and nervousness.

Drug Class: Phenothiazine Antiemetics; Typical Antipsychotic

Introduction

Phenothiazines are among the most commonly prescribed antiemetic agents available. They are available in a wide variety of preparations for oral, rectal, and IV administration, and they are generally less expensive than newer antiemetics on the market. These agents may also be used in treating psychiatric conditions such as schizophrenia and anxiety; however, they are generally not recommended for this use due to their questionable efficacy and potential for significant adverse events. Adverse reactions such as extrapyramidal reactions, tardive dyskinesia, orthostatic hypotension, and drug-induced Parkinson's syndrome are relatively common and more likely to develop in elderly patients and young children.

Mechanism of Action for the Drug Class

Antiemetic effect: Phenothiazines act centrally by inhibiting the dopamine receptors in the medullary chemoreceptor trigger zone and peripherally by blocking the vagus nerve in the GI tract. Antipsychotic effect: Phenothiazines block postsynaptic mesolimbic dopaminergic (D_1 and D_2) receptors in the brain.

Members of the Drug Class

In this section: Prochlorperazine
Others: Chlorpromazine, perphenazine, promethazine

■ Prochlorperazine

Brand Names

Compazine, Compro

Generic Name

Prochlorperazine

Dosage Forms

Tablets, spansule delayed-release capsules, suppository, IV/IM injection

Usage

- Nausea/vomiting (including chemotherapy-induced nausea and vomiting)*, schizophrenia, anxiety, psychosis/agitation related to Alzheimer's dementia (not recommended for this use), headaches (migraine, tension, vascular)

Dosing

- Antiemetic:
  ○ Oral (immediate release): 5–10 mg three to four times a day
  ○ Oral (sustained-release capsule): 10 mg every 12 hours or 15 mg daily
  ○ Rectal: 25 mg twice daily
  ○ IV/IM (deep): 2.5–10 mg every 3–4 hours (maximum 10 mg/dose, 40 mg/day)

Adverse Reactions: Most Common

- Hypotension, constipation, dry mouth, akathisia, dizziness, dystonia, EPS, drug-induced Parkinsonian disease

Adverse Reactions: Rare/Serious/Important

- Agranulocytosis, leukopenia, thrombocytopenia, ineffective thermoregulation, NMS, cholestatic jaundice, seizure, tardive dyskinesia

Major Drug Interactions

Prochlorperazine's Effect on Other Drugs

- Dofetilide: Increased serum concentration of dofetilide
- Phenytoin: May cause increase or decrease in serum phenytoin levels

Contraindications

- Bone marrow depression or history of blood dyscrasias; severe CNS depression; coma; Reye's syndrome; severe hypotension

Counseling Points

- This drug may impair mental alertness; use caution when driving or engaging in tasks that require alertness
- Notify physician if feelings of restlessness or involuntary/spastic muscle movements occur

Key Points

- The use of prochlorperazine is generally reserved for the acute treatment of generalized nausea and vomiting and nausea and vomiting related to chemotherapy
- Prochlorperazine has fallen out of favor as an antipsychotic agent due to the high incidence of adverse effects, including extrapyramidal reactions, drug-induced Parkinsonian disease, tardive dyskinesia, seizures, and anticholinergic side effects

1. Which of the following H$_2$ receptor antagonists is most likely to have significant drug interactions?
   A. Cimetidine
   B. Famotidine
   C. Ranitidine
   D. H$_2$ receptor antagonists have the same likelihood of causing drug interactions

2. MiraLAX is best described as what kind of laxative?
   A. Bulk-forming laxative
   B. Emollient laxative
   C. Lubricant
   D. Osmotic laxative

3. Which of the following medications is *not* used to treat the symptoms of GERD?
   A. Esomeprazole
   B. Famotidine
   C. Metoclopramide
   D. Ondansetron

4. A patient approaches the pharmacy complaining of watery diarrhea. After asking several questions you find out that she is also experiencing fever, abdominal pain, and has passed some blood in her stool. What is the best recommendation?
   A. Bismuth subsalicylate 30 ml every 6 hours as needed
   B. Loperamide 2 mg after each loose stool
   C. Refer her to a physician
   D. Simethicone 80 mg every 6 hours as needed

5. Which of the following uses for aluminum/magnesium hydroxides is incorrect?
   A. Adjunct agent in peptic ulcer disease
   B. Diarrhea
   C. Heartburn relief
   D. Hyperphosphatemia

6. Which of the following GI agents must be administered separately from other medications due to the risk of poor absorption?
   A. Maalox
   B. Metamucil
   C. Mylanta
   D. All of the above

7. Metoclopramide was recently issued a **black box warning** from the FDA due to recent data that suggested it increased the risk of what adverse effect?
   A. Bowel obstruction
   B. QT prolongation
   C. Renal failure
   D. Tardive dyskinesia

8. Which of the following agents will *not* decrease the absorption of itraconazole?
   A. Bismuth subsalicylate
   B. Maalox
   C. Protonix
   D. Zantac

9. Which of the following statements regarding PPIs is false?
   A. Long-term use of PPIs has been associated with increased risk of pneumonia.
   B. PPI therapy is available in over-the-counter formulations.
   C. PPIs are generally interchangeable; selection is usually based on cost.
   D. PPIs may be used as monotherapy in the treatment of *H. pylori*–associated ulcers.

10. 5-HT$_3$ receptor antagonists have been associated with all of the following side effects except
    A. Constipation/diarrhea
    B. Gallstone formation
    C. QT prolongation
    D. Sedation

11. Which of the following drugs acts peripherally on intestinal opioid receptors, to inhibit peristalsis and prolong transit time?
    A. Loperamide
    B. Ondansetron
    C. Psyllium
    D. Simethicone

12. Which of the following disease states is a contraindication to dicyclomine use?
    A. GI tract obstruction
    B. Myasthenia gravis
    C. Narrow-angle glaucoma
    D. All of the above

13. Compazine belongs to which of the following drug classes?
    A. Anticholinergics
    B. Phenothiazines
    C. Prokinetic agents
    D. 5-HT$_3$ receptor antagonists

14. Which of the following statements is true regarding H$_2$ antagonists and PPIs?
    A. H$_2$ antagonist-based regimens are more effective than PPI-based regimens for *H. pylori*–associated ulcers.
    B. Long-term use of H$_2$ antagonists has been associated with increased risk of *C. difficile* infection.
    C. Only H$_2$ antagonists are available over the counter.
    D. PPIs are preferred in NSAID-induced gastric ulcers if NSAID therapy is continued.

15. Which of the following statements regarding Pepto-Bismol is false?
    A. An active component of Pepto-Bismol is salicylate.
    B. Pepto-Bismol is not used in the treatment or prevention of traveler's diarrhea.
    C. Pepto-Bismol may temporarily darken the tongue or stools.
    D. Pepto-Bismol should be avoided in children with influenza or chicken pox.

CHAPTER 9

Hematologic Agents

Deborah DeEugenio, PharmD, BCPS, CACP

Drug Class: Anticoagulant, Coumarin Derivatives

Introduction

Warfarin is an oral anticoagulant used to reduce the formation of pathologic clots. Its exceptional efficacy is tempered by its narrow therapeutic index and significant drug–drug, drug–diet, and drug–disease interactions and need for intensive monitoring to ensure safety and efficacy. Its major adverse effect is bleeding.

Mechanism of Action for the Drug Class

Warfarin inhibits the carboxylation (activation) of the vitamin K–dependent clotting factors II, VII, IX, and X.

Members of the Drug Class

In this section: Warfarin
  Others: Acenocoumarol

Warfarin

Brand Names

Coumadin, Jantoven

Generic Name

Warfarin

Dosage Forms

Tablets, injection available for IV use (rarely used clinically)

Usage

- Prophylaxis and treatment of DVT and its extension and/or PE*
- Prophylaxis and treatment of stroke in high-risk patients with atrial fibrillation*
- Prophylaxis and treatment of the thromboembolic complications associated with cardiac valve replacement*
- Reduces risk of death, recurrent myocardial infarction, and thromboembolic events such as stroke and systemic embolization after myocardial infarction*

Dosing

Initiation of warfarin therapy should generally begin with the average dose requirement of 5 mg/day for the first few days with subsequent dosing based on the INR response. Patients expected to have lower dosage requirements (i.e., malnourished, active liver disease, on interacting medications) should be initiated on 2.5 mg/day.

- Pharmacokinetic Monitoring:
  - INR: Goal usually 2–3 for most indications, 2.5–3.5 for most mechanical cardiac valve replacements

Adverse Reactions: Most Common

- Bleeding

Adverse Reactions: Rare/Severe/Important

- Intracranial, retroperitoneal, or intraocular bleeding, purple toe syndrome, skin necrosis

Major Drug Interactions

Drugs Affecting Warfarin

- Amiodarone, fluconazole, metronidazole, ciprofloxacin, erythromycin, prednisone, sulfamethoxazole/trimethoprim: Potentiate INR
- Carbamazepine, chlordiazepoxide, rifampin: Decrease INR
- Aspirin, NSAIDs, concomitant anticoagulants: Increased risk of bleeding

Contraindications

Hemorrhagic tendencies (e.g., patients bleeding from the GI, respiratory, or GU tract; aneurysm; cerebrovascular hemorrhage; following spinal puncture and other diagnostic or therapeutic procedures with potential for significant bleeding; history of bleeding diathesis); recent or potential surgery of the eye or CNS; major regional lumbar block anesthesia or surgery resulting in large, open surfaces; blood dyscrasias; severe uncontrolled or malignant hypertension; pericarditis or pericardial effusion; subacute bacterial endocarditis; history of warfarin-induced necrosis; an unreliable, noncompliant patient; alcoholism; patient who has a history of falls or is a significant fall risk; unsupervised senile or psychotic patient; eclampsia/preeclampsia, threatened abortion, pregnancy.

Counseling Points

- Explain importance of blood test monitoring; INR testing required every 3 days to every 4 weeks
- Risk of bleeding: Monitor for blood in urine, stool, nosebleeds, hemoptysis
- Drug–drug, drug–herbal interactions: Inform your doctor when initiating or discontinuing any medication
- Drug–food interaction: Keep vitamin K intake consistent
- Alcohol: Binge drinking will increase INR
- Avoid or take precautions (e.g., helmet, protective clothing) when participating in contact sports or activities with high risk of trauma
- Have ID card in wallet or medical bracelet noting you are taking warfarin in case of emergency
- Warfarin is pregnancy category X: Discuss with your doctor before attempting to become pregnant or use appropriate contraception _don't take while pregnant_

Key Points

- Generally stop 5 days before surgical procedure
- Vitamin K is the antidote

Drug Class: Antiplatelet, Aspirin

Introduction

Aspirin is an oral antiplatelet agent used as an analgesic, antipyretic, anti-inflammatory, and most commonly for prevention of cardiovascular events. Aspirin is most commonly used to reduce arterial thrombosis, which may lead to myocardial infarction or stroke in high-risk patients. Aspirin's benefits are tempered by its dose-dependent risk of bleeding, especially gastrointestinal.

Mechanism of Action for the Drug Class

Aspirin irreversibly inhibits the cyclo-oxygenase enzyme, blocking the synthesis of cyclic prostanoids such as thromboxane A2, prostacyclin, and other prostaglandins. Aspirin's antiplatelet effects are due to the inhibition of thromboxane A2 synthesis, a potent mediator of platelet aggregation and vasoconstriction.

Members of the Drug Class

In this section: Aspirin
  Others: None

■ Aspirin

Brand Names
Various

Generic Name
Aspirin

Dosage Forms
Oral tablets: regular, chewable, or enteric-coated; suppository

Usage
- Pain
- Fever
- Various inflammatory conditions such as rheumatic fever, rheumatoid arthritis, and osteoarthritis
- Cardioprotection (prevention of CVA and MI) in high-risk primary prevention patients and in secondary prevention of MI, CVA, TIA, or following PCI or CABG*
- Prevention of in-stent thrombosis following PCI or CABG

Dosing
- Pain, fever:
  ○ 325–650 mg orally every 4–6 hours as needed
- Inflammation:
  ○ 3.2–6 g/day orally in divided doses
- TIA/CVA:
  ○ 50–325 mg orally daily
- MI/Post-PCI/post-CABG:
  ○ 81–325 mg orally daily
- Pharmacokinetic monitoring:
  ○ None (platelet aggregation tests exist but have not been standardized to measure antiplatelet effects)

Adverse Reactions: Most Common
- Dyspepsia, bleeding

Adverse Reactions: Rare/Severe/Important
- Gastrointestinal bleeding (dose-dependent)

Major Drug Interactions

Drugs Affecting Aspirin
- Diuretics, uricosurics: May decrease effectiveness
- Anticoagulants: Increase bleeding risk
- NSAIDs: Increase bleeding risk, and may reduce antiplatelet efficacy of aspirin

Aspirin's Effect on Other Drugs
- Lithium: Increase levels of lithium
- Methotrexate: Increase levels of methotrexate
- ACEI: decrease effectiveness of ACEI's

Contraindications

Hypersensitivity to salicylates, other NSAIDs, or any component of the formulation; asthma; rhinitis; nasal polyps; inherited or acquired bleeding disorders (including factor VII and factor IX deficiency); do not use in children (<16 years of age) for viral infections (chickenpox or flu symptoms), with or without fever, due to a potential association with Reye's syndrome; pregnancy (3rd trimester especially).

Counseling Points
- Risk of bleeding: Monitor for blood in urine and, stool; nosebleeds
- Take with food or after meals to reduce gastrointestinal upset
- Limit alcohol intake

Key Points
- Avoid use in children <18 years of age due to risk of Reye's syndrome
- Generally, stop 1 week before surgical procedure
- Use minimal required dose because gastrointestinal bleeding is a dose-dependent adverse effect

Drug Class: Antiplatelets, Thienopyridine

Introduction
Clopidogrel is an antiplatelet agent used predominantly in combination with aspirin to prevent arterial thrombosis especially following MI or PCI. Clopidogrel has largely replaced ticlopidine in clinical practice because of its reduced risk of hematologic adverse effects. Its major adverse effect is bleeding.

Mechanism of Action for the Drug Class
Clopidogrel irreversibly inhibits platelet aggregation by selectively blocking adenosine diphosphate (ADP) to its platelet receptor and the subsequent ADP-mediated activation of the glycoprotein GPIIb/IIIa complex, thereby inhibiting platelet aggregation.

Members of the Drug Class
In this section: Clopidogrel
   Others: Prasugrel, ticlopidine

◼ Clopidogrel

Brand Name
Plavix

Generic Name
Clopidogrel

Dosage Forms
Oral tablets

Usage
- Reduction of thrombotic events (myocardial infarction, stroke, and vascular death) in patients with atherosclerosis documented by recent stroke, recent myocardial infarction, or established peripheral arterial disease*
- For patients with acute coronary syndromes (unstable angina/MI), including patients who are to be managed medically and those who are to be managed with PCI or CABG*

Dosing
- Recent MI, recent stroke, or established peripheral arterial disease:
  - 75 mg orally daily
- Acute "coronary syndromes:"
  - 300–600 mg loading dose orally on day 1, then 75 mg orally daily
- Pharmacokinetic monitoring:
  - None (platelet aggregation tests exist but have not been standardized to measure antiplatelet effects)

Adverse Reactions: Most Common
- Bleeding

Adverse Reactions: Rare/Severe/Important
- Thrombotic thrombocytopenic purpura

Major Drug Interactions
Drugs Affecting Clopidogrel
- Proton pump inhibitors: May decrease effectiveness
- Anticoagulants, NSAIDs, aspirin: Increase bleeding risk

Contraindications
Active pathological bleeding such as peptic ulcer or intracranial hemorrhage.

Counseling Points
- Adherence is critical post-PCI or CABG because in-stent thrombosis has a high-fatality rate
- Report unusual bleeding, symptoms of dark or bloody urine, or petechiae

Key Point
- Stop 5–7 days before surgical procedure

Drug Class: Colony-Stimulating Factors

Introduction

Filgrastim and pegfilgrastim are colony-stimulating factors used most commonly for the prevention and treatment of neutropenia in cancer and HIV patients. Pegfilgrastim is a pegylated form of filgrastim with a longer duration of action.

Mechanism of Action for the Drug Class

Filgrastim and pegfilgrastim are human granulocyte colony-stimulating factors (G-CSFs), produced by recombinant DNA technology. Endogenous G-CSF is a lineage-specific colony-stimulating factor that is produced by monocytes, fibroblasts, and endothelial cells. G-CSF regulates the production of neutrophils within the bone marrow and affects neutrophil progenitor proliferation, differentiation, and selected end-cell functional activation. Pegfilgrastim has a longer duration of action than filgrastim.

Members of the Drug Class

In this section: Filgrastim, pegfilgrastim

Others: Eltrombopag, plerixafor, romiplostim, sargramostim

■ Filgrastim

Brand Name

Neupogen

Generic Name

Filgrastim

Dosage Forms

- Injection (IV, SUB-Q)

Usage

- Myelosuppressive chemotherapy: Decrease incidence of infection, as manifested by febrile neutropenia, in patients with nonmyeloid malignancies receiving myelosuppressive anticancer drugs associated with a significant incidence of severe neutropenia and fever*
- Bone marrow transplantation (BMT): Reduce duration of neutropenia and neutropenia-associated sequelae in patients with nonmyeloid malignancies undergoing myeloablative therapy followed by BMT*
- Peripheral blood progenitor cell (PBPC) collection and therapy in cancer patients: For mobilization of hematopoietic progenitor cells into the peripheral blood for leukapheresis collection*
- Patients with severe chronic neutropenia (SCN): Chronic administration to reduce the incidence and duration of sequelae of neutropenia in symptomatic patients with congenital, cyclic, or idiopathic neutropenia*
- Neutropenia in patients with human immunodeficiency virus (HIV)*

Dosing

- "Myelosuppressive chemotherapy:"
  - Initial dose: 5 μg/kg per day SUB-Q daily, short IV infusion (15–30 minutes), or continuous SUB-Q or IV infusion
- BMT:
  - 10 μg/kg per day IV infusion of 4 or 24 hours or 24-hour SUB-Q infusion
- PBPC:
  - 10 μg/kg per day SUB-Q, either as a bolus or continuous infusion
- SCN:
  - Congenital neutropenia: 6 μg/kg SUB-Q twice daily
  - Idiopathic or cyclic neutropenia: 5 μg/kg SUB-Q daily
- HIV with neutropenia:
  - 5–10 μg/kg per day SUB-Q for 2–4 weeks

■ Pegfilgrastim

Brand Name

Neulasta

Generic Name

Pegfilgrastim

Dosage Forms

- SUB-Q injection

Usage

- Myelosuppressive chemotherapy: Decrease incidence of infection, as manifested by febrile neutropenia, in patients with nonmyeloid malignancies receiving myelosuppressive anticancer drugs associated with a significant incidence of severe neutropenia and fever*
- PBPC collection and therapy in cancer patients: For mobilization of hematopoietic progenitor cells into the peripheral blood for leukapheresis collection*

Dosing

- Myelosuppressive chemotherapy
  - Initial dose: 6 mg SUB-Q once per chemotherapy cycle
- PBPC
  - 6–12 mg SUB-Q
- Monitoring
  - None (neutrophil count is monitored to assess response to therapy)

Adverse Reactions: Most Common

- Bone pain, reversible elevations in uric acid, lactate hydrogenase, alkaline phosphatase; nausea, vomiting

Adverse Reactions: Rare/Severe/Important

- Hypersensitivity, splenic rupture, ARDS, sickle cell crisis

Major Drug Interactions

Drugs Affecting Filgrastim/Pegfilgrastim

- Lithium: May potentiate release of neutrophils

Counseling Point

- Proper dosage and administration

Key Points

- Nonnarcotic analgesics relieve bone pain
- Round dose to nearest full vial or prefilled syringe
- Do not administer 14 days before to 24 hours after administration of cytotoxic chemotherapy

---

Drug Class: Erythropoietin, Recombinant Human

Introduction

Epoetin alfa and darbepoetin alfa are both injections used to treat anemia. Darbepoetin alfa has a longer duration of action.

Mechanism of Action for the Drug Class

Erythropoietin is a glycoprotein that stimulates red blood cell production. It is produced in the kidneys and stimulates the division and differentiation of committed erythroid progenitors in the bone marrow. Epoetin alfa and darbepoetin alfa are made by recombinant DNA technology and have the same biological effects as endogenous erythropoietin. Darbepoetin alfa has a longer terminal half-life than epoetin alfa.

■ Epoetin Alfa

Brand Names

Epogen, Procrit

Generic Name

Epoetin alfa

Dosage Forms

Injection (IV, SUB-Q)

Usage

- Treatment of anemia associated with CRF*
- Treatment of anemia in cancer patients on chemotherapy*
- Treatment of anemia related to zidovudine therapy in HIV*
- Reduction of allogeneic blood transfusion in surgery patients*

Dosing

- CRF
  - Initial dose: 50–100 units/kg three times weekly IV or SUBQ
  - Maintenance dose: Individualize dose to target Hct (NTE 12 g/dl)
- HIV
  - Initial dose: 100 units/kg IV or SUB-Q three times weekly for 8 weeks
  - Maintenance dose: Increase dosages in 50–100 units/kg increments to achieve target Hct

- Maximum dose: NTE 300 international units/kg dose three times weekly
- Cancer patients
  - Initial dose: 150 units /kg SUBQ three times weekly
  - Maximum dose: NTE 300 international units/kg dosed three times weekly
- Surgery
  - 300 units/kg per day SUB-Q for 10 days before surgery and for 4 days after surgery or 600 units/kg SUB-Q in once-weekly doses 21, 14, and 7 days before surgery plus a fourth dose on the day of surgery

■ Darbepoetin Alfa

Brand Name

Aranesp

Generic Name

Darbepoetin alfa

Dosage Forms

Injection (IV or SUB-Q)

Usage

- Treatment of anemia associated with CRF*
- Treatment of anemia in cancer patients on chemotherapy*

Dosing

- CRF:
  - Initial dose: 0.45 μg/kg as single IV or SUB-Q injection once weekly
  - Maintenance dose: Individualize dose to target hemoglobin (HGB) (NTE 12 g/dl)
- Cancer patients
  - Initial dose: 2.25 μg/kg SUB-Q weekly or 500 μg SUB-Q every 3 weeks
  - Maximum dose: Individualize dose to target HGB (NTE 12 g/dl)
- Pharmacokinetic Monitoring:
  - None

Adverse Reactions: Most Common

- Hypertension, headache, tachycardia, nausea, vomiting, diarrhea, shortness of breath, hyperkalemia

Adverse Reactions: Rare/Severe/Important
- Hypertension, hypersensitivity, thrombosis, seizures

Major Drug Interactions
- None

Counseling Points
- Proper dosage and administration
- Be aware of the signs and symptoms of an allergic drug reaction and take appropriate action

- Do not reuse needles, syringes, or drug products and dispose of them properly

Key Points
- Approximately 2–6 weeks for clinically significant change in Hct
- Iron stores should be assessed and iron supplementation given, as needed

---

Drug Class: Heparin, Unfractionated

Introduction

Unfractionated heparin (UFH) is an injectable anticoagulant used to prevent and treat arterial and venous thromboses. UFH's use is limited by its short half-life requiring a continuous infusion to maintain therapeutic levels, and its propensity to cause the life-threatening adverse effect heparin-induced thrombocytopenia. UFH has largely been replaced by newer heparin formulations such as low molecular weight heparins and fondaparinux. However, UFH is still the treatment of choice for patients with severe renal dysfunction or those needing invasive procedures that require temporary disruptions in anticoagulation. UFH is often used as a "bridge" to maintenance therapy with warfarin.

Mechanism of Action for the Drug Class

Binds to antithrombin and accelerates antithrombin's ability to inhibit factors IXa, Xa, XIa, XIIa, and IIa.

Members of the Drug Class

In this section: Unfractionated heparin
Others: None

■ Unfractionated Heparin

Brand Names
Various

Generic Names
Heparin, UFH

Dosage Forms
Injection, IV infusion for treatment doses (SUB-Q administration has poor absorption and it is very difficult to maintain therapeutic levels with this route); SUB-Q injection can be used for prophylaxis

Usage
- Thrombosis and embolism: Prophylaxis and treatment of venous thrombosis and its extension; PE; peripheral arterial embolism; atrial fibrillation with high risk of stroke*
- Coagulopathies: Diagnosis and treatment of acute and chronic consumption coagulopathies (disseminated intravascular coagulation)*

- Prophylaxis: Prevention of postoperative DVT and PE in high-risk medical and surgical patients*
- Clotting prevention: Prevention of clotting in arterial and heart surgery, blood transfusions, extracorporeal circulation, dialysis procedures, and blood samples*
- Prophylaxis of left ventricular thrombi and cerebrovascular accidents post-MI*
- "Bridge" to warfarin therapy to prevent CVA in patients with cardiac valve replacements*

Dosing
- IV infusion for treatment of thromboembolism
  ○ 80 units/kg (range: 50–100 units/kg) IV bolus, followed by 18 units/kg per hour (range: 15–25 units/kg per hour) continuous IV infusion. Adjust dosage to target aPTT.
- Acute coronary syndrome
  ○ 60–70 units/kg IV bolus (maximum 5000 units), followed by 12–15 units/kg per hour continuous IV infusion (maximum 1000 units/hour). Adjust dosage to target aPTT.
- Prophylaxis of Postoperative Thromboembolism:
  ○ 5000 units SUB-Q every 8 to 12 hours
- Pharmacokinetic Monitoring:
  ○ Partial thromboplastin time (PTT) or aPTT: Institution-specific values: Correlates with 0.3–0.7 anti-factor Xa units
  ○ Activated clotting time (ACT) used in cardiac catheterization lab and for CABG

Adverse Reactions: Most Common
- Bleeding

Adverse Reactions: Rare/Severe/Important
- HIT type I and type II, osteoporosis (with prolonged use), bleeding

Major Drug Interactions
Drugs Affecting Heparin
- Anticoagulants, antiplatelets, thrombolytics: Increase bleeding risk

Contraindications
History of HIT, severe thrombocytopenia; uncontrolled active bleeding except when due to disseminated intravascular

coagulation (DIC); suspected intracranial hemorrhage; not for I.M. use; not for use when appropriate blood coagulation tests cannot be obtained at appropriate intervals (applies to full-dose heparin only).

Counseling Point

- Risk of bleeding; monitor for blood in urine and stool; nosebleeds

Key Points

- Does not cross placenta in pregnancy; however, difficult to maintain therapeutic levels with SUB-Q administration and high risk of osteoporosis with extended use
- Protamine sulfate is antidote
- Has 1-hour half-life when aPTT is therapeutic; however, half-life increases exponentially when supratherapeutic, usually held for 4 hours before surgery if aPTT is initially therapeutic
- Monitor platelets frequently to assess for HIT
- Never administer IM due to risk of hematoma

Drug Class: Heparin, Low Molecular Weight

Introduction

Enoxaparin is a low molecular weight heparin (LMWH) that has a similar anticoagulant effect to UFH. However, enoxaparin is largely replacing UFH because it has better SUB-Q absorption and a longer half-life allowing once- or twice-daily SUB-Q administration and has a much lower risk of HIT and osteoporosis. Enoxaparin's major adverse effect is bleeding.

Mechanism of Action for the Drug Class

Binds to antithrombin and accelerates antithrombin's ability to inhibit factor Xa and IIa. Anti-factor Xa activity is greater than anti-factor IIa activity.

Members of the Drug Class

In this section: Enoxaparin
    Others: Dalteparin, tinzaparin

■ Enoxaparin

Brand Name

Lovenox

Generic Name

Enoxaparin

Dosage Forms

Injection (SUB-Q), can be given IV for Acute Coronary Syndrome.

Usage

- DVT/PE*
- DVT/PE treatment*
- Unstable angina/non-Q-wave MI*

Dosing

- DVT/PE prophylaxis
  - Hip or knee replacement surgery: 30 mg every 12 hours SUB-Q with initial dose given within 12–24 hours postoperatively for 7–10 days, 30 mg SUB-Q every 24 hours for renal insufficiency (estimated creatinine clearance [CrCl] 10–30 ml/minute)
  - Abdominal or high-risk surgery: 40 mg once-daily SUB-Q with initial dose given 2 hours prior to surgery for 7–10 days
  - Medically ill/immobility: 40 mg SUB-Q once daily continued for up to 14 days
- DVT/PE treatment
  - Outpatient DVT treatment: 1 mg/kg SUB-Q every 12 hours
  - Inpatient: DVT ± PE: 1 mg/kg SUB-Q every 12 hours or 1.5 mg/kg SUB-Q once daily
  - 1 mg/kg SUB-Q every 24 hours for renal insufficiency (estimated CrCl 10–30 ml/minute)
  - Initiate concomitant warfarin therapy when appropriate and continue enoxaparin for a minimum of 5 days and until a therapeutic anticoagulant effect has been achieved (INR: 2–3)
- Unstable angina/non-Q-wave MI
  - 1 mg/kg SUB-Q every 12 hours in conjunction with oral aspirin therapy (100–325 mg once daily); 1 mg/kg SUB-Q every 24 hours for renal insufficiency (estimated CrCl 10–30 ml/minute)
- Pharmacokinetic monitoring
  - Generally no monitoring
  - Anti-Xa units should be measured in special populations (pregnant, severe renal dysfunction, pediatrics, morbidly obese). Goal enoxaparin peak anti-Xa levels (drawn 4 hours post-dose at steady state) are usually 0.6–1 international units/ml for twice-daily dosing and probably >1 international units/ml for once-daily dosing.

Adverse Reactions: Most Common

- Bleeding, bruising at injection site

Adverse Reactions: Rare/Severe/Important

- HIT type I and type II: Lower incidence than with UFH; osteoporosis (with prolonged use), lower incidence than with UFH; bleeding

Contraindications

Thrombocytopenia associated with a positive in vitro test for antiplatelet antibodies in the presence of enoxaparin; hypersensitivity to pork products; active major bleeding; not for IM use.

Major Drug Interactions

Drugs Affecting Enoxaparin

- Anticoagulants, antiplatelets, thrombolytics: Increase bleeding risk

Counseling Points

- Contact physician if experiencing bleeding
- Injections are given around the navel, upper thigh, or buttocks
- Rotate injection sites daily
- Proper injection technique: Inject under the skin, not into muscle
- Expect a slight pain during injection and bruising at the injection site

Key Points

- Never administer IM due to risk of hematoma
- Protamine sulfate (1%): 1 mg partially neutralizes 1 mg enoxaparin

- Use cautiously in patients with severe renal impairment or very low or high body weight
- When neuraxial anesthesia or spinal puncture is employed, patients who are anticoagulated or scheduled to be anticoagulated with LMWHs or heparinoids for prevention of thromboembolic complications are at risk of developing an epidural or spinal hematoma that can result in long-term or permanent paralysis. Consider benefit versus risk.
- Discontinue 24 hours prior to surgery
- Safe for home use and often employed as a "bridge" to maintenance anticoagulation with warfarin
- Does not cross the placenta and is often used in pregnancy; anti-Xa monitoring is required
- Cannot be used in patients with a history of HIT

Drug Class: Thrombolytics

Introduction

Thrombolytics, like alteplase, are the only agents available that can dissolve formed pathologic clots. These agents are employed in life-threatening situations such as MI, CVA, and critical limb ischemia where the benefit outweighs the risk of life-threatening bleeding.

Mechanism of Action for the Drug Class

Alteplase is a tissue plasminogen activator produced by recombinant DNA technology. Alteplase has high affinity to fibrin-bound plasminogen that stimulates the conversion of plasminogen to plasmin, which dissolves fibrin clots.

Members of the Drug Class

In this section: Alteplase
    Others: Reteplase, tenecteplase

■ Alteplase

Brand Name

Activase

Generic Names

Alteplase, recombinant or tissue plasminogen activator (TPA)

Dosage Forms

IV injection

Usage

- Acute myocardial infarction*
- Acute ischemic stroke
- Pulmonary embolism*
- Peripheral arterial thromboembolism
- Central venous catheter occlusion*

Dosing

- Acute myocardial infarction
  - Accelerated infusion: If weight >67 kg, 100 mg total dose: 15 mg IV bolus, 50 mg infused IV over 30 minutes, 35 mg infused IV over 60 minutes. If weight ≤67 kg, 15 mg IV bolus, 0.75 mg/kg infused IV 30 minutes (NTE 50 mg); then 0.50 mg/kg infused IV over 60 minutes (NTE 35 mg).
  - 3-hour infusion: 100 mg given as 60-mg infused IV in the first hour, 20-mg infused IV over the second hour, and 20-mg infused IV over the third hour. For smaller patients (<65 kg), use a dose of 1.25-mg/kg infused IV over 3 hours as described.
- Acute ischemic stroke
  - 0.9 mg/kg (NTE 90-mg) infused IV over 60 minutes with 10% of the total dose administered as an initial IV bolus over 1 minute
- Pulmonary embolism
  - 100-mg infused IV over 2 hours
- Catheter occlusion
  - 2 mg/2 ml instilled into occluded catheter; up to two doses may be used
- Most commonly used for
  - All of the above indications
- Pharmacokinetic monitoring
  - None

Adverse Reactions: Most Common

- Bleeding

Adverse Reactions: Rare/Severe/Important

- Intracranial hemorrhage, life-threatening bleeding

Major Drug Interactions

Drugs Affecting Alteplase/TPA

- Anticoagulants, antiplatelets: Increase bleeding risk

Contraindications

Active internal bleeding; history of CVA; recent intracranial or intraspinal surgery or trauma; intracranial neoplasm; arteriovenous malformation or aneurysm; known bleeding diathesis; severe uncontrolled hypertension; suspected aortic dissection.

Counseling Point

- This medication has a life-threatening risk especially intracranial bleeding

Key Points

- Most beneficial if given within 12 hours of onset of MI symptoms or within 3 hours of onset of stroke symptoms
- There is an extensive list of contraindications and precautions that must be considered. These indicate situations where the risk of life-threatening bleeding may outweigh the benefit of therapy.

Review Questions

1. What is the antidote for Coumadin?
   A. Vitamin K
   B. Protamine
   C. Folic acid
   D. Potassium

2. What is warfarin's mechanism of action?
   A. Inhibits the cyclo-oxygenase enzyme
   B. Inhibits the carboxylation (activation) of the vitamin K–dependent clotting factors II, VII, IX, and X
   C. Binds to antithrombin to inactivate thrombin, factor Xa, and other clotting factors
   D. Regulates the production of neutrophils within the bone marrow

3. Which of the following is *not* an indication for aspirin therapy?
   A. MI
   B. TIA
   C. Post-PCI
   D. HTN

4. Aspirin use should be avoided in children <18 years old due to risk of
   A. MI
   B. Dyspepsia
   C. Reye's syndrome
   D. Brugada syndrome

5. Plavix is available in which dosage form in the United States?
   A. Oral tablet
   B. Intravenous injection
   C. Oral tablet and intravenous injection
   D. Suppository

6. What is the difference in mechanism of action between Neupogen and Neulasta?
   A. They have a similar mechanism of action, but Neulasta has a shorter duration of action
   B. They have a similar mechanism of action, but Neulasta has a longer duration of action
   C. Neulasta increases production of neutrophils, whereas Neupogen increases production of eosinophils
   D. They have the exact same mechanism of action

7. Which of the following is one of the uses for epoetin alfa?
   A. Treatment of neutropenia in HIV patients
   B. Treatment of anemia in chronic renal failure
   C. Treatment of HTN
   D. Prevention and treatment of DVT and PE

8. Which of the following routes of administration are appropriate for heparin unfractionated?
   A. IV, SQ
   B. IV, IM
   C. PO, IM
   D. IV, PO

9. Which of the following is *not* an adverse effect of heparin unfractionated?
   A. HIT
   B. Osteoporosis
   C. Bleeding
   D. Hypernatremia

10. Which of the following is an appropriate dosing regimen for Lovenox?
    A. 1 mg/kg SUB-Q every 12 hours
    B. 5000 units SUB-Q every 8 hours
    C. 5 mg orally daily
    D. 81 mg orally daily

11. How long before surgery or invasive procedures must Lovenox be withheld?
    A. 1 week
    B. 5 days
    C. 24 hours
    D. 4 hours

12. What medication class includes Activase?
    A. Antiplatelet
    B. Anticoagulant
    C. Thrombolytic
    D. Antihypertensive

13. What medication class includes clopidogrel?
    A. Antiplatelet
    B. Anticoagulant
    C. Thrombolytic
    D. Antihypertensive

14. What test is used for monitoring of warfarin therapy?
    A. INR
    B. PTT
    C. Anti-Xa
    D. ACT

15. Which of the following is *not* an adverse effect of Aranesp?
    A. Hypertension
    B. Headache
    C. Seizures
    D. Thrombocytopenia

CHAPTER 10

Lipid-Lowering Agents

Nima M. Patel, PharmD, BCPS

Drug Class: HMG-CoA Reductase Inhibitors
(Commonly Referred to as Statins)

Introduction

Statins are considered first-line treatment for patients with dyslipidemia, in most patients with atherosclerotic vascular disease, and in patients at risk of developing atherosclerosis. In numerous clinical trials across many patient populations, statins have shown significant reduction in morbidity and mortality. Significant toxicities include increase in liver function tests (LFTs) and myalgias that rarely lead to rhabdomyolysis. Statins are contraindicated in patients with active liver disease, pregnancy, and lactation because they are designated as pregnancy category X drugs.

Mechanisms of Action for the Drug Class

HMG-CoA reductase inhibitors competitively inhibit hydroxymethylglutaryl-coenzyme A (HMG-CoA) reductase to mevalonate, which is the rate-limiting step in cholesterol biosynthesis. In addition, low-density lipoprotein (LDL) cholesterol receptors are upregulated, enhancing the catabolic rate of LDL and reducing the plasma pool of LDL. The combination of these pharmacologic effects makes statins highly effective LDL-lowering agents. To a lesser extent, they may also increase high-density lipoprotein (HDL) cholesterol and decrease triglycerides (TGs).

Members of the Drug Class

In this section: Atorvastatin, fluvastatin, lovastatin, pravastatin, rosuvastatin, simvastatin

Other: Pitavastatin

Generic and Brand Names for the Drug Class

Atorvastatin (Lipitor), fluvastatin (Lescol), lovastatin ER (Mevacor, Altoprev), pravastatin (Pravachol), simvastatin (Zocor), rosuvastatin (Crestor)

Dosage Forms for the Drug Class

- Oral tablets

Usage for the Drug Class

- Adjunct to diet and exercise, commonly referred to as Therapeutic Lifestyle Changes (TLCs), for the treatment of various dyslipidemia disorders in patients with no evidence of cardiovascular disease (primary prevention) and in patients with documented coronary artery disease (secondary prevention)*
- Various dyslipidemias are described using the Fredrickson–Levy–Lees classification of hyperlipoproteinemia.* Using this classification system, statins are primarily indicated for treatment of mixed dyslipidemia known as Fredrickson types IIa and IIb.
- Adjunct for treatment of hypertriglyceridemia (Fredrickson type IV hyperlipidemia) and primary dysbetalipoproteinemia (Fredrickson type III hyperlipidemia)

Dosing for the Drug Class

- Before starting therapy, check baseline LFTs and fasting lipid profile. Baseline CPK in high-risk patients may be checked. Recheck LFTs in 3 months and periodically thereafter; if the patient has symptoms of myalgia, check CPK.
- Statins should be used in combination with TLC. Patients can be started with the following doses of statins, although doses should be individualized according to the percentage decrease in LDL cholesterol needed, the recommended goal of therapy, and the patient's response.
  - Rosuvastatin: 10 mg daily
  - Atorvastatin: 10 mg daily
  - Pravastatin: 40 mg daily
  - Fluvastatin, lovastatin, simvastatin: 20 mg daily
- Titration should occur 4–6 weeks later to a maximum of 80 mg/day for all statins except rosuvastatin, which is 40 mg/day

- Several studies have started patients on a maximum doses of statins without titration. This is especially noted for atorvastatin, 80 mg/day in the setting of acute coronary syndrome.
- Patients with GFR <30 ml/minute, atorvastatin can be used safely up to 80 mg/day.
- Fluvastatin, lovastatin, pravastatin, and simvastatin can be safely used up to 40 mg/day.
- Rosuvastatin doses should be limited to 10 mg/day for patients with GFR 15–29 ml/minute and should be avoided for patients with GFR <15 ml/minute due to lack of data.
- Pharmacokinetic/Pharmacodynamics Properties
  - The ability of a statin to lower LDL is very important in the treatment of dyslipidemia. Rosuvastatin and atorvastatin have the greatest ability to lower LDL by approximately 60% followed by simvastatin, lovastatin, pravastatin, and fluvastatin.
  - The pharmacokinetic property of a particular statin plays an important role on the choice of statin for an individual patient. Increased bioavailability, decreased protein binding, long half-life, lipophilicity, and metabolism are considered to be important characteristics that may influence the risk of developing statin-induced myopathies. Of all the properties just listed, metabolism is considered to be the most important due to the potential for drug interactions.
  - Atorvastatin, lovastatin, and simvastatin are metabolized by the CYP3A4 system.
  - Fluvastatin is metabolized by the CYP2C9 system.
  - Rosuvastatin is metabolized by limited 2C9 system metabolism.
  - Pravastatin is not metabolized by the CYP system; instead it is metabolized by hydroxylation, oxidation, and conjugation.

Adverse Reactions for the Drug Class: Most Common
- GI upset, myalgias (dose-related)

Adverse Reactions for the Drug Class: Rare/ Severe/Important
- Hepatotoxicity (dose-related), myopathy (dose-related), rhabdomyolysis (dose-related)

Major Drug Interactions for the Drug Class
Drugs Affecting Statins
- Enhanced toxicity with drugs that inhibit isoenzyme CYP3A4 and statins that are substrates of CYP3A4 (lovastatin, simvastatin, and atorvastatin). Dose limitations do exist for certain inhibitors (e.g., simvastatin doses should be limited to 20 mg/day with amiodarone). Whereas with protease inhibitors, the use of lovastatin and simvastatin should be avoided and atorvastatin doses should be limited to 20 mg/day because the extent of interaction between atorvastatin and CYP3A4 inhibitors is less than that with lovastatin and simvastatin.
- Rosuvastatin exposure can be increased via unknown mechanisms with protease inhibitors in combination with ritonavir, and therefore the dose of rosuvastatin in these combinations should be limited to 10 mg/day.
- Statins are substrates for P-glycoprotein; therefore, drugs that inhibit P-glycoprotein (e.g., cyclosporine) may increase statin levels. Cyclosporine is also a potent inhibitor of the CYP3A4 system, and therefore statin dosages in patients receiving cyclosporine have been limited (e.g., 5 mg/day for rosuvastatin, 10 mg/day for simvastatin and atorvastatin, and 20 mg/day for lovastatin).
- Fibric acid derivatives increase the risk for myopathy/rhabdomyolysis due to additive effects of both drugs. Gemfibrozil can reduce the elimination of a statin by inhibiting glucuronidation, an elimination pathway of all statins except fluvastatin. Therefore, the use of fenofibrate when combination therapy with a statin is required may be a better choice. Dose-limitation exists when gemfibrozil is used in combination with a statin (e.g., limit rosuvastatin to 10 mg with gemfibrozil).

Counseling Points for the Drug Class
- Report unexplained muscle pain, tenderness, or weakness, particularly if accompanied by malaise or fever
- It is best to take statins with a short-life such as lovastatin, simvastatin, pravastatin, and fluvastatin in the evening because of a greater lipid-lowering effect; hepatic cholesterol production increases overnight
- Take lovastatin with an evening meal because fat facilitates absorption
- One may take atorvastatin and rosuvastatin anytime during the day without regard to meals because of their longer half-lives and more potent LDL cholesterol lowering ability
- Avoid drinking grapefruit juice for statins metabolized by the CYP3A4 system

Key Points for the Drug Class
- When combination therapy of a statin and fibrate is necessary, fenofibrate may be a better choice due to an increased risk of myopathy with gemfibrozil and a statin
- Be vigilant about dose-limitation and avoidance of statins with concomitant use of inhibitors of the CYP3A4 system

Introduction

Fibric acid derivatives are mainly used for the treatment of hypertriglyceridemia. Fenofibrate and gemfibrozil belong to this class. Fenofibrate is the preferred agent when used in combination with statins due to the potential for fewer drug interactions. These drugs are contraindicated in patients with severe renal or hepatic disease including primary biliary cirrhosis, unexplained persistent elevated liver function abnormality, and preexisting gallbladder disease.

Mechanisms of Action for the Drug Class

The mechanism of action of fibric acid derivatives is complex and not well understood. These drugs stimulate peroxisome proliferator activated receptors (PPARα). Activation of PPARα leads to an increase in lipoprotein lipase activity and a reduction in the production of apoprotein CIII (an inhibitor of lipoprotein lipase) causing a decrease in total triglycerides and triglyceride-rich lipoprotein (VLDL). In addition, these drugs upregulate the synthesis of apolipoprotein A-I, the building block of HDL, and therefore cause an increase in HDL.

Usage for the Drug Class

- Fibric acid derivatives are indicated for adjunctive therapy to diet in the treatment of adult patients with very high levels of serum triglycerides (types IV and V hyperlipidemia) who present a risk of pancreatitis (TG >500 mg/dl) and who do not respond adequately to dietary control*
- Treatment of hypercholesterolemia to reduce LDL, TG, and apolipoprotein B, and to increase HDL in adults with primary hypercholesterolemia or mixed dyslipidemia (Fredrickson types IIa and IIb)

Dosing for the Drug Class

- Gemfibrozil is given 600 mg twice daily 30 minutes before the morning and evening meals.
- In patients with renal disease, gemfibrozil is the preferred agent according to the National Kidney Foundation recommendations.

Adverse Reactions for the Drug Class: Most Common

- Dyspepsia, GI-related side effects such as nausea/vomiting, diarrhea, constipation

Adverse Reactions for the Drug Class: Rare/Severe/Important

- Myalgias and more serious muscle-related adverse drug reactions such as myopathy and rhabdomyolysis, risk is increased when fibrates are combined with a statin. Hepatotoxicity, cholelithiasis, gallstones.

Major Drug Interactions for the Drug Class

Fibric Acid Derivatives' Effect on Other Drugs

- Warfarin: Increases INR, an empiric reduction in warfarin dosage may be considered to minimize bleeding risk
- HMG CoA reductase inhibitors: Increase the risk of myopathy and rhabdomyolysis (the risk is greater with gemfibrozil than fenofibrate; thus, for combination treatment with a statin, fenofibrate is preferred)
  ○ Note: Dose-limitation exists with certain statins (e.g., with lovastatin, dose should be limited to 20 mg/day in combination with gemfibrozil and fenofibrate)
- Repaglinide should be used cautiously with gemfibrozil because combinations result in increased hypoglycemic effects

Counseling Points for the Drug Class

- Report unexplained muscle pain, tenderness, or weakness, particularly if accompanied by malaise or fever
- Use in conjunction with diet and exercise for therapeutic effects

Key Points for the Drug Class

- When combination therapy with a statin and a fibrate is required, fenofibrate may be preferred because of an increased risk of myalgias rarely leading to myopathy and rhabdomyolysis with a gemfibrozil and statin combination
- LFTs should be monitored periodically
- Fenofibrate should be avoided in patients with severe kidney disease
- Fenofibrate and gemfibrozil can individually increase the INR, and a patient's warfarin dose may be empirically reduced to avoid elevated bleeding risk

Members of the Drug Class

In this section: Fenofibrate, gemfibrozil

■ Fenofibrate

Brand Name

TriCor

Generic Name

Fenofibrate

Dosage Forms

Capsules and tablets

Dosing

- Many different formulations of fenofibrate exist, and thus the dose ranges from 50-200 mg daily.
- Fenofibrate should be dose adjusted for renal dysfunction (i.e., maximum dose for CrCl 15-69 ml/minute is 67 mg/day if using TriCor).
- In patients with CrCl <15 ml/minute, fenofibrate should be avoided.

Gemfibrozil

Brand Name

Lopid

Generic Name

Gemfibrozil

Dosage Forms

- Oral tablets

Drug Class: Nicotinic Acid

Introduction

Niacin is a water-soluble B vitamin important for DNA repair and energy metabolism. When used in high doses of 1–2 g/day, niacin is an antilipemic agent. Because it is considered to be a vitamin, niacin is available as a dietary supplement, OTC, as well as prescription. Niacin is available in three main dosage forms: immediate-release, slow/timed-release, and extended-release. The differences in formulations relate to flushing and hepatotoxicity risk. Niacin is the best known agent to raise HDL. Niacin should not be used in patients with active liver disease or unexplained transaminase elevations.

Mechanisms of Action for the Drug Class

The exact mechanism is not fully understood. The process may involve inhibiting mobilization of free fatty acids from peripheral adipose tissue to the liver, which results in decreased hepatic production VLDL that decreases LDL production. Niacin reduces the amount of apolipoprotein A-I extracted and catabolized from HDL during hepatic uptake, resulting in increased HDL.

Niacin

Brand Names

Slo-Niacin, Niacor (IR), Niaspan ER (Rx), Niacin-Time

Generic Name

Niacin

Dosage Forms

Oral tablets, capsules

Usage

- Adjunctive treatment of dyslipidemias (types IIa and IIb or primary hypercholesterolemia) to lower the risk of recurrent MI and/or slow progression of coronary artery disease*
- Combination therapy with other antidyslipidemic agents when additional TG-lowering or HDL-increasing effects are desired*
- Treatment of hypertriglyceridemia in patients at risk of pancreatitis
- Treatment of pellagra (niacin deficiency)

Dosing

- Hyperlipidemia: Regular-release: 1.5–6 g/day in three divided doses with or after meals using a dosage titration schedule; extended-release: 500 mg: 2 g once daily at bedtime
- Pellagra: 50–100 mg three to four times/day, maximum of 500 mg/day

Adverse Reactions: Most Common

- Flushing (prostaglandin-mediated): Most common with immediate-release and least common with long-acting products; hyperglycemia, hyperuricemia, upper GI distress

Adverse Reactions: Rare/Severe/Important

- Hepatotoxicity: Rise in serum transaminase values are seen with all niacin formulations, but the worst cases have been reported with slow-release niacin and there is often a dose-related side effect when doses >2000 mg/day are administered. Slow-release products should not be recommended due to increased hepatotoxicity risk. Immediate-release products have the least hepatotoxicity; however, they must be dosed three times daily and can cause significant flushing.
- Most experts prefer Niaspan (niacin extended-release) because it causes less flushing than immediate-release niacin, is dosed once daily, and is associated with less liver toxicity than sustained-release, controlled-release, or timed-release niacin (e.g., Slo-Niacin).

Major Drug Interactions

Drugs Affecting Niacin

- The levels of niacin may be decreased by bile acid sequestrants (give niacin 1 hour before or 4–6 hours after giving bile acid sequestrant)

Counseling Point

- The adherence of this drug may be compromised due to the adverse effects of flushing. Proper counseling reduces the incidence of flushing. The flushing occurs because of the release of prostaglandin D_2 from the skin and therefore giving aspirin or ibuprofen 30 minutes before therapy helps diminish the side effects. Patients should be advised to take niacin on a full stomach and that flushing may be worsened by hot, spicy food; hot beverages; hot baths; and hot showers.

Key Points

- Niacin is the best known agent to raise HDL. The side effect of flushing may diminish adherence. Patients should be properly counseled on avoiding the side effects.

- The different formulations of niacin relate to the risk of hepatotoxicity and flushing. Products that claim to be "flush-free" or "no flush" are available OTC; however, these products fail to release free niacin, making them an ineffective antilipemic agent.

Drug Class: Cholesterol Absorption Inhibitors

Introduction

Ezetimibe is the only agent available in this class. It is specifically used in combination with a statin to lower LDL. An available combination product, Vytorin, contains simvastatin and ezetimibe. An additional approximately 25% lowering of the LDL can be seen when ezetimibe is combined with a statin, which makes it an attractive add-on agent to reach a lower LDL goal of <70 mg/dl. The drug lacks outcome data on the prevention of cardiovascular disease events.

Mechanisms of Action for the Drug Class

Inhibits absorption of cholesterol at the brush border of the small intestine via the sterol transporter, Niemann-Pick C1-Like1, leading to a decreased delivery of cholesterol to the liver, reduction of hepatic cholesterol stores, and an increased clearance of cholesterol from the blood.

■ Ezetimibe

Brand Name
Zetia

Generic Name
Ezetimibe

Dosage Forms
Oral tablets

Usage

- Monotherapy or in combination with HMG-CoA reductase inhibitors: Primary heterozygous familial and nonfamilial hypercholesterolemia (in combination with dietary therapy)*
- Mixed hyperlipidemia (in combination with fenofibrate)
- Homozygous familial hypercholesterolemia (in combination with atorvastatin or simvastatin)
- Homozygous sitosterolemia

Dosing

- Ezetimibe should be dosed 10 mg daily without regard to meals. Dosing adjustments are not necessary for renal or mild hepatic insufficiency. Not recommended for use in patients with moderate–severe hepatic impairment.

Adverse Reactions: Most Common

- When compared to placebo, ezetimibe is well-tolerated. Most common side effects reported were abdominal pain, diarrhea, arthralgia, cough, fatigue, and headache.

Adverse Reactions: Rare/Severe/Important

- Hypersensitivity reactions (including angioedema and rash), increased LFTs, drug-induced myopathy (very rarely with monotherapy), rhabdomyolysis (very rarely with monotherapy); the risk is increased in combination with a statin

Major Drug Interactions

Drugs Affecting Ezetimibe

- Bile acid sequestrants (cholestyramine/colestipol): May decrease ezetimibe bioavailability; administer 2 hours before or 4 hours after bile acid sequestrants. Note: No drug interaction results with the use of colesevelam.
- Cyclosporine: Ezetimibe serum levels may be increased. No monitoring is recommended for ezetimibe.
- Fibrates may increase cholesterol excretion into the bile, leading to cholelithiasis

Ezetimibe's Effect on Other Drugs

- Cyclosporine: Ezetimibe may increase serum levels of cyclosporine. Cyclosporine levels should be monitored.

Counseling Points

- Take at the same time every day, without regard for meals
- Report allergic reaction: Itching/hives, swelling in the face/hands, trouble breathing (angioedema)
- Report any muscle pain, tenderness, or weakness
- Report nausea, vomiting, loss of appetite, pain in your upper stomach (cholelithiasis)
- Use in conjunction with diet and exercise

Key Points

- In combination with a statin, LDL is lowered an additional approximately 25%
- Ezetimibe is also available as a combination product with the statin simvastatin. The brand name of this product is Vytorin.

Drug Class: Omega-3 Fatty Acids

Introduction

Omega-3 fatty acids are polyunsaturated fatty acids derived from marine and plant sources. Omega-3 fatty acids can decrease triglycerides by 50%, although in patients with very high triglycerides (>500 mg/dl) there is an increase in LDL. Omega-3 fatty acids are available as dietary supplements; however, there is a lower amount of EPA and DHA compared with the only prescription product, Lovaza. Lovaza is the purest form of omega-3 fatty acids and contains 85% of EPA and DHA in a 1000-mg capsule.

Mechanisms of Action for the Drug Class

The mechanism has not been completely defined. Possible mechanisms include inhibition of acyl CoA:1,2-diacyl-glycerol acyltransferase, increased hepatic β-oxidation, a reduction in the hepatic synthesis of triglycerides, or an increase in plasma lipoprotein lipase activity.

■ Omega-3 Fatty Acids

Brand Name
Lovaza

Generic Name
Omega-3 fatty acids

Dosage Forms
Oral capsules

Usage
- Adjunct to diet therapy in the treatment of hypertriglyceridemia (>500 mg/dl)*
- Prophylaxis to prevent a myocardial infarction (unlabeled use)
- Treatment of immunoglobulin (Ig)A nephropathy (unlabeled use)

Dosing
- Hypertriglyceridemia/treatment of IgA nephropathy: 4 g/day as a single daily dose or in two divided doses
- Prophylaxis to prevent a myocardial infarction: 1 g/day

Adverse Reactions: Most Common
- Generally well-tolerated, the most common side effect being a "fishy" burp smell called eructation, fishy aftertaste, and GI upset/nausea. Refrigeration of the capsules may help minimize these side effects.

Adverse Reactions: Rare/Severe/Important
- Increase in bleeding time, although this does not appear to exceed the normal range of bleeding time

Major Drug Interactions
Omega-3 Fatty Acids' Effect on Other Drugs
- May increase the levels/effects of antiplatelet agents, warfarin. More frequent monitoring of the INR may be necessary in patients taking warfarin.

Counseling Point
- OTC products differ in their EPA/DHA content. It is important to note the total amount of omega-3 fatty acids contained in each capsule rather than fish oil concentrate. Some products may require consumption up to 11 capsules to obtain same amount of omega-3 fatty acid content that is obtained from 4 capsules of Lovaza.

Key Point
- Omega-3 fatty acids are increasingly being used for prevention of myocardial infarction at doses of 1 g/day. Higher doses of 2–4 g/day are used to lower TG. Lovaza is the purest form of omega-3 fatty acids.

Drug Class: Bile Acid Sequestrants

Introduction

The three bile acid sequestrants (BASs) on the market are cholestyramine, colestipol, and colesevelam. Primary effect of these agents at optimal doses is to reduce LDL by 15–30%. However, in clinical practice, cholestyramine and colestipol are underused due to GI side effects and classic drug-binding interactions seen with these agents when drugs are given together. Colesevelam is much better tolerated and has fewer drug-binding interactions thus is generally the preferred agent in this class. These agents are contraindicated in patients with complete biliary obstruction and bowel obstruction. BASs may increase triglycerides, and therefore these agents should be avoided in patients with TG >400 mg/dL.

Mechanisms of Action for the Drug Class

Cholesterol is the precursor of bile acids, which are needed for emulsifying fat and lipid particles in food. Bile acids are secreted into the intestine through the bile, and most bile acids are reabsorbed in the intestines and returned to the liver by enterohepatic circulation. BAS binds to bile acids in the gut, which interrupts recycling through enterohepatic recirculation. Hepatic cells convert more cholesterol into bile acid, and there is an increase synthesis of LDL receptors leading to increased hepatic uptake of systemic LDL particles and lowered LDL.

Members of the Drug Class
In this section: Cholestyramine
    Others: Colesevelam, colestipol

■ Cholestyramine

Brand Names
Prevalite, Questran, Questran Light

Generic Name
Cholestyramine

Dosage Forms
Powder for oral suspension

Usage
- Adjunct to diet in the management of primary hypercholesterolemia*
- Pruritus associated with elevated levels of bile acids
- Diarrhea associated with excess fecal bile acids
- Binding toxicologic agents
- Adjunctive therapy for pseudomembranous colitis

Dosing
- 4 g one to two times a day to a maximum of 24 g/day (and a maximum of six times a day). BASs are not systemically absorbed, and dosage adjustment for renal insufficiency is not necessary.

Adverse Reactions: Most Common
- Constipation (increases with dose and age of the patient); other GI-related adverse reactions include abdominal pain, flatulence, nausea, vomiting, dyspepsia, and steatorrhea

Adverse Reactions: Rare/Severe/Important
- Theoretically patients taking BASs may be at an increased risk of bleeding from hypoprothrombinemia (secondary to vitamin K deficiency)

Major Drug Interactions
Cholestyramine's Effect on Other Drugs
- Delay or reduce the absorption of many drugs when cholestyramine is administered concomitantly. To avoid the drug interaction, give other medications 1 hour before or 4–6 hours after giving BASs.
  Note: Colesevelam does not have a decreased frequency for causing these interactions.
- Amiodarone, corticosteroids, digoxin, ezetimibe, fat-soluble vitamins (vitamins A, D, E, and K), gemfibrozil, HMG-CoA inhibitors, methyldopa, methotrexate, niacin, NSAIDs, propranolol (and potentially other β-blockers), sulfonylureas, thyroid hormones, thiazide and loop diuretics, thiazolidinedione, valproic acid, warfarin.
  Note: This list is not all inclusive.

Counseling Points
- Cholestyramine oral suspension packets should be mixed with 4–6 oz of beverage. Allow to stand 1–2 minutes before mixing. May also be mixed with highly fluid soups, cereals, applesauce, or pulpy fruits. To decrease the occurrence of flatulence, mix cholestyramine with noncarbonated pulpy juices and swallow it without engulfing air by using a straw.
- Separate the administration of other drugs by 1 hour before or 4–6 hours after cholestyramine

Key Point
- Patients should be counseled on drug-binding interactions and to separate dosing of other drugs from cholestyramine. GI-related adverse effects and the palatability of the drug may limit the use of the drug long-term.

Review Questions

1. What is the mechanism of action of statins?
   A. Competitive inhibition of HMG-CoA reductase to mevalonate
   B. Decreases hepatic production VLDL, which decreases LDL production
   C. Decreases TG by increased lipoprotein lipase activity
   D. Impairs dietary and biliary cholesterol absorption at the brush border of the intestine

2. Which niacin formulation has been associated with the least hepatotoxicity?
   A. Immediate-release
   B. Extended-release
   C. Sustained-release
   D. Timed-release

3. Which of the following is a major side effect of cholestyramine?
   A. Causes myopathy
   B. Decreases absorption of other concomitantly administered drugs
   C. Elevated liver function enzymes
   D. Increases glucose levels

4. Which of the following is an adverse event of statins?
   A. Gallstones
   B. Hyperglycemia
   C. Myopathy
   D. Peptic ulcer disease

5. Side effects of nicotinic acid include
   A. Cutaneous flushing
   B. Decrease absorption of other drugs
   C. Mental status changes
   D. Nephrotoxicity

6. Which of the following properties contribute to an increase of statin-induced myopathies?
   A. Drug–drug interaction via the CYP2C19 system
   B. High doses
   C. Hydrophilic property of the drug
   D. None of the above

7. Of the following statins, which is considered to be the highest in potency to lower LDL?
   A. Atorvastatin (Lipitor)
   B. Fluvastatin (Lescol)
   C. Lovastatin (Mevacor)
   D. Pravastatin (Pravachol)

8. The combination of gemfibrozil (Lopid) and simvastatin (Zocor) increases the risk for
   A. Diarrhea
   B. Dyspepsia
   C. Major coronary events
   D. Myopathy

9. Pravastatin (Pravachol) is metabolized by which metabolic pathway?
   A. CYP 2C9
   B. CYP 2D6
   C. CYP 3A4
   D. Hydroxylation, oxidation, conjugation

10. The following statement is true regarding lovastatin (Mevacor)
    A. Should be taken on an empty stomach for increased absorption
    B. Should be taken with food in the evening for increased absorption
    C. Should ideally be taken in the morning
    D. Should be taken twice daily

11. Fluvastatin (Lescol) is contraindicated for use in patients who are
    A. Allergic to penicillin
    B. Chronic asthmatics
    C. Diabetic
    D. Pregnant

12. What is the dose for omega-3 fatty acids (Lovaza) for prevention of myocardial infarction?
    A. 1 g/day
    B. 2 g/day
    C. 3 g/day
    D. 4 g/day

13. What is the effect of ezetimibe (Zetia) on cyclosporine?
    A. Ezetimibe (Zetia) decreases levels of cyclosporine
    B. The effects of ezetimibe (Zetia) on cyclosporine levels are not known
    C. Ezetimibe (Zetia) has no effect on the levels of cyclosporine
    D. Ezetimibe (Zetia) increases levels of cyclosporine

14. Bile acid sequestrants should not be utilized in patients with the following conditions:
    A. Complete biliary obstruction and bowel obstruction
    B. Currently on statin therapy
    C. Renal insufficiency
    D. Triglycerides <200 mg/dl

15. Simvastatin (Zocor) doses should be limited to _____ mg/day for patients who are concomitantly on treatment with amiodarone.
    A. 10
    B. 20
    C. 30
    D. 40

Miscellaneous Agents

Mirza Perez, PharmD, BCPS
Sarah Slabaugh, PharmD, RD

Drug Class: 5-Alpha Reductase Inhibitors

Introduction

The 5-alpha reductase inhibitors are agents that interfere with testosterone's stimulatory effect on prostate gland size. They are indicated for the management of moderate–severe benign prostatic hyperplasia (BPH). Their use may slow disease progression and decrease the risk of disease complications.

Mechanism of Action for the Drug Class

Competitively inhibit both tissue and hepatic 5-alpha reductase, resulting in inhibition of the conversion of testosterone to dihydrotestosterone.

Members of the Drug Class

In this section: Finasteride
  Other: Dutasteride

■ Finasteride

Brand Names

Propecia, Proscar

Generic Name

Finasteride

Dosage Forms

Tablets

Usage

Treatment of symptomatic BPH*, treatment of male pattern hair loss

Dosing

- BPH: 5 mg orally daily
- Male pattern baldness: 1 mg orally daily

Adverse Reactions: Most Common

- Rash, breast tenderness and swelling, reduced libido, ejaculation disturbances, erectile dysfunction

Adverse Reactions: Rare/Severe/Important

- Hypersensitivity, testicular pain, neoplasm of male breast

Contraindications

- Pregnancy, female gender, children

Major Drug Interactions

- No known significant drug interactions

Counseling Points

- Women of childbearing age should not touch or handle broken tablets
- Results of therapy may take several months
- This medication can be taken with or without meals

Key Point

- Pregnancy category X; female patients of childbearing age should not touch or handle broken tablets

Drug Class: Acne Products/Retinoic Acid Derivatives

Introduction

Retinoic acid derivatives are agents commonly used first-line in the treatment of mild–moderate acne. They are also used as maintenance therapy to minimize antibiotic use in acne treatment. The side-effect profile of isotretinoin requires special monitoring.

Mechanism of Action for the Drug Class

Reduces sebaceous gland size and secretion and regulates cell proliferation and differentiation.

Members of the Drug Class

In this section: Isotretinoin
 Others: Topical tretinoin

■ Isotretinoin

Brand Names

Accutane, Amnesteem, Claravis, Sotret

Generic Name

Isotretinoin

Dosage Forms

Capsules

Usage

Treatment of severe recalcitrant nodular acne unresponsive to conventional therapy*

Dosing

- 0.5–2 mg/kg per day in two divided doses for 15–20 weeks or until the total nodule count decreases by 70%, whichever occurs first

Adverse Reactions: Most Common

- Alopecia, cheilitis, dry skin, photosensitivity, pruritus, xerostomia, arthralgia, backache, conjunctivitis, epistaxis

Adverse Reactions: Rare/Severe/Important

- Elevated triglycerides, pancreatitis, neutropenia, hepatotoxicity, anaphylaxis, visual disturbances, hearing loss, aggressive behavior, depression, violent behavior

Major Drug Interactions

Drugs Affecting Isotretinoin

- Vitamin A derivatives: Additive toxicity (i.e., dry skin and mucous membranes)
- Ethanol: Increased risk of elevated triglycerides

Isotretinoin's Effect on Other Drugs

- Tetracyclines: May increase the risk of pseudotumor cerebri
- Contraceptives (estrogens and progestins): May decrease effectiveness of oral contraceptives

Contraindications

- Patients who are pregnant or who may become pregnant

Counseling Points

- Avoid pregnancy during treatment with isotretinoin
- Counsel men about the risks associated with impregnating a woman on isotretinoin
- Exacerbations of acne can occur during first week of treatment
- Report the following effects to physician immediately: Visual difficulties, abdominal pain, rectal bleeding, feelings of depression, and/or suicidal ideation
- Some night vision acuity may be lost during therapy
- Avoid prolonged exposure to the sun, use sunscreen, and wear protective clothing
- You can manage cheilitis (dry mouth, cracked skin around lips, nose, and eyes) with lip balms, sugarless candy, saline nasal spray, and artificial tears
- Periodic blood tests (liver enzymes, CBC, lipid panel, glucose) will be ordered to monitor side effects
- If you have swallowing difficulties, the capsule can be chewed and swallowed
- Use caution in patients with diabetes mellitus because impaired glucose control has been reported

Key Points

- Pregnancy category X
- All patients (male and female), prescribers, wholesalers, and dispensing pharmacists must register and be active in the iPLEDGE risk management program designed to eliminate fetal exposure to isotretinoin
  - For female patients:
    - No woman should be pregnant or become pregnant when prescribed isotretinoin
    - No woman should become pregnant for at least 1 month following isotretinoin treatment
    - Female patients must have two negative pregnancy tests before a prescription for isotretinoin is written. Additionally, they are required to have a pregnancy test each month during treatment.
    - Women must have selected and committed to use two forms of contraception for 1 month prior, during, and for 1 month after isotretinoin treatment
    - Patients should not donate blood while taking isotretinoin
  - For male patients:
    - Male patients should be aware of the possibility of birth defects in an unborn child exposed to isotretinoin
    - Male patients should not donate blood while taking isotretinoin
  - Pharmacists:
    - Pharmacists should dispense no more than a 30-day supply of isotretinoin
    - Pharmacists can only fill prescriptions for isotretinoin within 7 days of the date of the "qualification"
    - No refills are permitted

Drug Class: Aminoquinolines (Antimalarial)

Introduction

Hydroxychloroquine is a medication in the class of anti-malarials and is also used to treat RA and autoimmune conditions that are not related to malaria. It is important to be familiar with the side-effect profile of this medication to know how to minimize the effects.

Mechanism of Action for the Drug Class

Interferes with digestive vacuole function within sensitive malarial parasites by increasing the pH and interfering with lysosomal degradation of hemoglobin; inhibits locomotion of neutrophils and chemotaxis of eosinophils; impairs complement-dependent antigen-antibody reactions.

Members of the Drug Class

In this section: Hydroxychloroquine
    Others: Chloroquine, primaquine

■ Hydroxychloroquine

Brand Name
Plaquenil

Generic Name
Hydroxychloroquine

Dosage Forms
Tablets

Usage
Treatment of systemic lupus erythematosus (SLE)*, treatment of RA*, suppression and treatment of malaria

Dosing
- Malaria, chemoprophylaxis: 400 mg orally once weekly; begin 2 weeks before exposure; continue for 4 weeks after leaving endemic area; if suppressive therapy is not begun before the exposure, double the initial dose and give in two doses, 6 hours apart, and continue treatment for 8 weeks
- Malaria, acute attack: 800 mg orally initially, followed by 400 mg at 6, 24, and 48 hours
- RA: Initial: 400–600 mg orally daily; increase dose gradually until optimum response level is reached; usually after 4–12 weeks dose should be reduced by half to a maintenance dose of 200–400 mg/day
- SLE: 400 mg orally once or twice daily until remission; 200–400 mg once daily for maintenance therapy

Adverse Reactions: Most Common
- Skin pigmentation changes (blue/back), nausea, vomiting, diarrhea, myopathy, headache, corneal changes

Adverse Reactions: Rare/Severe/Important
- Torsades de pointes, agranulocytosis, retinopathy, ototoxicity (night blindness, blurred vision)

Major Drug Interactions
Drug Affecting Hydroxychloroquine
- Aurothioglucose: Additive risk of blood dyscrasias

Hydroxychloroquine's Effect on Other Drugs
- Digoxin: Increased serum digoxin concentrations
- Mefloquine: Increased risk of seizures and QT interval prolongation
- Metoprolol: Increased plasma levels of metoprolol

Counseling Points
- Obtain ophthalmic examinations every 3 months if using this medication over extended periods
- This medication may increase sensitivity to sunlight. Therefore, wear dark glasses and protective clothing, use sunblock, and avoid direct exposure to sunlight.
- GI side effects are short-lived and typically managed by taking the medication with food

Key Points
- Monitoring is needed to avoid severe side effects
- This agent is not preferred as first-line in prevention and treatment of malaria
- Hydroxychloroquine is considered the least potent synthetic DMARD and is the most common DMARD to be combined with methotrexate when required in RA

Drug Class: Anticholinergic/Anti-Parkinson's

Introduction

Benztropine is an anticholinergic agent used in the treatment of Parkinson's disease and in the treatment and prevention of extrapyramidal symptoms. Its use in the treatment of extrapyramidal symptoms has decreased since the introduction of atypical antipsychotic agents.

Mechanism of Action of the Drug Class

Decreases the activity of acetylcholine to balance out the production of dopamine and acetylcholine; may inhibit the reuptake and storage of dopamine, thereby prolonging the action of dopamine.

Members of the Drug Class

In this section: Benztropine
    Others: Orphenadrine, trihexyphenidyl

■ Benztropine

Brand Name
Cogentin

Generic Name
Benztropine

Dosage Forms
Tablets, injection

Usage
Adjunctive treatment of Parkinson's disease*, treatment of drug-induced extrapyramidal symptoms*

Dosing
- Drug-induced extrapyramidal symptoms: Oral/IM/IV: 1–4 mg once or twice daily
- Parkinsonism: Oral/IM/IV: 1–2 mg/day (range: 0.5–6 mg/day)

Adverse Reactions: Most Common
- Tachyarrhythmia, constipation, nausea, xerostomia, blurred vision, urinary retention

Adverse Reactions: Rare/Severe/Important
- Heat stroke, hyperthermia, paralytic ileus, confusion, increased intraocular pressure, mood or mental changes

Major Drug Interactions

Drugs Affecting Benztropine
- Agents with anticholinergic activity: Additive anticholinergic side effects
- Ethanol: Increased CNS depression

Benztropine's Effect on Other Drugs
- Potassium chloride: Increased risk of GI lesions

Contraindications
- Pyloric or duodenal obstruction, stenosing peptic ulcers, bladder neck obstructions, achalasia, myasthenia gravis, children <3 years of age

Counseling Points
- Because this drug may impair heat regulation, advise patient to use caution with activities that lead to an increased body temperature
- Patient may experience drowsiness, dizziness, and blurry vision
- Avoid alcohol during treatment with benztropine

Key Points
- Anticholinergic side effects of this medication are common. Therefore, benztropine should not be used long-term.
- Avoid use in older patients due to an increased risk of confusion and hallucinations
- Benztropine is most effective for relieving tremor and/or rigidity rather than bradykinesia

---

Drug Class: Antiemetic/Antivertigo

Introduction
This medication is an antihistamine used to treat and prevent nausea and vomiting due to motion sickness.

Mechanism of Action for the Drug Class
Centrally acting agent with anticholinergic, antihistaminic, and antiemetic activity; decreases the excitability of the labyrinth of the middle ear and blocks conduction of the middle ear vestibular pathways.

Members of the Drug Class
In this section: Meclizine
    Others: Cyclizine, dimenhydrinate, promethazine, scopolamine

■ Meclizine

Brand Names
Antivert, Bonine (OTC), Dramamine II (OTC)

Generic Name
Meclizine

Dosage Forms
Tablets, chewable tablets

Usage
Prevention and treatment of motion sickness and vertigo

Dosing
- Motion sickness: 12.5–50 mg orally 1 hour before travel; repeat, if necessary at 24-hour intervals
- Vertigo: 25–100 mg orally daily in divided doses, depending on clinical response

Adverse Reactions: Most Common
- Drowsiness, dry mouth, nausea, constipation, blurred vision, tinnitus

Adverse Reactions: Rare/Severe/Important
- Cholestatic jaundice, auditory and visual hallucinations

Major Drug Interactions

Drugs Affecting Meclizine
- CNS depressant agents: Additive sedation
- Anticholinergic agents: Additive anticholinergic effects

Counseling Points
- Meclizine may impair the ability to perform hazardous activities requiring mental alertness or physical coordination, including driving and operation of heavy machinery
- Avoid alcohol while using meclizine

Key Points
- Meclizine should only be used for mild–moderate motion sickness because other medications are more effective for severe conditions
- Meclizine should be used for prevention of motion sickness rather than treatment
- Drowsiness is a common side effect of meclizine

Drug Class: Antigout Agent

Introduction
Colchicine is an antimitotic drug that is highly effective at relieving acute gout attacks.

Mechanism of Action for the Drug Class
Reduces deposition of urate crystals by decreasing leukocyte motility, phagocytosis in joints, and lactic acid production.

■ Colchicine

Brand Names
Colcrys, Colsalide

Generic Name
Colchicine

Dosage Forms
Tablets

Usage
Treatment of acute gout attacks and prophylaxis*, treatment of familial Mediterranean fever

Dosing
- Gout treatment: 1.2 mg orally at first sign of a flare, followed by 0.6 mg 1 hour later; maximum: 1.8 mg over 1 hour
- Gout prophylaxis: 0.6 mg orally twice daily; maximum: 1.2 mg/day
- Familial Mediterranean fever: 1.2–2.4 mg orally daily
- Renal dosage adjustment:
  ○ Doses are adjusted for CrCl <80 ml/minute

Adverse Reactions: Most Common
- Nausea, vomiting, diarrhea

Adverse Reactions: Rare/Severe/Important
- Myelosuppression, neuromyopathy

Major Drug Interactions

Drugs Affecting Colchicine
- CYP3A4 and p-glycoprotein inhibitors (i.e., azole antifungals, cyclosporine, macrolides, diltiazem, verapamil, protease inhibitors): Increased colchicine concentrations and increased risk of toxicity
- Digoxin: Increased colchicine concentration
- P-glycoprotein inducers: Decreased colchicine concentration and effectiveness

Colchicine's Effect on Other Drugs
- HMG-CoA reductase inhibitors (rosuvastatin excluded): Increased risk of rhabdomyolysis
- Fibric acid derivatives: Increased risk of rhabdomyolysis

Contraindications
- Concomitant use of p-glycoprotein or strong CYP3A4 inhibitors in the presence of hepatic or renal impairment

Counseling Point
- A low purine diet and adequate hydration is recommended to decrease the frequency of gout attacks

Key Points
- Dose needs to be adjusted in patients with renal dysfunction
- Doses may be given at less frequent intervals if used in combination with CYP3A4 inhibitors
- The most common side effect of colchicine is diarrhea. Lower doses may help to decrease GI side effects.

Introduction

Allopurinol is a xanthine oxidase inhibitor used to prevent gout attacks and treat high uric acid levels in patients receiving chemotherapy.

Mechanism of Action for the Drug Class

Decreases the production of uric acid by blocking the action of xanthine oxidase, an enzyme that converts hypoxanthine to xanthine and xanthine to uric acid.

Members of the Drug Class

In this section: Allopurinol
   Other: Febuxostat

■ Allopurinol

Brand Name

Zyloprim

Generic Name

Allopurinol

Dosage Forms

Tablets, injection (powder for reconstitution)

Usage

Prevention of gout attacks*, treatment of secondary hyperuricemia associated with chemotherapy (tumor lysis syndrome), prevention of recurrent calcium oxalate calculi

Dosing

- Mild gout: 100–300 mg orally daily as a single or divided dose
- Moderate–severe gout: 400–600 mg orally daily as a single or divided dose; maximum: 800 mg/day
- Renal dosage adjustments:
  - Doses are adjusted with CrCl <20 ml/minute and individualized based on serum uric acid levels

Adverse Reactions: Most Common

- Maculopapular rash and pruritus

Adverse Reactions: Rare/Severe/Important

- Rash, Stevens–Johnson syndrome, toxic epidermal necrolysis, agranulocytosis, aplastic anemia, eosinophilia, myelosuppression, thrombocytopenia, hepatitis, renal failure

Major Drug Interactions

Drugs Affecting Allopurinol

- ACE inhibitors and thiazide diuretics: Increased risk of hypersensitivity
- Uricosurics: Decreased effectiveness of allopurinol
- Antacids: Decreased absorption of allopurinol

Allopurinol's Effect on Other Drugs

- Azathioprine: Inhibited metabolism of azathioprine; dose of azathioprine must be reduced by 50–75% to prevent severe myelosuppression
- Mercaptopurine: Inhibited metabolism of mercaptopurine; increased risk of myelosuppression
- Didanosine: Inhibited metabolism of didanosine
- Cyclosporine: Increased cyclosporine levels
- Amoxicillin/ampicillin: Increased risk of rash
- Warfarin: Enhanced anticoagulant effect of warfarin

Contraindications

- Concomitant use of didanosine

Counseling Points

- Immediately report any skin rash to physician
- Maintain adequate hydration while taking allopurinol
- Take allopurinol with food to minimize GI upset
- Report any fever, sore throat, painful urination, blood in urine, and/or swelling of mouth or lips to physician
- Avoid alcohol, caffeine, and large amounts of vitamin C during therapy
- Periodic blood tests (CBC, LFTs, uric acid level, and renal function tests) may be ordered to monitor for effectiveness and side effects

Key Points

- A common adverse reaction is rash that can occur at any time during therapy
- Reduce dosage in renal failure

Introduction

These are genetically engineered protein molecules that block the proinflammatory cytokine tumor necrosis factor (TNF)-α. These medications are used in the treatment of RA when other options fail to achieve adequate response. These agents are expensive and have many side effects.

Mechanism of Action for the Drug Class

Blocks TNF by binding to and blocking its action.

Adverse Reactions for the Drug Class: Most Common

- Injection site reaction, abdominal pain, vomiting, headache, rhinitis, upper respiratory infection

Adverse Reactions for the Drug Class: Rare/Severe/Important

- Basal cell carcinoma, erythema multiforme, Stevens-Johnson syndrome, epidermal necrolysis, anemia, leucopenia, pancytopenia, autoimmune hepatitis, tuberculosis, sepsis, malignant lymphoma, multiple sclerosis, optic neuritis

Major Drug Interactions for the Drug Class

Drugs Affecting TNF Inhibitors

- DMARDs (abatacept, anakinra, natalizumab): Increased risk of toxicities
- Live vaccines: Increased risk of developing vaccinial infections

Contraindications for the Drug Class

- Patients with sepsis and/or active infections (chronic or local)

Counseling Points for the Drug Class

- Stop medication and contact prescriber immediately if you experience stomach pain or cramping, unusual bleeding, persistent fever, rash, muscle weakness, and/or signs of respiratory infections
- Avoid receiving immunizations during therapy and for at least 3 months after therapy with TNF inhibitors

Key Points for the Drug Class

- Patients should be evaluated for latent tuberculosis infection with a tuberculin skin test before therapy
- Use caution in patients with chronic infections. If a patient develops a serious infection or sepsis, the medication should be discontinued.
- Rare reactivation of hepatitis B has occurred while receiving these agents. Evaluate before initiation and during treatment.
- Use caution in patients with heart failure because exacerbations may occur

Members of the Drug Class

In this section: Etanercept, infliximab, adalimumab
Others: Certolizumab pegol

■ Etanercept

Brand Name
Enbrel

Generic Name
Etanercept

Dosage Forms
Injection

Usage
Treatment of moderately to severely active RA*, moderately to severely active polyarticular juvenile idiopathic arthritis (JIA), psoriatic arthritis, active ankylosing spondylitis, moderate-to-severe chronic plaque psoriasis

Dosing
- RA: 25 mg SUB-Q twice weekly or 50 mg SUB-Q once weekly

■ Infliximab

Brand Name
Remicade

Generic Name
Infliximab

Dosage Forms
Injection

Usage
RA*, Crohn's disease*, ulcerative colitis, psoriatic arthritis and plaque psoriasis

Dosing
- Crohn's disease and ulcerative colitis: 5 mg/kg IV at 0, 2, and 6 weeks, followed by 5 mg/kg every 8 weeks thereafter
- RA (in combination with methotrexate): 3 mg/kg IV at 0, 2, and 6 weeks, then every 8 weeks thereafter

■ Adalimumab

Brand Name
Humira

Generic Name
Adalimumab

Dosage Forms
Injection

Usage
Moderate–severe RA*, severe Crohn's disease, plaque psoriasis, severe JIA

Dosing
- RA: 40 mg SUB-Q once every other week

Drug Class: Electrolyte Supplements

Introduction

Potassium is a major intracellular electrolyte essential for the conduction of nerve impulses. Appropriate amounts of potassium are needed for body functions.

Mechanism of Action for the Drug Class

Potassium is the major intracellular cation and is essential for the conduction of nerve impulses in the heart, brain, and skeletal muscle. Potassium maintains intracellular tonicity, contractility of cardiac, skeletal, and smooth muscle, acid/base balance, gastric secretion, and carbohydrate metabolism.

■ Potassium Chloride

Brand Names
K-Dur, K-Lor, Klor-Con, Klotrix, Kaochlor, Micro-K, Slow-K, K-Tab

Generic Name
Potassium chloride

Dosage Forms
Tablets, powder, liquid, injection

Usage
Treatment and prevention of hypokalemia*

Dosing
- Prevention of hypokalemia due to diuretic therapy: 20 to 40 mEq orally daily in one to two divided doses
- Treatment of hypokalemia:
  - Oral: Asymptomatic, mild: 40–100 mEq/day divided in two to five doses
  - Mild–moderate: 120–240 mEq/day divided in three to four doses; limit doses to 40–60 mEq/dose
  - IV: Serum potassium >2.5 mEq/L: 10 mEq/hour; maximum concentration: 40 mEq/L; maximum 24-hour dose: 200 mEq. Serum potassium <2 mEq/L: 40 mEq/hour (via central line).

Adverse Reactions: Most Common
- Nausea, vomiting, diarrhea, flatulence

Adverse Reactions: Rare/Severe/Important
- Cardiac arrest, EKG abnormalities, hyperkalemia, abdominal pain, GI ulcer

Major Drug Interactions
Drugs Affecting Potassium Chloride
- ACE inhibitors, angiotensin II receptor blockers, potassium-sparing diuretics, salt substitutes containing potassium: Increased risk of hyperkalemia

Contraindications
- Hyperkalemia, severe renal impairment with azotemia, patients with structural, pathologic, and/or pharmacologic GI delay or immobility

Counseling Points
- Sustained-release and wax matrix products need to be swallowed whole and should not be cut or crushed
- Liquid and powder preparations may be diluted in water or juice

Key Points
- Signs/symptoms of hypokalemia include weakness, fatigue, tetany, polydipsia
- Potassium chloride concentrate for injections must be diluted before use. Numerous fatalities have occurred with patients accidentally receiving undiluted potassium chloride concentration. Potassium chloride concentrate should only be stored in a pharmacy and diluted in appropriate volume before dispensing.
- Infusions of potassium chloride have the following maximum parameters:
  - Maximum infusion rate: 40 mEq/hour (central line)
  - Maximum concentration: 80 mEq/liter
  - Maximum 24-hour dose: 400 mEq
- IV doses should be incorporated into the patient's maintenance IV fluids
- Intermittent IV potassium administration should be reserved for patients with severe depletion and with concurrent EKG monitoring

---

Drug Class: Phosphodiesterase Inhibitors/Erectile Dysfunction Agents

Introduction
These agents are usually used first-line for the treatment of erectile dysfunction. They have a convenient route of administration, low incidence of side effects, and are effective.

Mechanism of Action for the Drug Class
Inhibits phosphodiesterase (PDE) 5 leading to increased levels of cyclic guanosine monophosphate and enhancing smooth muscle relaxation in the corpus cavernosum of the penis and smooth muscle of the pulmonary vasculature. Overall, these agents enhance the nitric oxide–induced relaxation of penile vascular smooth muscle.

Usage for the Drug Class
Treatment of erectile dysfunction*, pulmonary arterial hypertension

Adverse Reactions for the Drug Class: Most Common
- Headache, flushing, dizziness, rhinitis, visual abnormalities (inability to distinguish between blue and green colors)

Adverse Reactions for the Drug Class: Rare/Severe/Important
- Chest pain, myocardial infarction, prolonged QT interval, seizure, optic neuropathy, decreased hearing, sudden hearing loss, priapism

Major Drug Interactions
Drugs Affecting Phosphodiesterase Inhibitors
- Potent CYP3A4 inhibitors (i.e., protease inhibitors, erythromycin, azole antifungals): Increased levels of phosphodiesterase inhibitors

- Nitrates: Potentiates vasodilation whereby potentially fatal hypotension can occur
- Antihypertensives: Potentiates antihypertensive effect

Contraindications for the Drug Class
- Concomitant use of organic nitrates of any kind

Counseling Points for the Drug Class
- PDE5 inhibitors offer no protection against sexually transmitted diseases
- These agents are ineffective in the absence of sexual arousal
- Do not take if you are using any form of nitrate
- Be aware of signs of low blood pressure such as dizziness and unsteadiness
- Priapism (prolonged erection >6 hours) is a medical emergency. Seek immediate medical attention.
- Do not engage in sexual activity if clinically inadvisable

Key Point for the Drug Class
- Nitrates are contraindicated while using phosphodiesterase inhibitors

Members of the Drug Class
In this section: Sildenafil, tadalafil
   Other: Vardenafil

■ Sildenafil

Brand Names
Viagra, Revatio

Generic Name
Sildenafil

Dosage Forms
Tablets

Dosing
- Erectile dysfunction: 25–100 mg (50 mg usual dose) orally a half hour to 4 hours before anticipated sexual activity (25 mg in patients ≥65 years old); maximum dose: 100 mg daily
- Pulmonary arterial hypertension (Revatio only): 20 mg orally three times daily
- Renal dosage adjustment:
  - Dose is adjusted for CrCl <30 ml/minute
- Hepatic dosage adjustment:
  - Dose is adjusted for hepatic impairment and/or concomitant use of potent CYP3A4 inhibitors
- Concomitant α-blocker dose adjustment:
  - Initiate at the lowest dose possible and titrate carefully

■ Tadalafil

Brand Names
Cialis, Adcirca

Generic Name
Tadalafil

Dosage Forms
Tablets

Dosing
- Erectile dysfunction: 10 mg orally at least 30 minutes before anticipated sexual activity (maximum dose: 20 mg) or 2.5 mg orally daily (maximum dose: 5 mg)
- Pulmonary arterial hypertension (Adcirca) only: 40 mg orally daily
- Renal dose adjustment:
  - Dose is adjusted for CrCl <50 ml/minute
- Hepatic dosage adjustment:
  - Dose is adjusted for hepatic impairment and/or concomitant use of potent CYP3A4 inhibitors

---

Drug Class: Immunosuppressant Agents/Calcineurin Inhibitors

Introduction
These medications are the backbone of organ transplant immunosuppression.

Mechanism of Action for the Drug Class
Inhibit interleukin-2 production and subsequently T-cell differentiation and proliferation thus preventing allograft rejection.

Members of the Drug Class
In this section: Cyclosporine, tacrolimus

■ Cyclosporine

Brand Names
Gengraf, Neoral, Restasis, Sandimmune

Generic Name
Cyclosporine

Dosage Forms
Capsules, oral solution, injection

Usage
- Prevention of organ transplant rejection*, RA arthritis, psoriasis.
- Increase tear production (Restasis only)

Dosing
- Prevention of organ transplant rejection:
  - Oral: 8–18 mg/kg in two divided doses depending on type of transplant. Subsequent doses are adjusted based on serum concentrations.
  - IV: A third of the oral dose infused over 2–6 hours
- RA: 2.5 mg/kg per day in two divided doses; dose is titrated based on response (maximum dose: 4 mg/kg per day)

- Psoriasis: 2.5 mg/kg per day in two divided doses; dose is titrated based on response (maximum dose: 4 mg/kg per day)
- Renal dosage adjustment:
  - Adjust dose to maintain lower cyclosporine blood trough concentrations

Adverse Reactions: Most Common
- Hypertension, hirsutism, gingival hyperplasia, headache, tremor, burning sensation in eyes

Adverse Reactions: Rare/Severe/Important
- Hyperkalemia, hypomagnesemia, hepatotoxicity, coma, encephalopathy, leukoencephalopathy, seizure, hemolytic uremic syndrome, nephrotoxicity

Major Drug Interactions
Drugs Affecting Cyclosporine
- CYP3A4 inducers (i.e., phenytoin, phenobarbital, carbamazepine, rifampin, nevirapine, St. John's wort): Decreased cyclosporine blood concentrations
- CYP3A4 inhibitors (i.e., azole antifungals, amiodarone, macrolide antibiotics, diltiazem, verapamil, ritonavir, grapefruit juice): Increased cyclosporine toxicity
- Allopurinol: Increased cyclosporine toxicity
- Vancomycin, aminoglycosides, ACE inhibitors, colchicine: May potentiate renal dysfunction

Cyclosporine's Effect on Other Drugs
- HMG-CoA reductase inhibitors: Increased HMG-CoA reductase inhibitor concentrations that places patients at an increased risk of rhabdomyolysis
- Digoxin: Increased digoxin levels

Contraindications
- Psoriasis or RA patients with abnormal renal function, uncontrolled hypertension, or malignancy
- Concomitant use with pulsed ultraviolet actinotherapy or ultraviolet B therapy, methotrexate, or other immunosuppressant agents, coal tar, or radiation therapy in psoriasis patients

Counseling Points
- Take prescribed dose at the same time each day with meals
- When administering the solution, mix with water or orange juice in a glass, not plastic, container, then stir and drink all at once
- Avoid grapefruit and grapefruit juice, which can affect the metabolism of cyclosporine
- Avoid live attenuated vaccines
- Frequent laboratory monitoring will be needed

Key Points
- Sandimmune capsules and oral solution have decreased bioavailability when compared with Neoral

formulations. Sandimmune and Neoral are not bioequivalent. Recommend frequent cyclosporine blood trough concentration monitoring (every 4–7 days until stable blood trough levels are achieved) when switching between products.
- Cyclosporine dose adjustments should be made in small increments (about a 25% change at any one time)

◼ Tacrolimus
Brand Names
Prograf, Protopic

Generic Name
Tacrolimus

Dosage Forms
Capsules, ointment, injection

Usage
Prevention of organ transplant rejection*, prevention of graft-versus-host disease, moderate–severe atopic dermatitis

Dosing
- Prevention of organ transplant rejection:
  - Oral: 0.075–0.2 mg/kg per day in two divided doses depending on type of transplant
  - IV: 0.03–0.05 mg/kg per day as a continuous infusion

Adverse Reactions: Most Common
- Alopecia, erythema of skin, pruritus, constipation, diarrhea, nausea, vomiting, anemia, leukocytosis, thrombocytopenia, headache, insomnia, paresthesia, tremor

Adverse Reactions: Rare/Severe/Important
- Hypertension, prolonged QT interval, diabetes mellitus, hypomagnesemia, anaphylaxis, infectious disease, lymphoma, seizure, leukoencephalopathy, nephrotoxicity

Major Drug Interactions
Drugs Affecting Tacrolimus
- Potent CYP3A4 inhibitors: Increased tacrolimus toxicity
- Potent CYP3A4 inducers: Decreased concentration of tacrolimus

Counseling Points
- Take prescribed dose at the same time each day. Tacrolimus may be taken with or without food as long as you are consistent.
- Avoid grapefruit or grapefruit juice, which can affect the metabolism of tacrolimus
- Avoid live attenuated vaccines
- Frequent laboratory monitoring will be needed

Drug Class: Urinary Analgesic

Introduction
This medication is used for the treatment of symptoms associated with urinary tract infections.

Mechanism of Action for the Drug Class
This agent is an azo dye that provides local anesthetic and analgesic actions on the urinary mucosa for patients with a urinary tract infection.

■ Phenazopyridine

Brand Names
Pyridium, Azo-Standard [OTC], Prodium [OTC]

Generic Name
Phenazopyridine

Dosage Forms
Tablets

Usage
Symptomatic relief of dysuria*

Dosing
- Oral: 100–200 mg three times daily after meals for 2 days when used concomitantly with an antibiotic
- Renal dosage adjustment:
    ○ Dosing interval is adjusted for CrCl ≤80 ml/minute. Avoid use in patients with CrCl <50 ml/minute.

Adverse Reactions: Most Common
- Headache, pruritus, GI disturbances, anaphylactoid reaction

Adverse Reactions: Rare/Severe/Important
- Hemolytic anemia, hepatotoxicity, nephrotoxicity

Major Drug Interactions
- No known significant drug interactions

Contraindications
- Renal or hepatic disease

Counseling Points
- Take with food to lessen gastric irritation
- Phenazopyridine may discolor urine and sclera red or orange, leading to staining of contact lenses and undergarments. Tablets may also stain clothing. Any discoloration is harmless.

Key Points
- Phenazopyridine is only effective for relief of symptoms
- Phenazopyridine will discolor urine and can interfere with urine dipstick tests to diagnose urinary tract infections

Drug Class: Smoking Cessation Aids

Introduction
The most commonly used drugs in this class are the nicotine replacement agents. These are available in different dosage forms to allow better compliance depending on patients' preference.

Member of the Drug Class
In this section: Nicotine, Varenicline
    Others: None

■ Nicotine

Brand Names
Nicorette (gum), Thrive (gum), Commit (lozenge), Habitrol (patch), NicoDerm CQ (patch), Nicotrol OTC (patch), Nicotrol NS (nasal spray), Nicotrol Inhaler (inhaler)

Generic Name
Nicotine

Dosage Forms
Gum, lozenges, patches, nasal spray, oral inhaler

Mechanism of Action
Nicotine replacement agents provide smaller amounts of nicotine than those found in cigarettes in an effort to prevent or reduce withdrawal symptoms.

Usage
Smoking cessation aid for the relief of nicotine withdrawal symptoms and craving*

Dosing
- Nicorette gum:
    ○ Initial dose: 4-mg gum for persons smoking >25 cigarettes daily; 2-mg gum for persons smoking <25 cigarettes daily
    ○ Maintenance dose: 4-mg gum: 9–12 pieces a day; 2-mg gum: 9–12 pieces a day; may use 4-mg gum chews in patients not responding to 2-mg gum chews
    ○ Duration of therapy: 2–6 months; attempt to wean and stop therapy by month 4 or 6
    ○ Maximum dose: 4-mg gum, 20 pieces a day; 2-mg gum, 30 pieces a day

- Commit lozenge:
  - Initial dose: 2-mg lozenge for persons who normally smoke after 30 minutes of awakening in the morning; 4-mg lozenge for persons who normally smoke within 30 minutes of awakening; start with ≥9 lozenges/day for 6 weeks
  - Maintenance dose: ≥9 lozenges/day for up to 12 weeks
  - Maximum dose: 5 lozenges within 6 hours, 20 lozenges/day
- Habitrol and NicoDerm patch:
  - Initial dose: One 21-mg patch applied daily for 6 weeks
  - Maintenance dose: One 14-mg patch applied daily for 2–4 weeks, then one 7-mg patch applied daily for 2–4 weeks
- Nicotrol patch:
  - Initial dose: One 15-mg patch applied daily for 12 weeks
  - Maintenance dose: One 10-mg patch applied daily for 2–4 weeks, then one 5-mg patch daily for 2–4 weeks
- NicoDerm CQ patch:
  - Initial dose: One 21-mg patch applied daily (>10 cigarettes/day) or one 14-mg patch applied daily (<10 cigarettes/day)
  - Maintenance dose: One 21-mg patch applied daily for 6 weeks, then one 14-mg patch daily for 2 weeks, then one 7-mg patch daily for 2 weeks, then discontinue
  - Low-dose regimen: One 14-mg patch applied daily for 6 weeks, then one 7-mg patch daily for 2 weeks, then discontinue
- Nicotrol NS nasal spray:
  - Initial dose: One dose equals 1 mg (given as 2 sprays total, One in each nostril). Initial dose is one to two doses (1–2 mg)/hour with a minimum of 8 mg/day
  - Maintenance dose: Individualized for a duration of 3 months
  - Maximum dose: 5 mg (10 sprays)/hour, 40 mg (80 sprays)/day
- Nicotrol Inhaler oral inhaler:
  - Initial dose: 6–16 cartridges daily
  - Maintenance dose: Individualized for 3 months, then tapered over an additional 6–12 weeks
  - Maximum dose: 16 cartridges/day for 12 weeks before tapering

Adverse Reactions: Most Common
- Nausea, vomiting, palpitations, tachycardia, insomnia, headache, hypertension, insomnia
- Nicorette gum: Stomatitis, glossitis, pharyngitis, taste perversion, aphthous ulcers, gingivitis

Adverse Reactions: Rare/Severe/Important
- None

Contraindications
- Hypersensitivity

Counseling Points
- Nicorette gum:
  - Chew gum slowly until a tingling sensation occurs; then rest in buccal cavity. When tingling subsides, chew again until tingling returns. Intermittent chewing slows absorption and risk of side effects.
  - Avoid eating or drinking 15 minutes before chewing or while chewing
- Commit lozenges:
  - Avoid eating or drinking 15 minutes before using a lozenge or while using a lozenge
  - Do not chew or swallow the lozenge. Minimize swallowing while dissolving the lozenge.
- Nicotine patches:
  - Apply patch to clean, hairless, dry skin without cuts or scratches on upper body
  - Wash site of application with water only because soap will increase absorption
  - Dispose of patches and gum carefully and out of reach of children and pets
  - Nicotrol: Remove patch at bedtime
  - NicoDerm CQ: Wear patch 24 hours/day; when replacing new system, apply to a new site; avoid reusing same site more than once per week
- All types: Stop smoking completely while using nicotine aids

Key Points
- Caution using in patients with GI ulcers because nicotine may delay healing
- Avoid in patients immediately post myocardial infarction, with life-threatening arrhythmias, and/or with worsening angina

■ Varenicline

Brand Name
Chantix

Generic Name
Varenicline

Dosage Forms
Tablets

Mechanism of Action
Varenicline is a partial neuronal $\alpha_4 \beta_2$ nicotinic receptor agonist that prevents nicotine stimulation of mesolimbic dopamine system associated with nicotine addiction.

Usage
Treatment of smoking cessation*

Dosing
- 0.5 mg orally once daily from days 1 through 3, then 0.5 mg orally twice daily from days 4 through 7, then 1 mg orally twice daily
- Renal dosage adjustments:
  - Dose is adjusted in patients with CrCl <30 ml/minute

Adverse Reactions: Most Common

- Constipation, flatulence, nausea, vomiting, dream disorder, headache, insomnia

Adverse Reaction: Rare/Severe/Important

- Abnormal behavior, suicidal ideation

Major Drug Interactions

- No known significant drug interactions

Contraindications

- Specific contraindications have not been established

Counseling Points

- Start medication 1 week before quit date
- Report persistent symptoms (depression, suicide ideation, or emotional/behavioral changes)

Key Point

- Patients with a history of psychiatric disorders should not receive this medication

---

Drug Class: Overactive Bladder Agents/Anticholinergic and Antispasmodic

Introduction

Anticholinergic and antispasmodic drugs are agents used to suppress premature detrusor contractions, enhance bladder storage, and relieve urge urinary incontinence symptoms and complications.

Members of the Drug Class

In this section: Tolterodine, oxybutynin
    Others: None

■ Tolterodine

Brand Names
Detrol, Detrol LA

Generic Name
Tolterodine

Dosage Forms
Tablets, capsules

Mechanism of Action (Anticholinergic)
Competitively antagonizes muscarinic receptors causing the detrusor muscle to relax and thus reduce the frequency and intensity of contractions of the bladder.

Usage
Overactive bladder*

Dosing

- Immediate-release tablet: 1–2 mg orally twice daily depending on tolerability and response
- Extended-release capsule: 2–4 mg orally daily depending on tolerability and response
- Renal dosage adjustment:
  - Doses are adjusted for patients with CrCl ≤30 ml/minute
- Hepatic dosage adjustment:
  - Doses are adjusted in patients with severe hepatic impairment and/or when tolterodine is used concomitantly with potent CYP3A4 inhibitors

Adverse Reactions: Most Common

- Constipation, xerostomia, headache

Adverse Reactions: Rare/Severe/Important

- Anaphylactoid reaction, dementia, memory impairment, angioedema

Major Drug Interactions

Drugs Affecting Tolterodine

- Anticholinergic agents: Additive anticholinergic side effects
- CYP3A4 and 2D6 inhibitors: Increased anticholinergic side effects
- CYP3A4 and 2D6 inducers: Increased metabolism of tolterodine
- Warfarin: May increase the effects of warfarin

Contraindications

- Urinary retention, gastric retention, uncontrolled narrow-angle glaucoma

Counseling Points

- Do not crush or chew extended-release capsules
- Drink water or eat sugarless candy to lessen dry mouth effects
- Exercise caution with driving because this medication may cause sedation

Key Points

- Anticholinergic side effects are common with tolterodine
- Tolterodine is a major substrate of CYP3A4 and 2D6

■ Oxybutynin

Brand Names
Ditropan, Ditropan XL, Oxytrol

Generic Name
Oxybutynin

Dosage Forms
Gel, patch, syrup, tablets

Mechanism of Action (Antispasmodic)
Inhibits the action of acetylcholine on smooth muscle; direct antispasmodic effect on smooth muscle.

Usage
Overactive bladder*, neurogenic bladder*

Dosing
- Regular-release tablets: 5 mg orally two to three times daily up to maximum of 5 mg orally four times a day
- Extended-release tablets: Initial: 5–10 mg orally once daily; adjust dose in 5-mg increments at weekly intervals; maximum: 30 mg daily
- Topical gel: Apply contents of 1 sachet (100 mg/g) once daily
- Transdermal: Apply one 3.9 mg/day patch twice weekly (every 3–4 days)

Adverse Reactions: Most Common
- Anticholinergic (dry mouth, xerophthalmia, blurred vision, constipation, delirium), headache, dizziness, sedation

Adverse Reactions: Rare/Severe/Important
- Tachycardia, hallucinations, mydriasis

Major Drug Interactions
Drugs Affecting Oxybutynin
- Anticholinergic: Additive anticholinergic side effects

Contraindications
- Uncontrolled narrow-angle glaucoma, urinary retention, gastric retention or conditions with severely decreased GI motility

Counseling Points
- Transdermal: Apply to clean, dry skin on abdomen, hip, or buttocks. Select a new site for each new system, avoiding reapplication to the same site within 7 days.
- Topical gel: Apply to clean, dry, intact skin on abdomen, thighs, or upper arms/shoulders. Rotate site; do not apply to same site on consecutive days. Wash hands after use. Cover treated area with clothing after gel has dried to prevent transfer of medication to others. Do not bathe, shower, or swim until 1 hour after gel is applied.

Key Point
- Anticholinergic side effects are common

Review Questions

1. Which of the following adverse reactions can be caused by isotretinoin?
   A. Myalgias
   B. Photosensitivity
   C. Hypertriglyceridemia
   D. All of the above

2. Which of the following are indications for a 5-alpha reductase inhibitor?
   A. BPH
   B. Erectile dysfunction
   C. Male pattern hair loss
   D. A and C are correct

3. All of the following statements are true regarding hydroxychloroquine except
   A. Commonly used for the treatment of rheumatoid arthritis.
   B. Regular ophthalmic exams are recommended.
   C. There are no drug interactions with hydroxychloroquine.
   D. The use of sunscreen is recommended while on this medication.

4. Which of the following medications will interact with tolterodine?
   A. Azole antifungals
   B. Phenytoin
   C. Oxybutynin
   D. All of the above

5. Which of the following statements about Colcrys is false?
   A. Does not need to be renally adjusted.
   B. Is a major substrate of CYP3A4.
   C. Most common side effects is GI upset.
   D. Used for the treatment and prevention of gout attacks.

6. Which of the following adverse reactions can occur while receiving infliximab?
   A. Reactivation of hepatitis B
   B. Reactivation of TB
   C. Sepsis
   D. All of the above are correct

7. All of the following are true regarding potassium chloride except
    A. High doses require EKG monitoring
    B. GI upset is a common adverse reaction
    C. Potassium chloride concentrate for injections does not need to be diluted before use
    D. The maximum infusion rate is 40 mEq/hour (central line)

8. All of the following are counseling points about tadalafil except
    A. Do not take if you are using any form of nitrate
    B. Ineffective in the absence of sexual arousal
    C. It may decrease blood pressure and cause dizziness and unsteadiness
    D. Priapism (prolonged erection >6 hours) is common and does not need medical attention

9. All of the following are common adverse reactions of cyclosporine except
    A. Hypertension
    B. Malignancies
    C. Nausea and vomiting
    D. Nephrotoxicity

10. All of the following are important counseling points about Pyridium except
    A. It is a local anesthetic
    B. Take with food
    C. Therapy is usually for 2–3 days
    D. Urine discoloration is a sign of a severe adverse reaction

11. All of the following are important counseling points about varenicline except
    A. Dose is 0.5 mg orally once daily on days 1–3, 0.5 mg orally twice daily on days 4–7, then 1 mg orally twice daily
    B. Insomnia and headaches are common side effects
    C. It should be started the day you are planning to quit smoking
    D. Report any signs of depression

12. Which of the following doses of benztropine are correct for the treatment of drug-induced extrapyramidal symptoms?
    A. 1–4 mg/dose orally one to two times a day
    B. 0.5–2 mg/kg/day orally in two divided doses for 15–20 weeks
    C. 25–100 mg orally daily in divided doses
    D. 200–300 mg orally daily

13. All of the following statements about Cogentin are true except
    A. It has anticholinergic properties.
    B. Used in the treatment of Parkinson's disease.
    C. Used in the treatment of extrapyramidal symptoms.
    D. Used in the treatment of depression.

14. Which of the following is not part of the mechanism of action of Antivert?
    A. Anticholinergic
    B. Antiemetic
    C. Antihistaminic
    D. Anti-inflammatory

15. Which of the following agents is not an anti-TNF agent?
    A. Enbrel
    B. Humira
    C. Sandimmune
    D. Remicade

Ophthalmic Products

Jamila Stanton, PharmD, BCPS

Proper Administration of Ophthalmic Products

Proper instillation of all eye solutions, suspensions, and ointments is necessary for optimal efficacy and prevention of superinfection. Refer to the techniques provided here for all ophthalmic solutions, suspensions, and ointments. Follow these recommended procedures for application of ophthalmic solutions:

- Wash hands thoroughly before administration
- Tilt head back or lie down and gaze upward
- Place medication in conjunctival sac and close eyes; do not blink
- Apply light finger pressure on lacrimal sac (corner of eye near nose) for 1 minute following instillation; this is called "nasolacrimal occlusion" (NLO)
- If more than one type of ophthalmic solution is used, wait at least 5 minutes before administering second agent
- To avoid contamination, do not touch tip of container to eye or any surface

Recommended procedures for application of ophthalmic suspensions are as follows:

- Shake bottle before instillation
- Follow steps for application of ophthalmic solution

These are the recommended procedures for application of ophthalmic ointments:

- Wash hands thoroughly before administration
- Hold the ointment tube in your hand for a few minutes to warm ointment and facilitate flow
- When opening tube for the first time, squeeze out and discard the first 0.25 inches of ointment
- Tilt head backward or lie down and gaze upward
- Gently pull down lower lid to form a pouch
- Place 0.25–0.5 inch of ointment in sweeping motion inside the lower eyelid
- To avoid contamination, do not touch tip of container to eye or any surface
- Close the eye for 1 or 2 minutes and roll the eyeball in all directions
- If more than one type of ointment is needed, wait at least 10 minutes before administering second agent
- Vision may be blurry for up to 20 minutes following administration of ophthalmic ointments

---

Drug Class: Antibiotic, Ophthalmic

Introduction

Ophthalmic antibacterial agents are active against a variety of Gram-positive and Gram-negative organisms. They are generally used to treat ocular infections involving the conjunctiva or cornea, such as conjunctivitis, keratitis, corneal ulcers, and blepharitis. Many different combination preparations are available on the U.S. market, so particular caution should be exercised when dispensing these products with regard to the selected agent(s), strength, and formulation. In addition, the dosage and frequency of administration varies with each agent; individual package labeling is a useful reference for pharmacists. In general, the risk of superinfection is high when using topical ophthalmic antibiotics due to contamination of the container (dropper, tube, etc.). Proper administration technique is an important counseling point to help reduce the incidence of superinfection (see the beginning of the chapter for the proper administration technique of ophthalmic products). Patients being treated for bacterial conjunctivitis, the most common indication, should be advised not to wear contact lenses until the infection is completely resolved. Disposable lenses should be thrown away, and a new pair should be started. Non-disposable lenses should be thoroughly cleaned before reinsertion following an eye infection. Using a new contact lens case is also recommended.

Members of the Drug Class

In this section: Neomycin/polymyxin B sulfate/gramicidin (combination product), ciprofloxacin, ofloxacin, erythromycin, tobramycin (in combination)

Others: Multiple mono and combination products are available containing the following antibacterial agents: Chloramphenicol, gentamicin, bacitracin, levofloxacin, gatifloxacin, moxifloxacin, tetracycline, trimethoprim, sulfisoxazole, sulfacetamide

Neomycin/Polymyxin B Sulfate/Gramicidin

Brand Name
Neosporin

Generic Name
Neomycin/polymyxin B sulfate/gramicidin

Dosage Forms
Solution

Mechanism of Action
Interferes with bacterial protein synthesis by binding to 30S ribosomal subunits; binds to phospholipids and alters permeability of the bacterial membrane permitting leakage of intracellular contents.

Usage
Treatment of superficial infections due to strains of microorganisms susceptible to the antibiotic in conditions such as conjunctivitis and blepharitis*

Dosing
Instill 1 or 2 drops in the affected eye every 4–6 hours

Adverse Reactions: Most Common
- Superinfection, transient burning, stinging, irritation upon instillation

Adverse Reactions: Rare/Severe/Important
- Redness, irritation, swelling, decreased vision, sensitivity reaction

Counseling Points
- For ophthalmic use only
- To avoid contamination, do not touch tip of container to eye or any other surface

Key Points
- Combination antibiotics are used for a variety of ophthalmic infections
- Common adverse effects, including stinging, irritation, and burning, are usually transient and not harmful
- Products containing neomycin have been specifically linked to cutaneous sensitization reactions, which manifest as itching, reddening, and edema of the conjunctiva and eyelid or failure of infection to heal

■ Ciprofloxacin

Brand Name
Ciloxan

Generic Name
Ciprofloxacin

Dosage Forms
Solution, ointment

Mechanism of Action
Fluoroquinolones work by inhibiting the activity of DNA gyrase, an enzyme that is needed for replication of bacterial DNA.

Usage
Treatment of superficial ocular infections, including conjunctivitis and corneal ulcers, due to strains of microorganisms susceptible to the antibiotic*

Dosing
- Corneal ulcers:
  - Day 1: Instill 2 drops into the affected eye every 15 minutes for the first 6 hours and then 2 drops into the affected eye every 30 minutes for the remainder of the day
  - Day 2: Instill 2 drops into the affected eye hourly
  - Days 3–14: Instill 2 drops into the affected eye every 4 hours
- Bacterial conjunctivitis:
  - Days 1–2: Solution: Instill 1 or 2 drops in the conjunctival sac every 2 hours while awake
  - Days 3–7: Solution: Instill 1 or 2 drops in the conjunctival sac every 4 hours
  - Days 1–2: Ointment: Apply a 0.5-inch ribbon into the conjunctival sac three times a day
  - Days 3–7: Ointment: Apply a 0.5-inch ribbon into the conjunctival sac two times a day

Adverse Reactions: Most Common
- Localized discomfort and irritation, transient burning, stinging

Adverse Reactions: Rare/Severe/Important
- Redness, secondary infection, prolonged irritation, swelling, pain, itching, decreased vision, hypersensitivity

Contraindications
- Hypersensitivity to any quinolone antibiotic

Counseling Points
- For ophthalmic use only
- To avoid contamination, do not touch tip of container to eye or any other surface
- If you are being treated for bacterial conjunctivitis, do not wear contact lenses while using these medications

Key Points
- Bacterial conjunctivitis is usually self-limiting; however, use of topical antibiotics is common to help accelerate resolution, decrease spread, and prevent complications
- With a broad spectrum of activity and efficacy against Gram-positive and Gram-negative bacteria, fluoroquinolones are often overused, leading to bacterial resistance, a common concern among clinicians. They are, however, the drug of choice for treatment of corneal ulcers and conjunctivitis in contact lens wearers.

■ Ofloxacin

Brand Name
Ocuflox

Generic Name
Ofloxacin

Dosage Forms
Solution

Mechanism of Action
Fluoroquinolones work by inhibiting the activity of DNA gyrase, an enzyme that is needed for replication of bacterial DNA.

Usage
Treatment of superficial ocular infections, including conjunctivitis and corneal ulcers, due to strains of microorganisms susceptible to the antibiotic*

Dosing
- Bacterial corneal ulcer
  - Days 1 and 2: Instill 1–2 drops in the affected eye every 30 minutes while awake and every 4 to 6 hours during normal sleeping time
  - Days 3–7 to 9: Instill 1–2 drops every hour while awake
  - Days 7–9 through treatment completion: Instill 1–2 drops four times a day
- Bacterial conjunctivitis:
  - Days 1 and 2: Instill 1–2 drops in the affected eye every 2 to 4 hours
  - Days 3–7: Instill 1–2 drops four times a day

Adverse Reactions: Most Common
- Localized discomfort and irritation, transient burning, stinging

Adverse Reactions: Rare/Severe/Important
- Redness, secondary infection, prolonged irritation, swelling, pain, itching, decreased vision, hypersensitivity

Contraindications
- Hypersensitivity to any quinolone antibiotic

Counseling Points
- For ophthalmic use only
- To avoid contamination, do not touch tip of container to eye or any other surface
- If you are being treated for bacterial conjunctivitis, do not wear contact lenses while using these medications

Key Points
- Bacterial conjunctivitis is usually self-limiting; however, use of topical antibiotics is common to help accelerate resolution, decrease spread, and prevent complications
- With a broad spectrum of activity and efficacy against Gram-positive and Gram-negative bacteria, fluoroquinolones are often overused, leading to bacterial resistance, a common concern among clinicians. They are, however, the drug of choice for treatment of corneal ulcers and conjunctivitis in contact lens wearers.

■ Erythromycin

Brand Name
Ilotycin

Generic Name
Erythromycin

Dosage Forms
Ointment

Mechanism of Action
Macrolide antibacterial agents bind to the 50S subunit of the bacterial ribosome, inhibiting RNA-dependent protein synthesis.

Usage
Treatment of superficial ocular infections involving the conjunctiva or cornea caused by organisms susceptible to the antibiotic*, prophylaxis of ophthalmia neonatorum due to *Neisseria gonorrhoeae* or *Chlamydia trachomatis*

Dosing
Apply a 0.5-inch ribbon into the conjunctival sac of the affected eye two to six times daily depending on severity

Adverse Reactions: Most Common
- Blurred vision for the first few minutes after instillation, transient minor irritation and redness upon instillation

Adverse Reactions: Rare/Severe/Important
- Decreased vision, hypersensitivity

Counseling Points
- For ophthalmic use only
- To avoid contamination, do not touch tip of container to eye or any other surface
- Remove contact lenses during treatment for conjunctivitis with this medication

Key Points
- Erythromycin ophthalmic ointment is a first-line agent in treating simple cases of bacterial conjunctivitis
- Ointments are often preferred in children and those who have difficulty administrating medications. The ointment commonly stays on the lid and lashes, providing a therapeutic effect, even if the medication was not applied directly to the conjunctiva.
- Erythromycin is also used frequently in neonates for prophylaxis of ophthalmia neonatorum due to *N. gonorrhoeae* or *C. trachomatis*. Importantly, infants born to mothers with gonorrhea require treatment with systemic penicillin because topical erythromycin alone is inadequate.

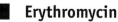

Drug Class: Combination Antibiotic and Corticosteroid, Ophthalmic

Introduction

Combination antibiotic/corticosteroid ophthalmic products are used in a variety of conditions in which a corticosteroid is indicated and in which superficial bacterial infection or risk of infection exists. The steroid component suppresses the inflammatory response; however, it is also likely to delay or slow wound healing. Because corticosteroids may inhibit the body's defense mechanisms against infection, a concomitant antimicrobial agent may be used when this inhibition is considered to be clinically significant. Topical ophthalmic steroids are not recommended for long-term use. Prolonged use may lead to elevated IOP and the development of glaucoma.

Members of the Drug Class

In this section: Tobramycin/dexamethasone

Others: Multiple combination products are available containing the following antibacterial agents: Neomycin, neomycin/polymyxin B, gentamicin, tobramycin, chloramphenicol, bacitracin; multiple combination products are available containing the following steroid components: hydrocortisone, prednisolone, dexamethasone

■ Tobramycin/Dexamethasone

Brand Name
TobraDex

Generic Name
Tobramycin/dexamethasone

Dosage Forms
Suspension, ointment

Mechanism of Action
Dexamethasone is a potent corticosteroid that inhibits an inflammatory response; tobramycin is an aminoglycoside antibiotic that provides action against susceptible organisms.

Usage
Steroid-responsive inflammatory ocular conditions with infection or risk of infection*

Dosing
- Suspension: Instill 1 or 2 drops into the conjunctival sac every 4–6 hours. Alternatively, for severe infections, instill 1 or 2 drops every 2 hours for the first 24–48 hours, and then decrease to administration every 4–6 hours.
- Ointment: Apply 0.5-inch ribbon to the conjunctival sac every 6–8 hours. Alternatively, for severe infections, apply 0.5-inch ribbon to the conjunctival sac every 3–4 hours for the first 24–48 hours, and then decrease administration to every 6–8 hours.

Adverse Reactions: Most Common
- Superinfection, eyelid itching and swelling

Adverse Reactions: Rare/Severe/Important
- Redness, irritation, decreased vision, hypersensitivity, elevated IOP leading to glaucoma (>10 days of use), secondary infections, perforation of cornea or sclera in patients predisposed to cornea or sclera thinning

Contraindications
- Viral, mycobacterial, and fungal infections of the cornea and conjunctiva

Counseling Points
- For ophthalmic use only
- Store suspensions upright and shake well before using
- To avoid contamination, do not touch tip of container to eye or any other surface
- Do not wear contact lenses during the use of this product
- Do not discontinue therapy prematurely without contacting your physician

Key Points
- Combination steroid/antibiotic preparations are used in the setting of steroid-responsive inflammatory ocular conditions with infection or high risk of infection
- Prolonged use of ophthalmic corticosteroids is associated with risk of elevated IOP, damage of the optic nerve, development of glaucoma, secondary infections, and thinning/perforation of the cornea or sclera

Drug Class: Prostaglandin Agonist, Ophthalmic

Introduction

Prostaglandin analogs are effective in the treatment of ocular hypertension and glaucoma as monotherapy and in combination with other topical agents. With limited systemic toxicities, potent IOP lowering, and once-daily administration, many clinicians use these agents as first-line therapy in the treatment of glaucoma. High cost, however, limits the use of these agents for many patients. Notable side effects include altered iris pigmentation, which occurs in 15–30% of patients and is not believed to be harmful.

Mechanism of Action for the Drug Class
Reduction in IOP is achieved by increasing aqueous humor outflow from the eye.

Members of the Drug Class
In this section: Latanoprost
    Others: Bimatoprost, travoprost

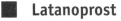 Latanoprost

Brand Name
Xalatan

Generic Name
Latanoprost

Dosage Forms
Solution

Usage
Elevated IOP in patients with open-angle glaucoma or ocular hypertension*

Dosing
Instill 1 drop in the affected eye once a day in the evening

Adverse Reactions: Most Common
- Increased pigmentation of the iris, eyelash changes, eyelid skin darkening, transient burning and stinging upon instillation, blurred vision, conjunctival hyperemia

Adverse Reactions: Rare/Severe/Important
- Excessive tearing, eyelid crusting, pain, discomfort, iritis/uveitis

Contraindications
- Hypersensitivity to latanoprost or benzalkonium chloride

Counseling Points
- For ophthalmic use only
- Latanoprost may cause a color change of the iris, increasing the amount of brown pigmentation. This change occurs slowly, may not be present for several months to a year, and is likely to be permanent. Latanoprost may cause darkening of the eyelid skin and changes to the eyelashes, including increased thickness, length, and darkening.
- Remove contact lens before instillation of the solution. You may reinsert contact lenses 15 minutes following latanoprost administration.
- If more than one type of ophthalmic solution is used, wait at least 5 minutes before administering second agent
- Notify physician if any ocular infections or lid reactions occur
- Storage considerations: Protect this medication from light. Store unopened bottles in the refrigerator. Once opened, you may store the bottle at room temperature for up to 6 weeks.

Key Points
- Prostaglandin analogs are effective agents for the treatment of elevated IOP and glaucoma. In some studies, they have demonstrated superior IOP lowering when compared with timolol twice a day, and they have been advocated by some as first-line agents in the management of glaucoma. The cost of these agents often limits their use in clinical practice.
- Once-daily dosing should not be exceeded because more frequent administration may decrease the intraocular pressure lowering effect of latanoprost
- Although systemic adverse effects are limited, local side effects are notable for changes in iris, eyelid, and eyelash pigmentation. Taking advantage of this unique side effect, a topical formulation of bimatoprost was recently approved by the Food and Drug Administration to enhance the length, thickness, and darkness of eyelashes for cosmetic purposes.

Drug Class: β-Adrenergic Blocking Agents, Ophthalmic

Introduction
Topical β-adrenergic blockers are among the most commonly used antiglaucoma medications. Timolol was the first available ophthalmic β-blocker and is often considered the gold standard in clinical trials comparing classes of glaucoma therapies. β-Blockers are generally considered first-line agents in the treatment of glaucoma, although systemic effects (bradycardia, bronchospasm, reduced blood pressure, negative inotropic effects) may limit their use in specific patient populations.

Mechanism of Action for the Drug Class
Ophthalmic β-adrenergic blocking agents decrease IOP by reducing aqueous humor production in the ciliary body of the eye. Nonselective β-blockers (timolol, levobunolol, carteolol, and metipranolol) affect β_1 and β_2 receptors, whereas selective β-blockers (betaxolol) affect only β_1 receptors.

Members of the Drug Class
In this section: Timolol, timolol-XE
    Others: Betaxolol, carteolol, levobunolol, metipranolol

■ Timolol, Timolol-XE

Brand Name
Timoptic

Generic Names
Timolol, timolol-XE

Dosage Forms
Solution, gel-forming solution

Usage
Treatment of elevated IOP in patients with open-angle glaucoma or ocular hypertension*

Dosing
- Solution: Instill 1 drop in the affected eye twice a day
- Gel-forming solution: 1 drop in the affected eye once daily

Adverse Reactions: Most Common
- Local effects include stinging and burning on application, dry eye, blepharitis, corneal anesthesia

Adverse Reactions: Rare/Severe/Important
- Local: Uveitis, keratitis, superinfection
- Systemic: Bradycardia, hypotension, exacerbation of CHF, bronchospasm, fatigue, dizziness, confusion, and depression. May also mask the signs and symptoms of hypoglycemia.

Contraindications
- Asthma, severe COPD, bradycardia, second- or third-degree AV block, overt heart failure, cardiogenic shock, previous hypersensitivity to β-blocking agents

Counseling Points
- For ophthalmic use only
- Using proper technique of nasolacrimal occlusion is particularly important to optimize efficacy and decrease systemic absorption and toxicities
- Before using, invert gel-forming solution and shake once. Administer other topical ophthalmic medications used concomitantly at least 10 minutes before the gel-forming solution.
- Remove contact lenses before using this medication; wait 15 minutes following administration to reinsert

Key Points
- Ophthalmic β-adrenergic blockers are generally equally effective in IOP lowering; however, they differ in duration of action, adverse effect potential, and cost. These agents are generally considered first-line therapy for the treatment of open-angle glaucoma.
- Because of the risk of systemic adverse events, these drugs are contraindicated in patients with severe pulmonary disease, bradycardia, second- or third-degree heart block, overt heart failure, and cardiogenic shock. If used, clinicians should exercise extreme caution; careful monitoring, use of the lowest effective dose, nasolacrimal occlusion, and a more β-selective agent can help to decrease the risk of systemic toxicities.

Review Questions

1. Which of the following ophthalmic products commonly causes a change in iris, eyelid, and eyelash pigmentation?
   A. Ciloxan
   B. Neosporin
   C. TobraDex
   D. Xalatan

2. When administering an ophthalmic suspension, which of the following is/are false?
   A. Apply light finger pressure to the outside corner of the eye after administration
   B. Medication should be placed in the conjunctival sac
   C. Never touch the applicator tip to the eye
   D. Shake well before administration

3. Neomycin has been specifically linked to cutaneous sensitization reactions. Which of the following manifestations is *not* common to this type of reaction?
   A. Double vision
   B. Edema of the eyelid
   C. Failure of infection to heal
   D. Itching

4. Which of the following prescriptions for timolol is correct?
   A. Timolol gel-forming solution: 1 drop in affected eye once a day
   B. Timolol gel-forming solution: 1 drop in affected eye twice a day
   C. Timolol solution: 1 drop in affected eye once a day
   D. Timolol solution: 2 drops in affected eye once a day

5. The long-term use of ophthalmic corticosteroids may result in which of the following serious complications?
   A. Glaucoma
   B. Ocular hypertension
   C. Secondary infection
   D. All of the above

6. Which of the following agents would *not* be used to treat an infection of the eye?
   A. Ciprofloxacin
   B. Latanoprost
   C. Norfloxacin
   D. Ofloxacin

7. Which of the following agents is a first-line option in the treatment of uncomplicated bacterial conjunctivitis?
   A. Ilotycin
   B. Ocuflox
   C. TobraDex
   D. Timoptic

8. Which of the following statements are true regarding latanoprost?
   A. Cost of latanoprost is not a concern for most patients.
   B. Latanoprost works to lower IOP by decreasing aqueous humor production.
   C. Latanoprost works to lower IOP by increasing aqueous humor outflow.
   D. Opened bottles must be stored in the refrigerator.

9. Which of the following statements is true regarding proper ophthalmic ointment instillation?
   A. Ointment should be instilled into the lower lid pouch.
   B. Short-term blurred vision is commonly seen after ointment administration.
   C. Wait 10 minutes before instillation of another ophthalmic medication.
   D. All of the above.

10. Which of the following agents should be used with caution in a patient with heart failure and diabetes?
    A. Erythromycin
    B. Latanoprost
    C. Neomycin/polymyxin/gramicidin
    D. Timolol

11. Which of the following statements is false regarding the combination product TobraDex?
    A. Contact lenses should not be worn while using this product.
    B. Store TobraDex suspension in the upright position.
    C. Tobramycin is helpful in cases when there is a high risk of bacterial infection.
    D. TobraDex is used to treat viral and fungal infections of the conjunctiva.

12. Nasolacrimal occlusion is important because it does which of the following?
    A. Decreases frequency of administration
    B. Decreases systemic toxicity
    C. Increases frequency of administration
    D. Increases systemic toxicity

13. Erythromycin is used as monotherapy for all of the following indications except
    A. Prophylaxis of ophthalmia neonatorum
    B. Treatment of infants born to mothers with gonorrhea
    C. Treatment of superficial ocular infections of the conjunctiva
    D. Treatment of superficial ocular infections of the cornea

14. Advantages of Xalatan include all of the following except
    A. Efficacy in closed- and open-angle glaucoma
    B. Few systemic side effects
    C. Once-daily administration
    D. Potent IOP lowering

15. Which of the following medications do not come in an ointment formulation?
    A. Ciprofloxacin
    B. Erythromycin
    C. Ofloxacin
    D. Tobramycin/dexamethasone

CHAPTER 13

Pulmonary and Allergy Agents

Christina Rose, PharmD, BCPS

Drug Class: Inhaled Anticholinergics

Introduction

Anticholinergic inhalers and nasal preparations are primarily used for chronic obstructive pulmonary disease (COPD), allergic and nonallergic rhinitis and nasal cold symptoms, respectively. Long-acting anticholinergic inhalation preparations are not used in the chronic treatment of asthma. Ipratropium may be used during acute asthma exacerbation but only in combination with short-acting β-adrenergic agonists. The most common adverse reaction associated with the inhalation preparations is dry mouth.

Mechanism of Action for the Drug Class

The drug class appears to produce bronchodilation by competitive inhibition of cholinergic receptors on bronchial smooth muscle. Local application to nasal mucosa inhibits mucous gland secretions.

Members of the Drug Class

In this section: Ipratropium, tiotropium
   Others: None

■ Ipratropium

Brand Name

Atrovent

Generic Name

Ipratropium

Dosage Forms

MDI hydrofluoroalkane (HFA) 17 µg/actuation, solution for nebulizer 0.02%, and nasal spray 0.03% and 0.06%

Usage

Maintenance treatment of bronchospasm associated with COPD*, allergic and nonallergic rhinitis (nasal spray 0.03%), common cold (nasal spray 0.06%)

Dosing

COPD:
- Initial dose:
  - Usual dose: 2 puffs inhaled by mouth four times a day
  - Maximum dose: 12 puffs per day

Solution for nebulizers:
- Usual dose: 200–500 µg inhaled by mouth three to four times a day
- Maximum dose: 2 mg/24 hours

Allergic/nonallergic rhinitis: Nasal spray 0.03%
- Usual dose: 2 puffs in each nostril two to three times a day
- Maximum dose: 12 puffs/24 hours

Common cold: Nasal spray 0.06%
- Usual dose: 2 puffs in each nostril three to four times a day
- Maximum dose: 16 puffs/24 hours

Adverse Reactions: Most Common

- Cough, dry mouth, chest pain/palpitations, nausea, dizziness, headache, dyspepsia, urinary retention, nasal irritation (nasal spray), epistaxis (nasal spray), taste perversion (nasal spray)

Adverse Reactions: Rare/Severe/Important

- Worsening of narrow-angle glaucoma

Major Drug Interactions

Drugs Affecting Ipratropium

- Other anticholinergics or drugs that have anticholinergic properties: May potentiate effects

Counseling Points

- Use proper administration technique
- You do not have to shake HFA inhalation aerosol products

- Directions for proper use of MDIs:
  1. The inhaler must be "primed" two times before taking the first dose from a new inhaler or when the inhaler has not been used for >3 days
  2. Insert the metal canister into the top of the mouthpiece and remove the protective dust cap from the mouthpiece
  3. Exhale deeply through your mouth
  4. Put the mouthpiece in your mouth and close your lips. Keep your eyes closed so no medicine will spray in your eyes.
  5. Inhale slowly through your mouth and at the same time firmly press once on the canister continuing to breathe deeply
  6. Hold your breath for 10 seconds or as long as you feel comfortable
  7. Exhale slowly
  8. Wait at least 15 seconds before repeating steps 1 through 7 for next inhalation
  9. Replace the dust cap after use
  10. Keep the mouthpiece clean. Wash it at least once a week. Shake it to remove excess water and let air-dry.
- Mouthpiece cleaning instructions:
  1. Remove and set aside the canister and dust cap from mouthpiece
  2. Wash the mouthpiece through the top and bottom with warm running water for at least 30 seconds. Do not use anything other than water to wash the mouthpiece.
  3. Dry the mouthpiece by shaking off the excess water and allow it to air-dry
  4. When the mouthpiece is dry, replace the canister. Make sure the canister is fully and firmly inserted into the mouthpiece.
- If using more than the prescribed amount, contact your healthcare provider
- Avoid contact with eyes. This can cause blurred vision and worsening glaucoma in glaucoma patients.
- Use with a proper spacing device

Key Points

- Used for COPD, rhinitis, and nasal symptoms of cold
- Most common adverse reaction is dry mouth and nasal irritation with nasal spray
- Use with caution in patients with glaucoma or urinary retention

■ Tiotropium

Brand Name
Spiriva

Generic Name
Tiotropium

Dosage Forms
Capsule dosage form containing 18 μg powder for inhalation delivered via a special dry powder inhaler device (HandiHaler) for oral inhalation only

Usage
Long-term management of COPD*

Dosing
COPD:
- Powder for inhalation:
  ○ Usual dose: Contents of 1 capsule (18 μg) inhaled orally once daily using HandiHaler

Adverse Reactions: Most Common
- Cough, dry mouth, dyspepsia, blurred vision, headache, sore throat, urinary retention

Adverse Reactions: Rare/Severe/Important
- Worsening of narrow-angle glaucoma

Major Drug Interactions
Drugs Affecting Tiotropium
- Other anticholinergics may potentiate effects

Counseling Points
- You must use proper administration technique
- Capsule is for inhalation only via the HandiHaler device; do not swallow
- Directions for proper use of HandiHaler device:
  1. Open the HandiHaler device. Pull the cap upward to expose the mouthpiece.
  2. Open the mouthpiece by pulling the mouthpiece ridge upward away from the base
  3. Remove capsule from blister pack. Do not open the capsule.
  4. Insert the capsule in the center chamber of the HandiHaler device. It does not matter which end of the capsule you put in the chamber.
  5. Close the mouthpiece until you hear a click, but leave the cap open
  6. Hold the HandiHaler device with the mouthpiece upright
  7. Press the green button until it is flat against the base and release
  8. Breathe out completely. Do not exhale into the mouthpiece.
  9. Hold the HandiHaler device by the gray base and raise the device to your mouth. Close your lips tightly around the mouthpiece.
  10. Breathe in slowly and deeply so you hear or feel the capsule vibrate
  11. Hold your breath as long as it is comfortable and at the same time take the inhaler out of your mouth
  12. To get the full dose of the medication, you must breathe out completely and repeat steps 9 through 11. Do not press the green button again.
  13. After you finish taking your daily dose, open the mouthpiece again. Tip out the used capsule and throw it away.
  14. Close the mouthpiece cap for storage of your HandiHaler

Key Points

- Used for chronic treatment of COPD
- Capsule should be inhaled via HandiHaler only
- Use with caution in patients with glaucoma or urinary retention

---

Drug Class: Antihistamines (First Generation: Sedating)

Introduction

The first-generation antihistamines are used primarily for hypersensitivity reactions, sleep disorders, and as an antiemetic. They are not typically used chronically for allergic rhinitis due to the potential for sedation. These agents are generally used on an as needed basis depending on the indication. Sedation is the most common adverse reaction associated with these agents, and concomitant drugs that cause sedation should be avoided when these agents are used.

Mechanism of Action for the Drug Class

Reversibly, competitively antagonize H1 receptors peripherally and centrally.

Adverse Reactions for the Drug Class: Most Common

Drowsiness, somnolence, dizziness, dyspepsia, headache, nausea, fatigue

Major Drug Interactions for the Drug Class

Drugs Affecting Antihistamines

- Alcohol and CNS depressants: Potentiate drowsiness
- Other anticholinergic drugs: Potentiate side effects

Members of the Drug Class

In this section: Diphenhydramine, hydroxyzine, promethazine

Others: Brompheniramine, chlorpheniramine, doxylamine

■ Diphenhydramine

Brand Name
Benadryl

Generic Name
Diphenhydramine

Dosage Forms
Capsules, tablets, chewable tablets, liquid, injection, topical cream

Usage
Allergic dermatitis*, hypersensitivity reactions*, sleep disorders*, allergic rhinitis, motion sickness

Dosing
Age 2–6 years:
- Not recommended for use in children <2 years of age due to dosing errors and accidental ingestion

- Usual dose: 6.25–12.5 mg orally every 4–6 hours
- Maximum dose: 37.5 mg/24 hours

Age 6–12 years:
- Usual dose: 12.5–25 mg orally every 4–6 hours
- Maximum dose: 150 mg/24 hours

Adults:
- Usual dose: 25–50 mg orally every 4–8 hours
- Maximum dose: 300 mg/24 hours

Adverse Reactions: Rare/Severe/Important
- None

Counseling Points
- Tolerance to CNS effects may develop quickly, so that sedation is no longer troublesome after a few days
- For motion sickness take dose 30 minutes to 1 hour before traveling

Key Points
- Diphenhydramine is commonly used for allergies, motion sickness, and sleep disorders
- Sedation is most common adverse reaction
- Not recommended for use in children <2 years of age
- May be inappropriate to use in the elderly due to anticholinergic effects

■ Hydroxyzine

Brand Names
Atarax, Vistaril

Generic Name
Hydroxyzine

Dosage Forms
Tablets, capsules, syrup, oral suspension, injection

Usage
Pruritus*, sedation*, anxiety

Dosing
Pruritus:
- Age 2–6 years:
  - Usual dose: 12.5 mg orally every 6 hours as needed
  - Maximum dose: 50 mg/24 hours
- Age 6–12 years:
  - Usual dose: 12.5–25 mg orally every 6 hours as needed
  - Maximum dose: 100 mg/24 hours

- Adults:
  - Usual dose: 25 mg orally every 4–6 hours
  - Maximum dose: 400 mg/24 hours

Sedation:
- Children:
  - Usual dose: 0.6 mg/kg orally as a single dose
  - Maximum dose: Not to exceed 50 mg as a single dose
- Adults:
  - Usual dose: 50–100 mg orally as a single dose
  - Usual dose: 50 mg IM as a single dose

Adverse Reactions: Rare/Severe/Important
- None

Counseling Point
- Tolerance to CNS effects may develop quickly, so sedation is no longer troublesome after a few days

Key Point
- Sedation is most common adverse reaction

■ Promethazine

Brand Name
Phenergan

Generic Name
Promethazine

Dosage Forms
Tablets, syrup, suppository, injection

Usage
Antiemetic*, motion sickness, treatment of allergic conditions, sedation

Dosing
Age >2 years (use the lowest most effective dose possible), oral/rectal/injection:
- Usual dose: 0.1–1 mg/kg/dose every 6 hours
- Maximum: 25–50 mg/dose (varies based on indication)

Adults, oral/rectal/injection:
- Usual dose: 25–50 mg at bedtime or 12.5–25 mg every 4–8 hours if needed
- Maximum dose: 150 mg/24 hours

Adverse Reactions: Rare/Severe/Important
- Photosensitivity, blood dyscrasias, injection site reactions (IM is preferred route of parenteral administration; IV administration may cause severe tissue damage)

Counseling Points
- Tolerance to CNS effects may develop quickly, so sedation is no longer troublesome after a few days
- Take with food, water, or milk to decrease GI upset
- For motion sickness take 30 minutes to 1 hour before traveling
- Use sugarless gum or candy, ice, or saliva substitute to decrease dry mouth

Key Points
- Most commonly used for hypersensitivity reactions, motion sickness, and as an antiemetic
- Promethazine is available in multiple dosage forms
- IV administration can cause severe tissue damage. Use IM route.

Drug Class: Antihistamines (Second Generation: Nonsedating)

Introduction
The second-generation antihistamines are used for allergic rhinitis and urticaria. They can be used to treat these chronic conditions due to the low risk of adverse events. Sedation is most common in cetirizine. All of these agents are available in combination with pseudoephedrine. The combination products should not be used in patients <12 years of age.

Mechanism of Action for the Drug Class
Reversibly, competitively antagonize H1 receptors peripherally and does not cross blood–brain barrier resulting in reduced sedation.

Usage for the Drug Class
Allergic rhinitis*, urticaria

Adverse Reactions for the Drug Class: Most Common
- Dizziness, dyspepsia, headache, nausea, xerostomia

Adverse Reactions for the Drug Class: Rare/Severe/Important
- None

Members of the Drug Class
In this section: Fexofenadine, loratadine, cetirizine
Others: Desloratadine

Fexofenadine

Brand Names
Allegra, Allegra D 12 hour (60 mg fexofenadine and 120 mg pseudoephedrine), Allegra D 24 hour (180 mg fexofenadine and 240 mg pseudoephedrine)

Generic Name
Fexofenadine

Dosage Forms
Tablets: 30, 60 mg; extended-release tablets: 180 mg; oral disintegrating tablets: 30 mg

Dosing
Age 6 months to <2 years:
- Usual dose: 15 mg orally twice daily
- Maximum dose: 15 mg orally twice daily

Age 2–11 years:
- Usual dose: 30 mg orally twice daily
- Maximum dose: 30 mg orally twice daily

Age >12 years and adults:
- Usual dose: 60 mg orally twice daily or 180 mg once daily
- Maximum dose: 60 mg orally twice daily or 180 mg once daily

Renal dosage adjustment:
- Dose adjustment is necessary in the renally impaired and the elderly

Note: Combination product with pseudoephedrine should not be used in patients <12 years of age

Major Drug Interactions
Drugs Affecting Fexofenadine
- Ketoconazole and erythromycin may increase fexofenadine levels (without evidence of QT prolongation)
- Concomitant use of aluminum- or magnesium-containing antacids decrease bioavailability of fexofenadine

Counseling Points
- Take at regular intervals
- Avoid aluminum- or magnesium-containing antacids
- Oral disintegrating tablets not recommended in children <6 years of age
- Avoid use of other CNS depressants and alcohol that may cause excess drowsiness

Key Points
- Should not cause drowsiness
- Available with pseudoephedrine for patients >12 years of age.

Loratadine

Brand Names
Claritin, Claritin D 12 hour (5 mg loratadine and 120 mg pseudoephedrine), Claritin D 24 hour (10 mg loratadine and 240 mg pseudoephedrine)

Generic Name
Loratadine

Dosage Forms
Tablets: 10 mg; Redi-tabs: 10 mg; syrup: 5 mg/5 ml

Dosing
Age 2–6 years:
- Usual dose: 5 mg orally once daily
- Maximum dose: 5 mg orally once daily

Age >6 years:
- Usual dose: 10 mg orally once daily
- Maximum dose: 10 mg orally once daily

Renal and hepatic dosage adjustment: Recommended to be adjusted to every other day dosing

Major Drug Interactions
- None

Counseling Points
- Take at regular intervals
- Redi-tabs are rapidly disintegrating tablets that dissolve on the tongue with or without water

Key Points
- Available with pseudoephedrine for patients >12 years of age
- Does not cause drowsiness

Cetirizine

Brand Names
Zyrtec, Zyrtec D 12 hour (5 mg cetirizine and 120 mg pseudoephedrine)

Generic Name
Cetirizine

Dosage Forms
Tablets: 10 mg; syrup: 5 mg/5 ml; chewable tablets: 5 mg and 10 mg

Dosing
Age 6–12 months:
- Usual dose: 2.5 mg orally once daily
- Maximum dose: 2.5 mg orally once daily

Age 12–23 months:
- Usual dose: 2.5 mg orally once daily
- Maximum dose: 2.5 mg orally twice daily

Age 2–5 years:
- Usual dose: 2.5 mg orally once daily
- Maximum dose: 5 mg orally once daily or 2.5 mg twice daily

Age >6 years and adults:
- Usual dose: 5–10 mg orally once daily
- Maximum dose: 10 mg orally once daily

Renal and hepatic dose adjustment: Dose adjustments are recommended in severe renal and hepatic disease

Adverse Reactions: Rare/Severe/Important
- None

Counseling Point
- May cause drowsiness or dizziness; observe caution when driving

Key Points
- Will cause more drowsiness compared with other agents in this class
- Available with pseudoephedrine for patients >12 years of age

---

Drug Class: Antitussives

Introduction
Antitussives are used in the treatment of nonproductive cough. Benzonatate is used for acute and chronic cough. Sedation is the most common side effect seen with these agents. Benzonatate capsules should not be crushed or chewed.

Mechanism of Action for the Drug Class
Suppress cough through a peripheral action, anesthetizing the stretch or cough receptors of vagal afferent fibers. May suppress cough reflexes in the medulla by a central mechanism.

Members of the Drug Class
In this section: Benzonatate, codeine, dextromethorphan, hydrocodone (these agents are covered in the combination cough/cold products section)
Others: Carbetapentane

■ Benzonatate

Brand Name
Tessalon

Generic Name
Benzonatate

Dosage Forms
100-mg capsules

Usage
Symptomatic relief of nonproductive cough*

Dosing
- Usual dose (age >10 years): 100 mg orally three times a day
- Maximum dose (age >10 years): 600 mg/24 hours

Adverse Reactions: Most Common
- Constipation, drowsiness, dizziness, headache, confusion, bronchospasm

Adverse Reactions: Rare/Severe/Important
- Oropharyngeal anesthesia if capsules are chewed or dissolved in mouth; burning sensation in eyes

Major Drug Interactions
Drugs Affecting Benzonatate
- Alcohol and CNS depressants: Potentiate drowsiness

Counseling Point
- Swallow whole; do not chew or dissolve capsule in mouth

Key Points
- Used for cough
- Do not break or puncture capsule. Swallow whole.

Drug Class: β-2 Agonist/Anticholinergic Combination Inhaler

Introduction
The primary use of these combination inhalers is in the chronic treatment of COPD when bronchospasms are still occurring despite treatment with a single bronchodilator. This agent may also be used for the treatment of bronchospasms or exacerbations associated with COPD and asthma. These agents can be used on a scheduled or as needed basis depending on the indication. The most common adverse events associated with these agents are dry mouth and nervousness. Patients with a history of a soy or peanut allergy should avoid this combination product.

Mechanism of Action of the Drug Class
See individual agents

Members of the Drug Class
In this section: Albuterol and Ipratropium
Others: None

■ Albuterol and Ipratropium
Brand Names
Combivent (Ipratropium bromide 18 μg and albuterol sulfate 103 μg per actuation), DuoNeb (ipratropium bromide 0.5 mg and albuterol base 2.5 mg per 3 ml)

Generic Names
Albuterol and ipratropium

Dosage Forms
MDI, solution for nebulization

Usage
Maintenance treatment of bronchospasms associated with COPD*, acute asthma exacerbation

Dosing
- MDI usual dose: 2 puffs inhaled orally four times a day and can be used on an as needed basis
- MDI maximum dose: 12 puffs/24 hours
- Solution for nebulization: 3 ml nebulized and inhaled orally every 4–6 hours

Adverse Reactions: Most Common
- Cough, nervousness, blurred vision, palpitations, tachycardia, tremor, headache, CNS stimulation

Adverse Reactions: Rare/Severe/Important
- Hypokalemia, hypertension, worsening of narrow-angle glaucoma

Major Drug Interactions
- See albuterol and ipratropium monographs

Counseling Points
- You must use proper administration technique:
  1. Shake inhaler for 10 seconds and remove the dust cap

2. If this is the first time you are using the inhaler or if you have not used it for >24 hours, shake the canister for 10 seconds and spray away from your eyes three times
3. Exhale slowly and deeply
4. Hold the inhaler upright and place the mouthpiece between your lips. Be careful not to block the opening with your tongue or teeth.
5. Press down on the inhaler once as you start a slow, deep inhalation
6. Continue to inhale slowly and deeply through your mouth. Try to inhale over at least 5 seconds.
7. Hold your breath for 10 seconds or as long as you feel comfortable
8. Exhale slowly
9. Wait approximately 1–2 minutes before repeating steps 1 through 8 for the next inhalation
- If using more than the prescribed amount, contact your healthcare provider
- Avoid contact with eyes
- Use with the proper spacing device
- Protect the nebulization solution from light

Key Points
- Commonly used in COPD
- Low potential for adverse reactions except dry mouth with inhalation
- Use in caution in patients with glaucoma or urinary retention
- Avoid use with soy and peanut allergies

Drug Class: β-2 Agonist/Corticosteroid Inhalers

Introduction
The β-2 agonist/corticosteroid inhaler combinations are used for the chronic treatment of asthma and COPD. Different strengths of corticosteroids are available depending on the patient's asthma severity. It is important to counsel patients on the proper use of the inhaler and instruct the patient to rinse mouth with water after each use. Patients should also be informed that these inhalers should not be used to treat acute bronchospasm or shortness of breath, and these agents need to be used regularly to achieve maximal effect. Coughing, dry mouth, and oral candidiasis are the most common adverse effects seen with these agents.

Mechanism of Action for the Drug Class
See individual agents

Usage for the Drug Class
Chronic treatment of asthma and COPD*

Adverse Reactions of the Drug Class: Most Common
- Hoarseness, pharyngitis, dry mouth, coughing, headache, hyperglycemia
- Hypokalemia, hypertension, oral candidiasis, palpitations, tachycardia, tremor, CNS stimulation

Adverse Reactions of the Drug Class: Rare/Severe/Important
- Edema, adrenal insufficiency, upper and lower respiratory tract infections

Counseling Points for the Drug Class
- Rinse mouth out with water after each use
- Use every day regularly
- Do not use for acute attacks
- You must have a rescue inhaler available for breakthrough attacks
- You must use proper administration technique

Key Points for the Drug Class

- Used in the chronic treatment of COPD and asthma
- Should not be used for the treatment of exacerbations
- Use as prescribed to see maximal benefit
- It may take 1–4 weeks to see maximal benefit
- Rinse mouth out with each use to avoid oral candidiasis

Members of the Drug Class

In this section: Fluticasone and salmeterol, budesonide and formoterol

Others: None

■ Fluticasone and Salmeterol

Brand Name

Advair

Generic Names

Fluticasone and salmeterol

Dosage Forms

Powder for inhalation via Diskus inhaler (available in three strengths of fluticasone and all contain 50 μg of salmeterol: 100/50, 250/50, and 500/50)

Dosing

- Initial dose for asthma: 100 μg fluticasone/50 μg salmeterol, 1 puff inhaled orally every 12 hours
- Usual dose: Titrate to the most effective dose that controls symptoms
- Maximum dose: 500 μg fluticasone/50 μg salmeterol (2 inhalations daily)

Major Drug Interactions

- See salmeterol and fluticasone monographs

Counseling Points

- You must use proper administration technique:
  1. Activate dry powder inhaler by sliding the activator
  2. Breathe out deeply
  3. Inhale contents of powder completely

■ Budesonide and Formoterol

Brand Name

Symbicort

Generic Names

Budesonide and formoterol

Dosage Forms

MDI (various doses of budesonide in combination with 4.5 μg of formoterol fumarate dehydrate: 80/4.5 and 160/4.5)

Dosing

- Two inhalations by mouth twice daily

Major Drug Interactions

- See budesonide and formoterol monographs

Counseling Point

- Counsel on proper inhalation technique

Drug Class: β-2 Agonists, Inhaled

Introduction

The inhaled β-2 agonists are primarily used for the treatment and prevention of bronchospasms in patients with obstructive airway disease. They can be used chronically or in the treatment of an exacerbation of the disease. Short-acting β-2 agonists are commonly used on an as-needed basis when feeling short of breath. The inhaled preparation of albuterol is used more commonly than the systemic preparations. The tablets and syrup are associated with an increased frequency of adverse reactions and are no longer recommended for the treatment of asthma. Long-acting agents should only be used twice daily and not on an as needed basis. Patients should be counseled on the proper use of these medications. The most common adverse reactions are palpitations, tachycardia, and tremor. Adverse reactions are more common with the short-acting β-2 agonists than with the long-acting agents.

Mechanism of Action for the Drug Class

β Agonists (type 1 and/or 2) produce bronchodilation by relaxing smooth muscles of the bronchioles.

Adverse Reactions for the Drug Class: Most Common

- Palpitations, tachycardia, tremor, headache, CNS stimulation

Adverse Reactions for the Drug Class: Rare/Severe/Important

- Hyperglycemia, hypokalemia, hypertension; use caution in patients with cardiac arrhythmias, uncontrolled hypertension, uncontrolled hyperthyroidism, or diagnosed or suspected pheochromocytoma because these agents may exacerbate the condition

Major Drug Interactions for the Drug Class

Drugs Affecting β-Agonists

- Nonselective β-blockers (ophthalmic and systemic): May blunt the bronchodilating effects of albuterol

β-Agonist Effect on Other Drugs

- None

Members of the Drug Class

In this section: Albuterol, formoterol, levalbuterol, salmeterol
   Others: Arformoterol, metaproterenol, pirbuterol, terbutaline

■ Albuterol

Brand Names
Ventolin, Proventil

Generic Name
Albuterol

Dosage Forms
HFA inhaler, nebulizer solution, oral tablet extended-release tablets, syrup

Usage
Relief and prevention of bronchospasm associated with asthma and COPD*, acute attacks of bronchospasm, exercise-induced bronchospasm

Dosing
Relief and prevention of bronchospasm:
- HFA:
  - Usual dose (age <5 years: Adults): 2 puffs inhaled orally every 4–6 hours as needed
- Nebulizer solution:
  - Usual dose (age <5 years): 0.63–2.5 mg inhaled via nebulizer every 4–6 hours as needed
  - Usual dose (age >5 years: Adults): 1.25–5 mg inhaled via nebulizer every 4–8 hours as needed
- Oral tablets and syrup:
  - Usual dose (age 2–6 years): 0.1–0.2 mg/kg/dose every 8 hours
  - Maximum dose (age 2–6 years): 12 mg/24 hours
  - Usual dose (age 6–12 years): 2 mg orally every 6–8 hours
  - Maximum dose (age 6–12 years): 24 mg/24 hours
  - Usual dose (age >12 years): 2–4 mg orally every 6–8 hours
  - Maximum dose (age >12 years): 32 mg/24 hours
- Extended-release tablets:
  - Usual dose (age 6–12 years): 4 mg orally every 12 hours
  - Maximum dose (age 6–12 years): 24 mg/24 hours
  - Usual dose (age >12 years and adults): 4 mg orally every 12 hours
  - Maximum dose (age >12 years and adults): 32 mg/24 hours

Dose for exercised-induced asthma:
- MDI usual dose (age <5 years): 1–2 puffs inhaled by mouth 5 minutes before exercise
- MDI usual dose (age >5 years and adults): 2 puffs inhaled by mouth 5–30 minutes before exercise

Counseling Points
- You must use proper administration technique (see ipratropium HFA)

- If using more than the prescribed amount, contact your healthcare provider
- If using more than two times a week and not on any anti-inflammatory inhalers, check with healthcare provider
- Swallow extended-release tablets whole; do not crush or chew

Key Points
- Albuterol is a short-acting β-2 selective agonist
- Oral tablets and syrup are not recommended for the immediate relief of bronchospasms or for the chronic treatment of asthma
- Use with caution in patients with cardiac arrhythmias, uncontrolled hypertension, uncontrolled hyperthyroidism, or diagnosed or suspected pheochromocytoma

■ Formoterol

Brand Names
Foradil, Perforomist Solution for Nebulization

Generic Name
Formoterol

Dosage Forms
Powder for oral inhalation (as a capsule 12 μg), solution for nebulization (20 μg/2 ml)

Mechanism of Action
β-Agonists produce bronchodilation by relaxing smooth muscles of the bronchioles. Formoterol is a long-acting β-2 agonist.

Usage
Chronic maintenance of asthma*, maintenance treatment of COPD*, prevention of exercise-induced bronchospasm, prevention of nocturnal symptoms of asthma

Dosing
- Oral powder for inhalation: 12 μg capsule inhaled by mouth twice daily
- Solution for nebulization: 20 μg inhaled twice daily
- Exercise-induced asthma: 12 μg capsule inhaled by mouth 30 minutes before exercise

Adverse Reactions: Rare/Severe/Important
- May increase the risk of asthma-related deaths

Counseling Points
- Do not use for acute attacks
- Do not use more frequently than recommended dose
- Learn how to use Aerolizer inhaler properly
- Do not use spacer with Aerolizer

Key Points
- Formoterol is a long-acting β-2 agonist
- Should only be used in combination with inhaled corticosteroids in asthma
- Adverse effects are minimal compared with short-acting β-2 agonists

■ Levalbuterol

Brand Name
Xopenex

Generic Name
Levalbuterol

Dosage Forms
MDI (Xopenex HFA 45 µg/spray and solution for nebulization available as 0.31, 0.63, or 1.25 mg/3 ml)

Usage
Treatment of bronchospasms in children and adults with asthma and adults with COPD*

Dosing
HFA:
- Children age >4 years and adults: 2 puffs inhaled by mouth every 4–6 hours

Solution for nebulization:
- Children age ≤4 years: 0.31–1.25 inhaled by nebulizer every 4–6 hours as needed
- Children age 5–11 years: 0.31–0.63 mg inhaled via nebulizer every 8 hours as needed
- Children age = 12 years and adults: 0.63–1.25 mg inhaled via nebulizer every 8 hours as needed

Note: May use higher doses in patients with asthma and COPD exacerbations

Adverse Reactions: Rare/Severe/Important
- Paradoxical bronchospasms

Counseling Points
- You must use proper administration technique (see ipratropium HFA)
- If using more than the prescribed amount, contact your healthcare provider
- If using more than two times a week and not on any anti-inflammatory inhalers, check with healthcare provider

Key Points
- Levalbuterol is the active R-isomer of albuterol
- Levalbuterol is a short-acting β-2 agonist used to treat bronchospasms
- Levalbuterol is thought to have fewer adverse reactions compared with albuterol but that has never been proven in clinical studies

■ Salmeterol

Brand Name
Serevent

Generic Name
Salmeterol

Dosage Forms
Inhalation (Diskus Powder for inhalation 50 µg/puff)

Mechanism of Action
β-Agonists produce bronchodilation by relaxing smooth muscles of the bronchioles. Salmeterol is a long-acting β-2 agonist.

Usage
Chronic maintenance of asthma*, maintenance treatment of COPD*, prevention of nocturnal symptoms of asthma, prevention of exercise-induced bronchospasm

Dosing
- Usual dose: 1 inhalation twice daily (morning and evening)
- Exercise-induced asthma: 1 inhalation 30 minutes before exercise

Adverse Reactions: Rare/Severe/Important
- Anaphylaxis due to lactose component in oral inhalation powder may increase the risk of asthma-related deaths

Drug Interactions
- Inducers or inhibitor of CYP3A4: Will have an effect on salmeterol concentrations

Counseling Points
- Do not use for acute attacks
- You must use proper administration technique (see Advair monograph for instructions)
- Do not wash Diskus and keep it dry
- Do not use more frequently than recommended dose

Key Points
- Salmeterol is a long-acting β-2 selective agonist
- Should only be used as additional therapy for patients not adequately controlled on other asthma-controller medications

---

Drug Class: Combination Cough/Cold Products

Introduction

Combination cold and cough products either contain guaifenesin that acts as an expectorant or an antihistamine to alleviate upper respiratory cold symptoms and a narcotic or narcotic derivative as a cough suppressant. These agents should be used short-term to treat symptoms of a cough and cold. The preparations containing narcotics are scheduled controlled substances and have abuse potential. The most common adverse effects of these agents include sedation. Cough and cold preparations are no longer recommended in children <2 years of age due to the potential for dosing errors. There is no evidence that cough-suppressant therapy can prevent coughing. These drugs do not resolve the underlying pathophysiology that is responsible for the coughing. In patients with cough due to upper respiratory infection, cough suppressants have limited efficacy and are not recommended for this use. In patients with chronic bronchitis, cough suppressants such as codeine and dextromethorphan are recommended for the short-term symptomatic relief of coughing. In patients with acute cough due to the common cold, OTC combination cold medications, with the exception of older antihistamine–decongestants, are not recommended due to the lack of supportive evidence. Expectorants have not been consistently shown to be effective either.

Members of the Drug Class

In this section: Benzonatate (covered in an earlier section), guaifenesin and codeine, guaifenesin with dextromethorphan, hydrocodone and chlorpheniramine, promethazine with codeine,

Others: Carbetapentane

■ Guaifenesin and Codeine

Brand Names

Cheratussin AC (multiple others available)

Generic Names

Guaifenesin and codeine

Dosage Forms

Liquid

Mechanism of Action

Guaifenesin enhances the removal of mucus by decreasing the viscosity and surface tension. Codeine depresses the cough center in the medulla.

Usage

Temporary relief of cough and chest congestion*

Dosing

- 10 ml orally every 4 hours (maximum: 60 ml in 24 hours)

Adverse Reactions: Most Common

- CNS depression, constipation, headache, respiratory depression, urinary retention

Adverse Reactions: Rare/Severe/Important

- Excessive sedation, respiratory depression, urolithiasis

Major Drug Interactions

Drug Affecting Guaifenesin with Codeine

- CNS depressants: May enhance the effect and increase adverse reactions

Counseling Points

- Avoid alcohol, which may increase the sedative effects
- Follow each dose with a full glass of water
- Sugar-free formulations are available

Key Points

- Schedule V controlled substance

- Using more than the recommended amount can cause CNS depressant effects and respiratory depression
- Should be administered under close supervision to individuals with a history of drug abuse or dependence

■ Guaifenesin with Dextromethorphan

Brand Names

Robitussin DM (multiple others available)

Generic Names

Guaifenesin with dextromethorphan

Dosage Forms

Liquid, tablets, capsules, extended-release tablets

Mechanism of Action

Guaifenesin enhances the removal of mucus by decreasing the viscosity and surface tension. Dextromethorphan depresses the cough center in the medulla.

Usage

Temporary relief of cough and chest congestion*

Dosing

- Usual dose: Guaifenesin 200–400 mg and dextromethorphan 10–20 mg orally every 4–6 hours as needed
- Maximum dose: Guaifenesin 2400 mg and dextromethorphan 120 mg orally in 24 hours

Adverse Reactions: Most Common

- Drowsiness, dizziness, headache, lightheadedness, confusion

Adverse Reactions: Rare/Severe/Important

- None

Major Drug Interactions

Drugs Affecting Guaifenesin with Dextromethorphan

- MAO inhibitors and other serotonin modulators: May cause hypertension, hyperpyrexia, agitation, confusion, hallucinations (serotonin syndrome)

Counseling Point

- Follow each dose with a full glass of water

Key Points

- Use caution in patients <2 years of age. Ensure doses are appropriate.
- Sugar-free formulations are available

■ Hydrocodone and Chlorpheniramine

Brand Name

Tussionex

Generic Names

Hydrocodone and chlorpheniramine

Dosage Forms

Liquid (hydrocodone 10 mg and chlorpheniramine 8 mg per 5 mL)

Mechanism of Action

Chlorpheniramine reversibly, competitively antagonizes H1 receptors peripherally. Hydrocodone depresses the cough center in the medulla.

Usage

Temporary relief of cough and cold associated with allergy*

Dosing

Age 6–12 years:
- Usual dose: 2.5 ml orally every 12 hours
- Maximum dose: 5 ml/24 hours

Age >12 years:
- Usual dose: 5 ml orally every 12 hours
- Maximum dose: 10 ml/24 hours

Adverse Reactions: Most Common

- Drowsiness, blurred vision, constipation, dry mouth, headache, fatigue, dizziness, nausea

Adverse Reactions: Rare/Severe/Important

- Physical dependence (hydrocodone component), respiratory depression (hydrocodone component)

Major Drug Interactions

Drugs Affecting Hydrocodone and Chlorpheniramine
- Alcohol and CNS depressants: Potentiate drowsiness; other anticholinergic drugs potentiate side effects

Counseling Points

- Shake suspension well before using
- May cause drowsiness; use caution when driving
- Take only as prescribed

Key Points

- Schedule III controlled substance
- Should be administered under close supervision to individuals with a history of drug abuse or dependence

◼ Promethazine with Codeine

Brand Names

Phenergan with Codeine

Generic Names

Promethazine with Codeine

Dosage Forms

Liquid (Promethazine 6.25 mg and codeine 10 mg per 5 mL)

Mechanism of Action

Promethazine reversibly, competitively antagonizes H1 receptors peripherally. Codeine depresses the cough center in the medulla.

Usage

Temporary relief of cough due to allergy and cold*

Dosing

Age 6–11 years:
- Usual dose: 2.5–5 ml orally every 4–6 hours
- Maximum dose: 30 ml/24 hours

Adults:
- Usual dose: 5 ml orally every 4–6 hours
- Maximum dose: 30 ml in 24 hours

Adverse Reactions: Most Common

- Drowsiness, blurred vision, constipation, dry mouth, headache, fatigue, dizziness, nausea, photosensitivity

Adverse Reactions: Rare/Severe/Important

- Physical dependence (codeine component), respiratory depression (codeine component)

Major Drug Interactions

Drugs Affecting Promethazine with Codeine
- Alcohol and CNS depressants: Potentiate drowsiness
- Other anticholinergic drugs: Potentiate side effects

Counseling Points

- May cause drowsiness; exercise caution when driving
- Avoid prolonged exposure to sunlight
- Take only as prescribed

Key Points

- Schedule V controlled substance
- Should be administered under close supervision to individuals with a history of drug abuse or dependence
- Use in children <6 years of age is contraindicated due to risk of respiratory depression
- Not recommended for use in patients with chronic respiratory disease

---

Drug Class: Corticosteroids, Inhaled

Introduction

Inhaled corticosteroids are used for the chronic treatment of asthma. Their exact mechanism of action is unknown but thought to decrease inflammatory cells and cause smooth muscle relaxation. The lowest possible dose should be used to avoid adverse reactions. The most common adverse reactions include hoarseness, dry mouth, and oral candidiasis. Patients should be counseled on the proper use of the inhalation devices, to rinse out their mouth after each use, and to use as directed, not as a rescue inhaler.

Mechanism of Action for the Drug Class

Exact mechanism is unknown. May decrease the number of inflammatory cells, inhibit bronchoconstrictor mechanisms, produce direct smooth muscle relaxation and decreased airway hyperresponsiveness.

Usage for the Drug Class
Chronic maintenance of asthma*

Adverse Reactions for the Drug Class: Most Common
- Hoarseness, pharyngitis, dry mouth, coughing, headache, oral candidiasis

Adverse Reactions for the Drug Class: Rare/Severe/Important
- Edema, adrenal insufficiency, growth suppression in children, hyperglycemia

Counseling Points for the Drug Class
- Rinse mouth out with water after each use to prevent oral thrush
- It may take 1–4 weeks to see maximal benefit
- Use every day regularly
- Do not use for acute attacks
- You must have a rescue inhaler available for breakthrough attacks
- Learn the proper administration technique for each inhalation device

Key Points for the Drug Class
- Used in the chronic treatment of asthma
- Should not be used for the treatment of exacerbations
- It may take 1–4 weeks to see maximal benefit
- Rinse mouth out with each use
- Fluticasone and budesonide should be avoided with CYP3A4 inhibitors, specifically protease inhibitors. Cushing's syndrome has been reported with concomitant use of these agents.

Members of the Drug Class
In this section: Beclomethasone, budesonide, fluticasone, triamcinolone
   Others: Ciclesonide, flunisolide, mometasone

■ Beclomethasone

Brand Name
QVAR

Generic Name
Beclomethasone

Dosage Forms
Inhalation (MDI) 40 µg/inhalation (100-metered actuations) (7.3 g); 80 µg/inhalation (100-metered actuations) (7.3 g)

Dosing
Age 5–11 years:
- Low daily dose: 40–80 µg inhaled by mouth twice daily
- Medium daily dose: 80–160 µg inhaled by mouth twice daily
- High daily dose: >160 µg inhaled by mouth twice daily

Age >12 years and adults
- Low daily dose: 40–120 µg inhaled by mouth twice daily

- Medium daily dose: 120–240 µg inhaled by mouth twice daily
- High daily dose: >240 µg inhaled by mouth twice daily

Major Drug Interactions
- None

■ Budesonide

Brand Names
Pulmicort Flexhaler, Pulmicort Respules

Generic Name
Budesonide

Dosage Forms
Powder for oral inhalation (Flexhaler 90 µg and 180 µg per inhalation); suspension for nebulization: Pulmicort Respules: 0.25 mg/2 ml; 0.5 mg/2 ml; 1 mg/2 ml

Dosing
Flexhaler:
- Age 5–11 years:
  - Low daily dose: 60–200 µg inhaled twice daily
  - Medium daily dose: 200–400 µg inhaled twice daily
  - High daily dose: >600 µg inhaled twice daily
- Age >12 years and adults:
  - Low daily dose: 60–300 µg inhaled twice daily
  - Medium daily dose: 300–600 µg inhaled twice daily
  - High daily dose: >600 µg inhaled twice daily

Suspension for nebulization:
- Age 0–4 years:
  - Low daily dose: 0.25–0.5 mg divided once or twice daily
  - Medium daily dose: 0.5–1 mg divided twice daily
  - High daily dose: >1 mg divided twice daily
- Age 5–11 years:
  - Low daily dose: 0.25–0.5 mg divided once or twice daily
  - Medium daily dose: 1 mg divided once or twice daily
  - High daily dose: 2 mg divided once or twice daily

Major Drug Interactions
CYP3A4 inhibitors may potentiate the adverse effects of budesonide.

Counseling Points
- Learn the proper use of the Flexhaler
- Use Pulmicort Respules only with a jet nebulizer; do not mix with other inhaled medications in the nebulizer

■ Fluticasone

Brand Name
Flovent HFA

Generic Name
Fluticasone

Dosage Forms

Inhalation (MDI) HFA CFC free 44, 110, 200 µg/inhalation, powder for oral inhalation (Flovent Diskus) 50, 100, 250, and 500 µg

Dosing

HFA/MDI:

- Age 0–4 years:
  - Low dose: 88 µg inhaled twice daily
  - Medium dose: 88–176 µg inhaled twice daily
  - High dose: >176 µg inhaled twice daily
- Age 5–11 years:
  - Low dose: 44–88 µg inhaled twice daily
  - Medium dose: 88–176 µg inhaled twice daily
  - High dose: >176 µg inhaled twice daily
- Age >12 years and adults:
  - Low dose: 44–132 µg inhaled twice daily
  - Medium dose: 132–220 µg inhaled twice daily
  - High dose: >220 µg inhaled twice daily

Diskus:

- Age 5–11 years:
  - Low dose: 50–100 µg inhaled twice daily
  - Medium dose: 100–200 µg inhaled twice daily
  - High dose: >200 µg inhaled twice daily
- Age >12 years and adults:
  - Low dose: 50–150 µg inhaled twice daily
  - Medium dose: 150–250 µg inhaled twice daily
  - High dose: >250 µg inhaled twice daily

Major Drug Interactions

Drugs Affecting Fluticasone

- Ketoconazole or CYP3A4 inhibitors: Increase fluticasone levels (clinical effect unknown)

- Protease inhibitors: Decrease the metabolism of fluticasone; reports of Cushing's syndrome developing from this combination have been found in the literature

Key Point

- Monitor for drug interactions with CYP3A4 inhibitors and inducers. Drug therapy may need to be adjusted in patients with some drug interactions.

■ Triamcinolone

Brand Name

Azmacort

Generic Name

Triamcinolone

Dosage Forms

Inhalation

Dosing

MDI:

- Age 5–11 years:
  - Low dose: 150–300 inhaled twice daily
  - Medium dose: 300–450 µg inhaled twice daily
  - High dose: 450 µg inhaled twice daily
- Age >12 years and adults:
  - Low dose: 150–375 µg inhaled twice daily
  - Medium dose: 375–750 µg inhaled twice daily
  - High dose: >750 µg inhaled twice daily

Major Drug Interactions

- None

Key Point

- Product comes with an attached spacing device

Drug Class: Corticosteroids, Intranasal

Introduction

Intranasal corticosteroids are primarily used for rhinitis and occasionally for the prevention of nasal polyps. The maximal benefit of these agents may not be seen for 1–2 weeks. The most common adverse reactions include epistaxis and nasal irritation. All patients should be counseled on the proper administration technique of intranasal products and instructed to blow nose before use.

Mechanism of Action for the Drug Class

Exact mechanism is unknown. May decrease the number of inflammatory cells, inhibit bronchoconstrictor mechanisms, produce direct smooth muscle relaxation and decreased airway hyperresponsiveness.

Usage for the Drug Class

Relief of symptoms of seasonal and perennial rhinitis*, prevention of nasal polyps

Adverse Reactions for the Drug Class: Most Common

- Headache, dizziness, epistaxis, throat discomfort, nasal irritation

Adverse Reactions for the Drug Class: Rare/Severe/Important

- None

Major Drug Interactions for the Drug Class

- None

Counseling Points for the Drug Class

- Blow nose before each use
- Avoid blowing nose 10–15 minutes after use
- It may take 1–2 weeks to see maximal benefit

Key Points for the Drug Class

- Used most commonly for seasonal and allergic rhinitis
- Administer by nasal inhalation only
- Caution spraying into eyes

Members of the Drug Class

In this section: Beclomethasone, budesonide, fluticasone, mometasone, triamcinolone

Others: Ciclesonide, flunisolide

■ Beclomethasone

Brand Name

Beconase AQ

Generic Name

Beclomethasone

Dosage Forms

Nasal inhalation

Dosing

- Age 6–12 years:
  - Usual dose: 1 spray into each nostril twice daily
  - Maximum dose: 8 sprays/24 hours
- Age >12 years:
  - Usual dose: 1–2 sprays into each nostril twice daily
  - Maximum dose: 8 sprays/24 hours

■ Budesonide

Brand Name

Rhinocort Aqua

Generic Name

Budesonide

Dosage Forms

Nasal inhalation

Dosing

- Usual dose age >6 years: 1 spray into each nostril daily
- Maximum dose age >12 years: 4 sprays into each nostril/ 24 hours
- Maximum dose 6–11 years: 2 sprays into each nostril/ 24 hours

■ Fluticasone

Brand Names

Flonase, Veramyst

Generic Name

Fluticasone

Dosage Forms

Nasal inhalation, intranasal suspension

Dosing

Flonase:
- Age 4–12 years:
  - Usual dose: 1 spray into each nostril once daily; may increase to 2 sprays into each nostril once daily
  - Maximum dose: 4 sprays/24 hours

Veramyst:
- Age 2–12 years:
  - Usual dose: 1 spray into each nostril once daily; may increase to 2 sprays into each nostril once daily
  - Maximum dose: 4 sprays/24 hours

Flonase and Veramyst:
- Adults:
  - Usual dose: 2 sprays into each nostril once daily
  - Maximum dose: 4 sprays/24 hours

■ Mometasone

Brand Name

Nasonex

Generic Name

Mometasone

Dosage Forms

Nasal inhalation

Dosing

- Usual dose (age 2–11 years): 1 spray into each nostril daily
- Usual dose (age >12 years): 2 sprays into each nostril once daily

■ Triamcinolone

Brand Name

Nasacort AQ

Generic Name

Triamcinolone

Dosage Forms

Nasal inhalation

Dosing

- Age 2–5 years:
  - Usual dose: 1 spray into each nostril once daily
  - Maximum dose: 1 spray into each nostril once daily
- Age 6–12 years:
  - Usual dose: 1 spray into each nostril once daily
  - Maximum dose: 4 sprays/24 hours
- Age >12 years:
  - Usual dose: 2 sprays into each nostril once daily
  - Maximum dose: 4 sprays/24 hours

Drug Class: Decongestants

Introduction

Topical decongestants are used for temporary relief of nasal congestion due to a cold or rhinitis. Oxymetazoline should not be used >3 days due to the risk of rebound congestion. Patients with coronary heart disease and hypertension should use this agent with caution. The most common adverse effects include restlessness, nasal dryness, and sneezing.

Mechanism of Action of the Drug Class

Stimulate α-adrenergic receptors of vascular smooth muscle resulting in relief of nasal congestion. Intranasal administration results in constriction of dilated blood vessels in the nasal mucosa, reducing blood flow to engorged edematous tissue. These effects promote drainage of the sinuses, relieving nasal stuffiness, and improving nasal ventilation.

Members of the Drug Class

In this section: Oxymetazoline
Others: Naphazoline, tetrahydrozoline

■ Oxymetazoline

Brand Names

Afrin, Dristan

Generic Name

Oxymetazoline

Dosage Forms

Nasal solution (OTC)

Usage

Temporary relief of nasal congestion due to common cold*, sinusitis, and allergies; adjunctive therapy for middle ear infections associated with acute or chronic rhinitis

Dosing

- Age >6 years, 0.05% solution:
  - Usual dose: 2–3 drops or sprays in each nostril twice daily
  - Maximum dose: 2 doses/24 hours

Adverse Reactions: Most Common

- Anxiety, insomnia, nausea, sneezing

Adverse Reactions: Rare/Severe/Important

- Rebound congestion, high blood pressure, palpitations

Major Drug Interactions

Drugs Affecting Oxymetazoline

- Tricyclic antidepressants, MAO inhibitors: Potentiate the pressor effects of oxymetazoline

Counseling Points

- Wipe tip of applicator clean after each use
- Do not share container with another individual
- Do not use medication >3 days without physician recommendation due to potential occurrence of rebound congestion

Key Points

- Use with caution in patients with coronary heart disease, angina, hypertension, enlarged prostate, diabetes mellitus, glaucoma, and hyperthyroidism
- Do not use >3 days unless prescribed by a physician

Drug Class: Expectorants

Introduction

Expectorants are used to thin respiratory secretions to make a cough more productive. These agents should be used for short-term treatment of a cough. If a cough persists >1 week, patients should be referred to a physician. Adverse effects are rare with guaifenesin.

Mechanism of Action for the Drug Class

Enhances the removal of viscous mucus by reducing adhesiveness and surface tension.

Members of the Drug Class

In this section: Guaifenesin
Others: None

■ Guaifenesin

Brand Names

Robitussin, Mucinex, Brontex

Generic Name

Guaifenesin

Dosage Forms

Tablets, extended-release tablets, syrup

Usage

Productive cough associated with common cold and bronchitis*

Dosing

Tablets and syrup:

- Age <2 years:
  - 12 mg/kg/day in six divided doses
- Age 2–6 years:
  - Usual dose: 50–100 mg by mouth every 4 hours
  - Maximum dose: 600 mg/24 hours
- Age 6–12 years:
  - Usual dose: 100–200 mg by mouth every 4 hours
  - Maximum dose: 1200 mg/24 hours
- Age >12 years:
  - Usual dose: 200–400 mg by mouth every 4 hours
  - Maximum dose: 2400 mg/24 hours

Extended-release tablets, adults:

- Usual dose: 600–1200 mg by mouth twice daily
- Maximum dose: 2400 mg/24 hours

Adverse Reactions: Most Common

- Diarrhea, drowsiness, dizziness, headache

Adverse Reactions: Rare/Severe/Important

- Urolithiasis with large doses

Major Drug Interactions

- None

Counseling Points

- Follow each dose with a full glass of water

- Do not chew and crush extended-release dosage formulations
- Sugar-free formulations are available

Key Points

- Supporting data are very limited and effectiveness is controversial
- Guaifenesin is usually used in combination with decongestants, antihistamines, and antitussives
- Use cautiously in children. Ensure that doses are correct to avoid an overdose.

Drug Class: Leukotriene Inhibitors

Introduction

Leukotriene inhibitors are used in adults and children with persistent asthma. They are administered orally, which improves patient compliance with asthma therapy. These agents are not the preferred first-line treatment for persistent asthma. Montelukast is also used for allergic rhinitis. Montelukast interacts with drug therapies affecting the CYP450 2C9 and 3A4 enzyme systems. Adverse reactions are minor and include headache, nausea, and diarrhea. Serious reactions that have been reported include elevated liver enzymes, eosinophilia, and neuropsychiatric symptoms.

Mechanism of Action for the Drug Class

Selectively block leukotriene receptors thereby decreasing airway edema, relaxing smooth muscles, and inhibiting inflammatory responses.

Members of the Drug Class

In this section: Montelukast
   Others: Zafirlukast

■ Montelukast

Brand Name

Singulair

Generic Name

Montelukast

Dosage Forms

Tablets, chewable tablets, oral granules

Usage

Prophylaxis and chronic treatment of asthma*, seasonal allergic rhinitis (patients >2 years of age), perennial allergic rhinitis (patients >6 months of age)

Dosing

- Age 6 months–5 years:
  - Usual dose: 4 mg (chewable tablet or packet of granules) by mouth once daily in the evening

- Age 6–14 years with asthma or allergic rhinitis:
  - Usual dose: 5 mg by mouth once daily in the evening
- Age >15 years and adults with asthma or allergic rhinitis:
  - Usual dose: 10 mg by mouth once daily in the evening
  - Usual dose in exercise-induced asthma: 10 mg by mouth at least 2 hours before exercise. (Additional doses should not be taken in the same 24 hours.)
  - Maximum dose: 10 mg once daily by mouth in the evening

Adverse Reactions: Most Common

- Headache, nausea, diarrhea, LFT abnormalities (asymptomatic)

Adverse Reactions: Rare/Severe/Important

- Churg–Strauss syndrome (eosinophilic vasculitis), neuropsychiatric symptoms (agitation, aggression, hallucinations, suicidal behavior), pyuria

Major Drug Interactions

Drugs Affecting Montelukast

- CYP450 inducers (phenobarbital and rifampin): Decrease bioavailability by 40%

Counseling Points

- Not for acute attacks
- Use regularly everyday
- Granules may be mixed with applesauce, formula, breast milk, ice cream

Key Points

- Use as adjunct treatment for asthma
- Montelukast should not be used in patients with severe liver disease
- Doses may have to be adjusted when used with drugs that inhibit or induce CYP450 2C9 and 3A4 enzyme systems
- Monitor patients for neuropsychiatric symptoms

Drug Class: Xanthine Derivatives

Introduction

Theophylline has been used for the treatment of asthma and COPD for decades. Currently, the role of theophylline is limited for these indications due to the introduction of inhaled bronchodilators and the potential for serious adverse reactions with xanthine derivatives. Theophylline is now considered as last-line or adjunct therapy for these indications. Theophylline has a narrow therapeutic range, and changes in dosing should only occur after a serum concentration is obtained.

Mechanism of Action for the Drug Class

Exact mechanism is unknown. Directly relaxes smooth muscle in the bronchial airways by inhibiting phosphodiesterase. May stimulate the medullary respiratory center and promotes catecholamine release.

Members of the Drug Class

In this section: Theophylline
  Others: Aminophylline

■ Theophylline

Brand Names
Various

Generic Name
Theophylline

Dosage Forms
Tablets, extended-release tablets and capsules, syrup, injection

Usage
Symptomatic treatment or prevention of bronchial asthma*, chronic bronchitis, or emphysema; apnea in infants

Dosing
- Dosing must be individualized based on age, weight, smoking history, and liver function
- Adults 16–60 years of age without risk factors for impaired theophylline clearance: 300 mg/day in divided doses every 6–8 hours for 3 days, then increase to 400 mg/day in divided doses every 6–8 hours for 3 days; maintenance dose: 600 mg/day in divided doses every 6–8 hours
- Dose using ideal body weight or actual body weight, whichever is less
- Different forms of theophylline have different bioavailability. Aminophylline contains about 80% theophylline.
- Dose needs to be decreased in hepatic dysfunction

- Pharmacokinetic monitoring
  - Therapeutic blood level is 5–15 µg/ml (target concentration: 10 µg/ml)
  - Theophylline is primarily eliminated through hepatic metabolism
  - Serum concentrations should be monitored before making any dose adjustments

Adverse Reactions: Most Common
- Gastroesophageal reflux, headache, increased urination, insomnia, nausea, nervousness

Adverse Reactions: Rare/Severe/Important
- Tachycardia, seizures, arrhythmias

Major Drug Interactions
Drugs Affecting Theophylline
- Phenytoin, phenobarbital, rifampin, ketoconazole, smoking: Decrease serum theophylline concentration
- Allopurinol, verapamil, cimetidine, erythromycin, clarithromycin, ciprofloxacin, enoxacin, thyroid hormones: Increase serum theophylline levels

Theophylline's Effect on Other Drugs
- Lithium: Decreases lithium levels

Counseling Points
- Take liquid or immediate-release formulations on an empty stomach
- Do not break, chew, or crush extended-release formulations
- Capsules may be sprinkled on small amount of food and swallowed whole without chewing
- Avoid smoking, which may change metabolism of theophylline
- Avoid dietary stimulants (coffee, tea, chocolate)

Key Points
- Theophylline should only be used as an adjunctive treatment in COPD and asthma
- Dosing must be individualized based on age, organ function, smoking history, and concomitant drug therapy
- Dose adjustment should not be made without drug concentration monitoring
- Most patients achieve a therapeutic effect with low likelihood of adverse effects at concentrations of 8–12 µg/ml
- Theophylline interacts with drugs that inhibit or induce CYP450 2E1, 1A2, and 3A4
- Charbroiled foods may increase elimination of theophylline

1. Which inhaled corticosteroid should be avoided with atazanavir therapy?
   A. Triamcinolone
   B. Beclomethasone
   C. Fluticasone
   D. All of the above

2. Which of the following cold and cough preparations is *not* considered a controlled substance?
   A. Cheratussin AC
   B. Promethazine with codeine
   C. Robitussin DM
   D. Tussionex

3. Which of the following inhaled medications should be avoided in patients with a peanut allergy?
   A. Combivent
   B. Formoterol
   C. Levalbuterol
   D. Tiotropium

4. Which of the following is a long-acting inhaled β-2 agonist?
   A. Atrovent
   B. Serevent
   C. Spiriva
   D. Xopenex

5. Which of the agents for asthma is only available in an oral dosage form?
   A. Albuterol
   B. Budesonide
   C. Montelukast
   D. Theophylline

6. Which of the following second-generation antihistamines are available in combination with pseudoephedrine?
   A. Cetirizine
   B. Fexofenadine
   C. Loratadine
   D. All of the above

7. Which of the following antihistamines is not available as an over-the-counter (OTC) product?
   A. Allegra
   B. Benadryl
   C. Claritin
   D. Zyrtec

8. SM was admitted to the hospital for a COPD exacerbation. At home she was taking albuterol MDI as needed, Advair inhaled twice daily, and theophylline extended–release tablets 200 mg twice daily. Her steady-state theophylline concentration was found to be 19.5 μg/ml. What would be the most appropriate next step?
   A. Decrease the dose. Theophylline concentrations >15 μg/ml are associated with a higher likelihood of adverse reactions.
   B. Switch the patient to an aminophylline infusion.
   C. Increase theophylline dose to 300 mg twice daily because the patient is having an asthma exacerbation.
   D. Recommend to keep the theophylline dose the same.

9. The physician would like to start SM on an aminophylline continuous infusion. What dose of aminophylline (in mg/hour) would be equivalent to theophylline extended-release 200 mg twice daily?
   A. 8.3 mg/hour
   B. 13.3 mg/hour
   C. 16.6 mg/hour
   D. 20.8 mg/hour

10. Which of the following agents can be used to treat acute shortness of breath caused by asthma?
    A. Foradil
    B. Ipratropium
    C. Symbicort
    D. Xopenex

11. Which of the following agents is intramuscular, the preferred route of administration, due to potential tissue damage when given intravenously?
    A. Benadryl
    B. Hydroxyzine
    C. Phenergan
    D. Theophylline

12. Which of the following adverse reactions can be caused by the use of Pulmicort?
    A. Tachycardia
    B. Thrush
    C. Tremors
    D. Seizures

13. Which agent should patients be counseled to discontinue after 3 days of use?
    A. Afrin
    B. Guaifenesin
    C. Mometasone nasal spray
    D. Tussionex

14. Which inhaled agent is dosed once daily?
    A. Albuterol
    B. Formoterol
    C. Ipratropium
    D. Tiotropium

15. Why should you counsel patients to avoid crushing or chewing benzonatate capsules?
    A. Benzonatate capsules are extended-release
    B. Benzonatate capsules can be chewed
    C. Benzonatate capsules can cause oral numbness if chewed
    D. Benzonatate capsules can cause oral thrush

CHAPTER 14

Topical Products

Susan Kent, PharmD, CGP

Drug Class: Analgesic, Topical

Introduction

The lidocaine topical patch offers a unique option for chronic pain syndromes. Systemic adverse reactions with appropriate use are unlikely, due to the small dose absorbed.

Mechanism of Action for the Drug Class

Lidocaine is an amide-type local anesthetic agent and is suggested to stabilize neuronal membranes by inhibiting the ionic fluxes required for the initiation and conduction of impulses, producing an analgesic effect.

Members of the Drug Class

In this section: Lidocaine topical patch
   Others: Benzyl alcohol, capsaicin, lidocaine (jelly, spray, gel, cream, ointment)

■ Lidocaine Topical Patch

Brand Name
Lidoderm

Generic Name
Lidocaine

Dosage Forms
Extended-release 5% topical patch

Usage
- Relief of chronic pain in postherpetic neuralgia (PHN)*
- Treatment of pain and other chronic pain syndromes, often in an effort to avoid or minimize use of opioid agents and related adverse effects*
- Relief of allodynia (painful hypersensitivity)

Dosing
- PHN: Apply patch to most painful area. Up to 3 patches may be applied in a single application. Patch may remain in place for up to 12 hours in any 24-hour period. It should only be applied to intact skin.

- Severe hepatic disease or impaired elimination recommendations:
  ○ It is not known if lidocaine is metabolized in the skin; however, lidocaine is rapidly metabolized in the liver to various metabolites and is excreted by the kidneys. Smaller areas of treatment are recommended in a debilitated patient or a patient with impaired elimination.

Adverse Reactions: Most Common
- Application site reactions are generally mild and transient, resolving within minutes to hours

Adverse Reactions: Rare/Severe/Important
- Allergic and anaphylactoid reactions associated with lidocaine, although rare, can occur. Transdermal patch may contain conducting metal (e.g., aluminum); remove patch before MRI to avoid burns.

Major Drug Interactions
- Antiarrhythmic drugs: Use with caution in patients receiving class I antiarrhythmic agents. Toxic effects are additive and potentially synergistic.
- Local anesthetics: When lidocaine is used concomitantly with other products containing local anesthetic agents, the amount absorbed from all formulations must be considered

Counseling Points
- Apply to intact skin only; patches may be cut into smaller sizes with scissors before removal of the release liner
- If irritation or a burning sensation occurs during application, remove the patch(es) and do not reapply until the irritation subsides
- Wash hands after handling lidocaine and avoid eye contact
- Store and dispose of patches out of the reach of children, pets, and others
- Never reuse a patch

Key Points

- Apply up to 3 patches, only once for up to 12 hours within a 24-hour period. Patches may be cut to accommodate a smaller area of intact skin.
- Use caution in severe hepatic impairment, pregnant or nursing women, and in patients prescribed medications to treat irregular heartbeat

- The penetration of lidocaine into intact skin after patch application is sufficient to produce an analgesic effect but less than the amount necessary to produce a complete sensory block

---

Drug Class: Antibiotic, Topical (Metronidazole)

Introduction

Topical metronidazole is a member of the imidazole class of antibacterial agents and is used in the treatment of inflammatory lesions of acne rosacea and bacterial vaginosis.

Mechanism of Action for the Drug Class

Metronidazole is classified as an antiprotozoal and antibacterial agent active against susceptible organisms. After diffusing into an organism, metronidazole interacts with DNA to cause a loss of helical DNA structure and strand breakage, resulting in inhibition of protein synthesis and cell death in susceptible organisms.

Members of the Drug Class

In this section: Metronidazole
    Others: Tinidazole (nitroimidazole)

Metronidazole

Brand Name
MetroGel

Generic Name
Metronidazole

Dosage Forms
Gel, topical, vaginal

Usage
- Treatment of inflammatory papules and pustules of acne rosacea*
- Treatment of bacterial vaginosis (BV)*

Dosing
- Apply topically and rub in a thin film twice a day to entire affected area

- One applicator-full (about 37.5 mg metronidazole) intravaginally once or twice daily for 5 days; apply once in morning and evening if using twice daily; if daily, use at bedtime

Adverse Reactions: Most Common
- Burning, skin irritation, dryness, headache; vulva/vaginal irritation, vaginal discharge, fungal infection

Adverse Reactions: Rare/Severe/Important
- Redness, leukopenia

Major Drug Interactions
- Oral metronidazole has been reported to potentiate the anticoagulant effect of warfarin resulting in a prolongation of prothrombin time. The effect of topical metronidazole on prothrombin time is not known.

Counseling Points
- For external use only. Avoid contact with eyes or mouth.
- Wash hands and affected areas before application of metronidazole topical or vaginal gel
- Patients may use cosmetics after application of metronidazole topical gel
- Discontinue use and notify physician at first sign of skin rash or allergic reaction

Key Points
- Apply gel to entire affected areas twice daily; use vaginal applicator as directed by physician, once or twice daily; cleanse areas to be treated before gel application
- Monitor for skin rash or allergic reaction
- Metronidazole is a nitroimidazole and should be used with care in patients with evidence of, or history of, blood dyscrasia

Drug Class: Antibiotic, Topical (Mupirocin)

Introduction

Mupirocin is an antibiotic produced from *Pseudomonas fluorescens* that is structurally unrelated to any other topical or systemic antibiotics. Mupirocin is used topically in the treatment of impetigo caused by *Staphylococcus aureus* and beta-hemolytic streptococci including *Streptococcus pyogenes*. Mupirocin cream was shown to be at least as effective as oral cephalexin for the treatment of secondarily infected traumatic skin lesions.

Mechanism of Action for the Drug Class

Binds to bacterial isoleucyl transfer-RNA synthetase resulting in the inhibition of protein synthesis.

Members of the Drug Class

In this section: Mupirocin
   Others: None; mupirocin is structurally unrelated to other systemic or topical antibiotics

■ Mupirocin

Brand Name

Bactroban

Generic Name

Mupirocin

Dosage Forms

2% cream, ointment

Usage

- Cream: Secondary infected skin lesions due to susceptible strains of *S. aureus* and *S. pyogenes**
- Ointment: Treatment of impetigo*

Dosing

- Cream: Apply a small amount to the affected area three times daily for 10 days
- Ointment: Apply a small amount to the affected area three times daily

Adverse Reactions: Most Common

- Burning, stinging, erythema

Adverse Reactions: Rare/Severe/Important

- Superinfection

Major Drug Interactions

Drugs Affecting Mupirocin

- None known

Mupirocin's Effect on Other Drugs

- May decrease the levels/effect of typhoid vaccine

Counseling Points

- For external use only. Avoid contact with eyes or mouth.
- You may cover treated area with gauze dressing
- Notify physician of any local side effects and if no improvement seen in 3–5 days

Key Points

- Effective for the treatment of skin lesions due to *S. aureus* and *S. pyogenes* (cream) and impetigo (ointment)
- Follow appropriate dosing and duration of treatment depending on indication
- Be aware of sound-alike/look-alike issues with Bactrim, bacitracin, and baclofen

Drug Class: Antibiotic, Topical (Chlorhexidine Gluconate)

Introduction

Chlorhexidine gluconate is used topically as an anti-infective skin cleanser for surgical hand antisepsis, preoperative skin preparation, routine hand hygiene in healthcare personnel, and skin wound and general skin cleansing. It is active against Gram-positive and Gram-negative organisms, facultative anaerobes, aerobes, and yeast.

Mechanism of Action for the Drug Class

The bactericidal effect of chlorhexidine is a result of the binding of this cationic molecule to negatively charged bacterial cell walls and extramicrobial complexes.

Members of the Drug Class

In this section: Chlorhexidine gluconate
   Other: Benzalkonium chloride

■ Chlorhexidine Gluconate

Brand Names

Avagard 1%, Betasept 4%, Hibiclens 4%

Generic Name

Chlorhexidine gluconate

Dosage Forms

Solution, lotion, sponge/brush, swab

Usage

- Skin cleanser for line placement, skin wounds, pre-operative skin preparation*
- Germicidal hand rinse*

Dosing

- Surgical scrub: Scrub 3 minutes and rinse thoroughly; wash for an additional 3 minutes
- Hand sanitizer (Avagard): Dispense 1 pumpful in palm of one hand; dip fingertips of opposite hand into solution and work it under nails. Spread remainder evenly over hand and just above elbow, covering all surfaces. Repeat on other hand. Dispense another pumpful in each hand and reapply to each hand up to the wrist. Allow to dry before gloving.
- Hand wash: Wash for 15 seconds and rinse
- Hand rinse: Rub 15 seconds and rinse

Adverse Reactions: Most Common

- Skin erythema, roughness and/or dryness, sensitization

Adverse Reactions: Rare/Severe/Important

- Allergic reactions

Major Drug Interactions

- None known

Counseling Points

- Keep out of eyes, ears, and mouth; avoid use in children <2 months of age due to increased absorption and/or irritation
- Do not apply to wounds that involve more than superficial layers of skin
- Avoid contact with meninges (do not use on lumbar puncture sites)
- Solutions may be flammable (contain isopropyl alcohol); avoid exposure to open flame and/or ignition source until completely dry
- Avoid application to hairy areas, which may significantly delay drying time

Key Points

- Chlorhexidine gluconate is used topically as an anti-infective skin cleanser
- It is active against Gram-positive and Gram-negative organisms, facultative anaerobes, aerobes, and yeast
- Follow specific washing times per product for adequate skin cleansing and eradication of bacteria

---

Drug Class: Antibiotic, Topical (Clindamycin Phosphate)

Introduction

Clindamycin is a derivative of lincomycin and is categorized as a lincosamide antibiotic. It is used topically for the treatment of inflammatory acne vulgaris and intravaginally for the treatment of BV.

Mechanism of Action for the Drug Class

Clindamycin appears to inhibit protein synthesis in susceptible organisms by binding to 50S ribosomal subunits. The exact mechanisms by which clindamycin reduces lesions of acne vulgaris are not fully understood; however, the effect appears to be related to the antibacterial activity of the drug. The drug inhibits the growth of susceptible organisms on the surface of the skin and reduces the concentration of free fatty acids in sebum. Free fatty acids are comedogenic and are believed to be a possible cause of the inflammatory lesions of acne. However, other mechanisms also appear to be involved.

Members of the Drug Class

In this section: Clindamycin phosphate

Others: Benzoyl peroxide (acne), metronidazole (BV), lincomycin (IV only)

■ Clindamycin Phosphate

Brand Names

Cleocin-T, Clindagel, Evoclin, Clindesse, Cleocin

Generic Name

Clindamycin phosphate

Dosage Forms

Topical gel, lotion, foam, solution, pledget, vaginal suppository/cream

Usage

- Treatment of severe acne (*Propionibacterium acnes*)*
- Treatment of bacterial vaginosis (*Gardnerella vaginalis*)*
- Treatment of susceptible bacterial infections, mainly those caused by anaerobes, streptococci, pneumococci, and staphylococci

Dosing

- Gel, pledget, lotion, solution: Apply a thin film twice daily
- Foam: Apply once daily
- Suppositories: Insert 1 ovule (100 mg clindamycin) daily into vagina at bedtime for 3 days

- Vaginal Cream:
  - Cleocin: 1 full applicator inserted intravaginally once daily before bedtime for 3 or 7 consecutive days in nonpregnant patients or for 7 consecutive days in pregnant patients
  - Clindesse: 1 full applicator inserted intravaginally as a single dose at any time during the day in non-pregnant patients

Adverse Reactions: Most Common

- Dermatologic: Dryness, burning, itching, scaliness, erythema, or peeling of skin; oiliness
- Genitourinary: Vaginal candidiasis, vaginitis, pruritus, vaginal pain

Adverse Reactions: Rare/Severe/Important

- Dermatologic: Pseudomembranous colitis, diarrhea, abdominal pain, hypersensitivity reactions
- Genitourinary: Atrophic vaginitis, local edema, menstrual disorders, pyelonephritis, urinary tract infection

Major Drug Interactions

- Neuromuscular blocking agents: Clindamycin has been shown to have neuromuscular blocking properties that may enhance the neuromuscular blocking action of other agents. Use with caution in patients receiving such agents because clindamycin can be absorbed systemically following intravaginal application.

Counseling Points

- Topical gel, lotion, or solution: Wash hands thoroughly before applying or wear gloves. Apply thin film of gel, lotion, or solution to affected area. Wash hands thoroughly. Wait 30 minutes before shaving or applying makeup.
- Topical foam: Do not dispense directly onto hands or face. Pick up small amounts of foam with fingertips and gently massage into affected areas until foam disappears. Wash hands thoroughly. Wait 30 minutes before shaving or applying makeup.
- Vaginal: Wash hands before using. At bedtime: If using applicator, gently insert full applicator into vagina and expel cream. Wash applicator with soap and water following use. If using suppository, remove foil and insert high into vagina. Remain lying down for 30 minutes following administration. Avoid intercourse during therapy. Vaginal products may weaken condoms or contraceptive diaphragms.

Key Points

- Clindamycin is active against *Gardnerella vaginalis* and *Propionibacterium acnes* and is effective in the treatment of bacterial vaginosis and acne vulgaris
- Wash hands thoroughly before applying product or wear gloves
- Report persistent burning, swelling, itching, excessive dryness, or worsening of condition

---

Drug Class: Antifungal, Topical (Ketoconazole)

Introduction

Ketoconazole, a synthetic azole antifungal agent, is an imidazole derivative and active against both dermatophytes and *Candida* species.

Mechanism of Action for the Drug Class

Alters the permeability of the cell wall by blocking fungal cytochrome P450. Ketoconazole is usually fungistatic in action.

Members of the Drug Class

In this section: Ketoconazole

Others: Clotrimazole, miconazole, nystatin, terbinafine, tolnaftate

■ Ketoconazole

Brand Name

Nizoral

Generic Name

Ketoconazole

Dosage Forms

Cream, foam, gel, shampoo

Usage

- Treatment of a variety of cutaneous fungal infections:
  - Cutaneous candidiasis*
  - Tinea pedis, tinea cruris, and tinea corporis*
  - Dandruff*
  - Seborrheic dermatitis*
  - Tinea versicolor*

Dosing

Fungal infections:

- Tinea infections: Rub cream gently into the affected area once daily
  - Duration of treatment: tinea corporis, cruris: 2 weeks; tinea pedis: 6 weeks
- Tinea versicolor: Apply shampoo twice weekly for 4 weeks with at least 3 days between each shampoo

Seborrheic dermatitis:
- Cream: Rub gently into the affected area twice daily for 4 weeks
- Foam: Apply to affected area twice daily for 4 weeks
- Gel: Rub gently into the affected area once daily for 2 weeks
- Shampoo: Apply twice weekly for 4 weeks with at least 3 days between each shampoo

Adverse Reactions: Most Common
- Severe skin irritation, pruritus, stinging

Adverse Reactions: Rare/Severe/Important
- Painful allergic reactions (local swelling and inflammation), contact dermatitis

Counseling Points
- For external use only; not for ophthalmic, oral, or intravaginal use
- Although improvement and symptom relief usually occur within the first week of therapy, tinea corporis and cruris should be treated for 2 weeks
- Tinea pedis should be treated for 6 weeks; cutaneous candidiasis should be treated for 2 weeks
- Report severe or persistent adverse effects or if condition worsens

Key Points
- Apply exactly as directed
- Wash hands thoroughly before and after applying
- Keep away from eyes or mouth

Drug Class: Antifungal, Topical (Terconazole)

Introduction
Terconazole, a triazole derivative, is a synthetic azole antifungal agent used intravaginally for the treatment of vulvovaginal candidiasis.

Mechanism of Action for the Drug Class
Terconazole exhibits fungicidal activity against *Candida albicans* by disrupting normal fungal cell membrane permeability.

Members of the Drug Class
In this section: Terconazole
    Other: Clotrimazole, miconazole, nystatin, terbinafine, tolnaftate

■ Terconazole

Brand Name
Terazol

Generic Name
Terconazole

Dosage Forms
Vaginal cream, suppository

Usage
Treatment of uncomplicated vulvovaginal candidiasis*

Dosing
- Vaginal cream 0.4%: Insert 1 applicator-full vaginally once a day at bedtime for 7 consecutive days
- Vaginal cream 0.8%: Insert 1 applicator-full vaginally once a day at bedtime for 3 consecutive days
- Vaginal suppositories: Use 1 suppository vaginally at bedtime for 3 consecutive days

Adverse Reactions: Most Common
- Burning and irritation, itching

Adverse Reactions: Rare/Severe/Important
- Abdominal pain, fever

Major Drug Interactions
- Efficacy of intravaginal terconazole is not affected by concomitant use of oral contraceptives
- Administration of intravaginal terconazole does not appear to affect estradiol or progesterone concentrations in women receiving low-dose oral contraceptives

Counseling Points
- For vaginal use only
- Open applicator just before administration to prevent contamination
- Clean applicator after use with mild soap solution and rinse with water
- Complete full course of therapy as directed
- Refrain from intercourse during period of treatment; sexual partner may experience penis irritation
- Suppositories may cause breakdown of rubber/latex products such as condoms and diaphragms; avoid concurrent use
- Inform prescriber if you are or intend to become pregnant. Consult prescriber if breastfeeding.

Key Points
- Terconazole is a topical azole antifungal agent used intravaginally for the treatment of vulvovaginal candidiasis
- Advise patients to finish complete course, even if symptoms have resolved
- Microbiological studies should be repeated in patients not responding to terconazole to confirm the diagnosis and rule out other pathogens

Drug Class: Combination Antibiotic, Topical

Introduction

Erythromycin and benzoyl peroxide is a combination topical antibiotic product used for the treatment of acne vulgaris.

Mechanism of Action for the Drug Class

Erythromycin is a macrolide antibiotic which is active against strains of susceptible organisms. Erythromycin inhibits RNA-dependent protein synthesis at the chain elongation step; it binds to the 50S ribosomal subunit resulting in blockage of transpeptidation. Benzoyl peroxide is an antibacterial and keratolytic agent that releases free-radical oxygen and oxidizes bacterial proteins in the sebaceous follicles decreasing the number of anaerobic bacteria and decreasing irritating-type free fatty acids.

Members of the Drug Class

In this section: Erythromycin and benzoyl peroxide
  Others: Clindamycin/benzoyl peroxide, benzoyl peroxide/hydrocortisone

■ Erythromycin and Benzoyl Peroxide

Brand Name

Benzamycin

Generic Names

Erythromycin and benzoyl peroxide

Dosage Forms

Gel

Usage

Treatment of mild to moderate acne vulgaris*

Dosing

- Apply to affected area twice daily, morning and evening

Adverse Reactions: Most Common

- Peeling, erythema, edema

Adverse Reactions: Rare/Severe/Important

- Sunburn, bleaching of hair and colored fabric, abdominal pain, cramps, diarrhea

Counseling Points

- For external use only. Avoid contact with eyes and mouth.
- Do not use any other topical acne preparation unless otherwise directed by physician. Report any adverse effects or if condition worsens.
- Keep product refrigerated after reconstitution; discard after 3 months

Key Points

- Clean skin before use; apply twice daily to affected area
- Patients should not use any other topical acne preparation concomitantly
- Benzamycin may bleach hair or colored fabric
- Follow manufacturer's reconstitution and storage recommendations

Drug Class: Combination Antifungal and Corticosteroid, Topical

Introduction

The combination of clotrimazole and betamethasone is used to treat fungal skin infections, such as athlete's foot, jock itch, and ringworm.

Mechanism of Action for the Drug Class

Clotrimazole is a synthetic antifungal agent that is active against most strains of dermatophytes. Clotrimazole binds to phospholipids in the fungal cell membrane altering cell wall permeability resulting in loss of essential intracellular elements. Betamethasone is a synthetic corticosteroid used to relieve redness, swelling, itching, and other discomforts of fungal infections. Betamethasone controls the rate of protein synthesis; depresses the migration of polymorphonuclear leukocytes, fibroblasts; reverses capillary permeability and lysosomal stabilization at the cellular level to prevent or control inflammation.

Members of the Drug Class

In this section: Clotrimazole and betamethasone dipropionate
  Others: Nystatin/triamcinolone

■ Clotrimazole and Betamethasone Dipropionate

Brand Name

Lotrisone

Generic Names

Clotrimazole and betamethasone dipropionate

Dosage Forms

Cream, lotion

Usage

- Treatment of symptomatic inflammatory tinea pedis, tinea cruris, and tinea corporis*
- Allergic or inflammatory diseases

Dosing

- Massage into affected area twice daily, morning and evening

Adverse Reactions: Most Common

- Itching, skin irritation

Adverse Reactions: Rare/Severe/Important

- Erythema, dry skin

Major Drug Interactions

Potential pharmacologic interaction with other corticosteroid-containing preparations

Counseling Points

- For external use only. Avoid contact with eyes and mouth.
- Shake lotion well before use

- Use for the full-prescribed treatment duration even though symptoms may have improved
- Notify physician if there is no improvement after 1 week for tinea cruris or tinea corporis or after 2 weeks for tinea pedis
- Do not bandage, cover, or wrap the treated area. Do not use on open wounds.

Key Points

- Follow duration of treatment according to specific type of fungal infection
- Do not exceed application of 45 g of cream/week or 45 ml lotion/week
- This medication should *not* be used >2 weeks for tinea corporis or tinea cruris or >4 weeks for tinea pedis
- This medication is *not* recommended for the treatment of diaper dermatitis

---

Drug Class: Corticosteroid, Topical (Clobetasol Propionate)

Introduction

Clobetasol propionate is a very high potency synthetic fluorinated corticosteroid.

Mechanism of Action for the Drug Class

Following topical application, corticosteroids produce anti-inflammatory, antipruritic, and vasoconstrictor actions. The activity of this class is thought to result at least in part from binding with a steroid receptor and controls the rate of protein synthesis; depresses the migration of polymorphonuclear leukocytes, fibroblasts; reverses capillary permeability and lysosomal stabilization at the cellular level to prevent or control inflammation.

Members of the Drug Class

In this section: Clobetasol propionate
  Others: Betamethasone dipropionate, diflorasone (very high potency)

■ Clobetasol Propionate

Brand Names

Temovate, Olux

Generic Name

Clobetasol propionate

Dosage Forms

Aerosol (foam), cream, gel, lotion, ointment, shampoo, solution

Usage

- Short-term relief of the inflammatory and pruritic manifestations of moderate to severe corticosteroid-responsive dermatoses, including plaque psoriasis and scalp psoriasis*
- Oral mucosal inflammation (unlabeled)

Dosing

- Apply to affected area twice daily, morning and evening, for up to 2 weeks
- Scalp psoriasis: Apply thin film of shampoo to dry scalp once daily; leave in place for 15 minutes; then add water, lather, and rinse thoroughly

Adverse Reactions: Most Common

- Skin burning, tingling, cracking, pruritus

Adverse Reactions: Rare/Severe/Important

- Acneiform eruptions, allergic contact dermatitis

Counseling Points

- For external use only; follow specific product directions
- Apply the smallest amount that will cover affected area. Do not apply to face, groin, or axilla areas. Total dose should not exceed 50 g/week (or 50 ml/week).
- Foam: Turn can upside down and spray a small amount (golf-ball size) of foam into the cap or another cool surface. If fingers are warm, rinse with cool water and dry before handling (foam will melt on contact with warm skin). Massage foam into affected area.
- Spray: Spray directly onto affected area of skin. Gently and completely rub into skin after spraying.

Key Points

- For external use only; do not apply to face, axilla, or groin areas

- Discontinue when control achieved; treatment beyond 2 consecutive weeks is not recommended. Total dosage should not exceed 50 g/week.
- The treated skin area should not be bandaged or wrapped unless directed by a physician

- Adverse systemic effects including hyperglycemia, fluid and electrolyte changes, and HPA suppression may occur when used on large surface areas, for prolonged periods, or with an occlusive dressing

Drug Class: Corticosteroid, Topical (Fluocinonide)

Introduction

Fluocinonide is a fluorinated topical corticosteroid considered to be of high potency.

Members of the Drug Class

In this section: Fluocinonide

Others: Betamethasone dipropionate/valerate, triamcinolone acetonide (high-potency)

■ Fluocinonide

Brand Name

Vanos

Generic Name

Fluocinonide

Dosage Forms

Cream, gel, ointment, solution

Usage

- Atopic dermatitis*
- Corticosteroid-responsive dermatoses*
- Plaque psoriasis*
- Epidermolysis bullosa
- Oral lichen planus

Dosing

- Pruritus and inflammation (0.05%): Apply thin layer to affected area two to four times daily depending on the severity of the condition
- Plaque-type psoriasis (0.1%): Apply a thin layer once or twice daily to affected areas for maximum of 2 consecutive weeks and 60 g/week

Adverse Reactions: Most Common

- Dry skin, pruritus, sensation of burning of skin, headache

Adverse Reactions: Rare/Severe/Important

- Cushing's syndrome, hyperglycemia, adrenal suppression, allergic contact dermatitis

Counseling Points

- For external use only. Do not use for eyes, mucous membranes, or open wounds.
- Use exactly as directed and for no longer than the period prescribed
- Before using, wash and dry area gently. Apply in a thin layer.
- Do not use occlusive dressing unless advised by prescriber. Avoid prolonged or excessive use around sensitive tissues, genital, or rectal areas.
- Avoid exposing treated area to direct sunlight
- Inform prescriber if condition worsens or fails to improve

Key Points

- Therapy should be discontinued when control is achieved; if no improvement is seen, reassessment of diagnosis may be necessary
- Higher strength (0.1%) should not be used on the face, groin, or axilla
- Duration of therapy: Use of the 0.1% cream for >2 weeks is not recommended

Drug Class: Corticosteroid, Topical (Hydrocortisone)

Introduction

Hydrocortisone is a low-to-medium potency corticosteroid used for the relief of inflammatory and pruritic manifestations of corticosteroid-responsive dermatoses.

Members of the Drug Class

In this section: Hydrocortisone

Others: Desonide, fluocinolone acetonide (low-to-medium potency)

◼ Hydrocortisone

Brand Names
Various (Hytone, Cortaid, Anusol-HC, Proctocort, Cortenema)

Generic Name
Hydrocortisone

Dosage Forms
- Topical: Cream, gel, lotion, ointment, solution
- Rectal: Cream, foam, enema, suppository

Usage
- Minor skin irritations*
- Itching and rash due to eczema, dermatitis, insect bites, poison ivy, oak and sumac, soaps, detergents, cosmetics, or jewelry*
- Scalp dermatitis*
- Seborrheic or atopic dermatitis*
- Anogenital pruritus*
- Psoriasis*
- Late phase of allergic contact dermatitis*
- Oral lesions

Dosing
- Dermatoses: Apply appropriate product sparingly one to four times daily; apply aerosol foam to affected area two to four times daily
- Oral lesions: Apply a small amount of paste to the lesion two or three times daily after meals and at bedtime

Adverse Reactions: Most Common
- Eczema, pruritus, stinging, dry skin

Adverse Reactions: Rare/Severe/Important
- Allergic contact dermatitis, burning, HPA axis suppression, hypopigmentation, metabolic effects

Counseling Points
- For dermatologic use only; avoid contact with eyes
- Nonprescription preparations should not be used for *self-medication* for >7 days
- If the condition worsens or symptoms persist, discontinue and consult a clinician
- Before applying, wash area gently and thoroughly; apply a thin film to cleansed area and rub in gently until medication vanishes
- Avoid use of occlusive dressings over topical application unless directed by a prescriber
- Avoid exposing affected area to sunlight

Key Points
- Consider location of the lesion and the condition being treated when choosing a dosage form
- Creams are suitable for most dermatoses, but ointments may also provide some occlusion and are usually used for the treatment of dry, scaly lesions
- Lotions are probably best for treatment of weeping eruptions, especially in areas subject to chafing. Lotions, gels, and aerosols may be used on hairy areas, particularly the scalp.
- Patients applying a topical corticosteroid to a large surface area and/or to areas under occlusion should be evaluated periodically for evidence of HPA axis suppression

---

Drug Class: Corticosteroid, Topical (Mometasone Furoate)

Introduction
Mometasone is a medium-potency topical corticosteroid that has anti-inflammatory, antipruritic, and vasoconstrictive properties.

Members of the Drug Class
In this section: Mometasone furoate

Others: Hydrocortisone butyrate 0.1%, betamethasone valerate 0.1% cream; fluocinolone acetonide 0.025% (medium potency)

◼ Mometasone Furoate

Brand Name
Elocon

Generic Name
Mometasone furoate

Dosage Forms
Lotion, cream, ointment

Usage
Relief of inflammatory and pruritic manifestations of corticosteroid-responsive dermatoses*

Dosing
- Apply a thin film of lotion, cream, or ointment to affected areas once daily

Adverse Reactions: Most Common
- Burning, pruritus

Adverse Reactions: Rare/Severe/Important
- Dryness, irritation

Counseling Points

- For external use only. Avoid contact with eyes, mouth, and open wounds.
- Wash and dry affected area gently before applying product
- Report severe or persistent adverse effects or if no improvement in 2 weeks
- Discontinue use and notify physician at first sign of allergic reaction or skin rash
- The treated skin area should *not* be covered with any occlusive dressing

Key Points

- Topical mometasone furoate products are applied sparingly in thin films and are rubbed into the affected area, usually once daily
- The treated skin area should *not* be covered with any occlusive dressing because this can increase percutaneous penetration of mometasone

---

Drug Class: Corticosteroid, Topical (Triamcinolone Acetonide)

Introduction

Triamcinolone acetonide is a synthetic fluorinated corticosteroid that has anti-inflammatory, antipruritic, and vasoconstrictive properties.

Members of the Drug Class

In this section: Triamcinolone acetonide
Others: Hydrocortisone valerate, fluocinolone acetonide (medium potency)

■ Triamcinolone Acetonide

Brand Name

Kenalog

Generic Name

Triamcinolone acetonide

Dosage Forms

Aerosol, cream, lotion, ointment, paste

Usage

- Inflammatory dermatoses responsive to steroids, including contact/atopic dermatitis*
- Adjunctive treatment and temporary relief of symptoms associated with oral inflammatory lesions and ulcerative lesions resulting from trauma

Dosing

- Apply a thin film sparingly and rub gently into the affected area two to four times daily
- Spray: Apply to affected area three to four times daily
- Oral topical: Press a small dab (about 0.25 inch) to the lesion until a thin film develops; use only enough to coat the lesion with a thin film; do not rub in

Adverse Reactions: Most Common

- Dryness, burning, itching, irritation

Adverse Reactions: Rare/Severe/Important

- Acneiform eruptions, allergic contact dermatitis

Counseling Points

- For external use only; do not use for eyes or mucous membranes or open wounds
- Oral topical (Kenalog in Orabase): Apply at bedtime or after meals if applications are needed throughout the day. Do not use if fungal, viral, or bacterial infections of the mouth or throat are present. If lesion not improved in 7 days, notify prescriber.
- Ointment: Apply a thin film sparingly. Do not use on open skin or wounds. Do not occlude area unless directed.
- Spray: Avoid eyes and do not inhale if spraying near face. Occlusive dressing may be used if instructed; monitor for infection.

Key Points

- Follow specific product directions for application; for external use only
- Avoid eyes, mucous membranes, or open wounds
- Avoid prolonged or excessive use around sensitive tissues, genital, or rectal areas
- Inform prescriber if condition worsens (skin irritation/contact dermatitis) or fails to improve

1. Which of the following agents is available as a topical patch?
   A. Metronidazole
   B. Terconazole
   C. Lidocaine
   D. Hydrocortisone

2. All of the following agents are indicated for the treatment of acne except
   A. Metronidazole
   B. Ketoconazole
   C. Clindamycin
   D. Erythromycin and benzoyl peroxide

3. Metronidazole is available in which of the following dosage forms?
   A. Ointment
   B. Topical patch
   C. Topical solution
   D. Gel

4. Which of the following agents is used to treat secondary infected skin lesions due to susceptible strains of *S. aureus* and *S. pyogenes*?
   A. Bactroban
   B. Betasept
   C. Terazol
   D. Vanos

5. Chlorhexidine gluconate is associated with which of the following usage instructions?
   A. Apply to face twice daily
   B. Wash for 15 seconds and rinse
   C. Apply a small amount of paste three times daily
   D. One full applicator inserted intravaginally

6. Which of the following are correct dosing instructions for Cleocin vaginal cream?
   A. 1 full applicator inserted intravaginally once daily before bedtime for 3 consecutive days in non-pregnant patients
   B. 1 full applicator inserted intravaginally once daily before bedtime for 2 consecutive days in non-pregnant patients
   C. 1 full applicator inserted intravaginally once daily before bedtime for 3 consecutive days in pregnant patients
   D. 1 full applicator inserted intravaginally as a single dose at anytime during the day in pregnant patients

7. Which of the following drug regimens is most appropriate to treat tinea pedis?
   A. Ketoconazole cream: Rub into affected area once daily for 2 weeks
   B. Terconazole cream: Rub into affected area once daily for 2 weeks
   C. Ketoconazole cream: Rub into affected area once daily for 6 weeks
   D. Terconazole cream: Rub into affected area once daily for 6 weeks

8. Which of the following statements is correct regarding Terazol?
   A. Efficacy of intravaginal Terazol is decreased by the use of concomitant oral contraceptives.
   B. Terazol suppositories have no effect on rubber/latex products and can be used with condoms and diaphragms.
   C. Terazol is available as a shampoo.
   D. Burning and irritation are the most common adverse reactions of Terazol.

9. A patient approaches the pharmacy counter with a new prescription for Lidoderm. All of the following are correct counseling points except
   A. No more than 3 patches may be applied in a 24-hour period
   B. The patch should not be cut into smaller sizes before application
   C. Application site reactions are generally mild and transient
   D. It is useful for chronic pain associated with post-herpetic neuralgia

10. Fluocinonide is also known as
    A. Elocon
    B. Temovate
    C. Kenalog
    D. Vanos

11. You are asked to counsel a patient with poison ivy on the proper use of hydrocortisone cream. You suggest all of the following except
    A. Apply a thin film to cleansed area and rub in gently
    B. Use an occlusive dressing on the affected area to protect it
    C. Nonprescription preparations should not be used for self-medication >7 days
    D. Common side effects include dry skin, pruritus, and stinging

12. Correct dosing of Nizoral shampoo for tinea versi-color is
    A. Apply shampoo daily for 2 weeks
    B. Apply shampoo weekly for 4 weeks
    C. Apply shampoo twice weekly for 4 weeks
    D. Apply shampoo twice weekly for 2 weeks

13. Which of the following is available as a paste for oral lesions?
    A. Kenalog
    B. Elocon
    C. Temovate
    D. Vanos

14. Which of the following is a very high-potency topical corticosteroid?
    A. Hydrocortisone
    B. Clobetasol
    C. Fluocinonide
    D. Mometasone

15. All of the following are correct regarding Benzamy-cin except
    A. Apply twice daily for mild–moderate acne vulgaris
    B. Benzamycin requires refrigeration once recon-stituted
    C. Other topical acne preparations may be used concurrently
    D. Bleaching of hair or colored fabrics may occur

Natural Products, Dietary Supplements, and Nutrients

Patrick McDonnell, PharmD

General Statement: Natural Products, Dietary Supplements, and Nutrients

Herbs and botanicals have been used for centuries for the treatment and prevention of disease. Egyptian papyrus, as well as Babylonian stone tablets list "prescriptions" for certain herbals remedies.

These products, defined legally as "dietary supplements" in the United States and also referred to as "natural health products" in the United States and Canada, consist of single or many ingredients. Under the Food and Drug Administration's (FDA) 1994 Dietary Supplement Health and Education Act, a *dietary supplement* is defined as a product taken by mouth that contains a "dietary ingredient" intended to supplement the diet. The "dietary ingredients" in these products may include vitamins, minerals, herbs or other botanicals, amino acids, and substances such as enzymes, organ tissues, glandulars, and metabolites. Although far from complete, data on the safety and efficacy of individual ingredients are more comprehensive for nutrients than for herbals and the others. It should be kept in mind that in the United States, these products, which number in the tens of thousands, are marketed with limited regulatory oversight. For example, there is no review of product safety, efficacy, or quality. The FDA does regulate the labeling and types of claims made on these products, however.

Monographs in this chapter are for some of the most commonly used dietary supplement ingredients. The products available that contain each ingredient are too numerous to list beyond a few examples from the U.S. marketplace. Indications listed are common uses not necessarily supported by clinical evidence. Dosing ranges for nutrients are based on the highest Dietary Reference Intake level for nonpregnant, nonlactating adults. Dosing for other ingredients is based more on current usage than on dose-finding trials. Additionally, dosing of an ingredient may differ between products containing them and may not necessarily be well supported in the literature. Although generally well-tolerated, dietary supplement products can produce adverse effects and interactions. These are based predominantly on case reports and may be reflective of the ingredient itself or the quality of the product it is delivered in. Dietary supplement ingredients do not receive formal pregnancy category ratings, and in most cases they have not been evaluated in pregnancy or lactation. Patients should always consult with their healthcare provider before taking any nonprescription medication or herbal/dietary supplement.

Natural Supplement: Chondroitin

Introduction

Derived from animal cartilage, a popular and relatively safe natural supplement used to reduce the pain of arthritis.

Mechanism of Action for the Drug Class

This mixture of polysulfated glycosaminoglycans (e.g., chondroitin-4-SO_4, chondroitin-6-SO_4) serves as a substrate for cartilage synthesis and may inhibit leukocyte elastase and improve joint mobility.

■ Chondroitin

Brand Names
Cosamin, Cosamin DS, Cosamin Protek, Others

Generic Name
Chondroitin

Dosage Forms
Tablets, capsules, liquid extract

Usage

- Pain relief from osteoarthritis*
- Maintenance of joint cartilage

Dosing

- 200–400 mg orally twice daily to three times daily, or up to 1200 mg orally daily
- Renal dosage adjustment: Not known

Adverse Reactions

- Most common: GI complaints (nausea, diarrhea, mild epigastric pain)
- Headache

Adverse Reactions: Rare/Severe/Important

- Myelosuppression (very rare)

Major Drug Interactions

- Theoretical interaction with anticoagulants because chondroitin's structure is similar to heparinoid compounds

Counseling Points

- Animal sources of chondroitin (bovine, porcine, shark) may pose risk of transmitting infectious agents; use products from trusted manufacturers
- Often found in combination products with glucosamine, although frequently in amounts lower than label claims
- Multi-ingredient products containing manganese may provide doses of this mineral above the tolerable upper limit for adults (11 mg)

Key Point

- Best to avoid during pregnancy and lactation until safety data are available

---

Natural Supplement: Co-Enzyme Q

Introduction

A popular antioxidant, co-enzyme Q is particularly popular in consumers using this agent for "heart health."

Mechanism of Action for the Drug Class

A mitochondrial enzyme, synthesized endogenously and containing 10 isoprenoid subunits, that is involved in electron transport and ATP generation.

■ Co-Enzyme Q

Brand Names

Heart Actives, Heart Support, Pure CoQ-10, Q-Gel, Q-Sorb, and Others

Generic Names

Co-enzyme Q, co-enzyme-Q_{10}, CoQ, CoQ_{10}, ubiquinone, ubidecarenone

Dosage Forms

Tablets, capsules, liquid extract

Usage

- Antioxidant activity for several disorders:
  - Cardiovascular (cardiomyopathy, heart failure, hypertension)*
  - HIV infection
  - Cancer
  - Parkinson's disease
  - Improve exercise performance

Dosing

- Typically 50–200 mg daily:
  - 50 mg twice daily for heart failure
  - 60 mg twice daily for hypertension
  - 50 mg three times daily for angina
  - 200 mg daily for HIV infection

Renal dosage adjustment: Not known

Adverse Reactions: Most Common

- GI complaints (anorexia, nausea, vomiting)

Adverse Reactions: Rare/Severe/Important

- Neurologic complaints (headache, dizziness, fatigue)
- Maculopapular rash
- Thrombocytopenia
- Elevated LFTs
- Hypotension

Major Drug Interactions

- Decreases effect of warfarin (theoretical)
- HMG-CoA reductase inhibitors and β-blockers reduce serum co-enzyme Q concentration

Counseling Points

- Supplied exogenously through many foods, and synthesized endogenously (sharing some synthetic pathways with cholesterol), but significance of source to co-enzyme Q status not yet clear
- Use only with medical supervision for cardiovascular disorders
- Take with food

Key Point

- Best to avoid during pregnancy and lactation until safety data are available

Natural Supplement: Creatine

Introduction

Popular among the younger consumers, creatine supplements are widely used to enhance muscle strength and athletic performance.

Mechanism of Action for the Drug Class

Endogenously synthesized and stored predominantly in skeletal muscle as creatine-phosphate; serves as a high-energy phosphate source during anaerobic metabolism.

■ Creatine

Brand Names

CRE Active, Creatine Blast, Creatine Fuel, Creatine Powder, CreaVATE, and many others

Generic Names

Creatine, creatine monohydrate, N-amidinosarcosine, N-(amino-imino-methyl)-N-methylglycine

Dosage Forms

Capsules, powder

Usage

- Improves muscle strength, athletic performance, and recovery during exercise*

Dosing

- Initial or loading dose of 5 g four times daily for 2–5 days followed by 2–5 g daily for 1–5 weeks; may also be in varying doses as an ingredient in many different exercise or "body-building" supplements

- Renal dosage adjustment: Not known, but avoid use in renal dysfunction

Adverse Reactions: Most Common

- GI complaints (nausea, abdominal pain, diarrhea)

Adverse Reactions: Rare/Severe/Important

- Renal failure

Major Drug Interactions

- When used with other drugs that may affect renal hemodynamics (NSAIDs, ACE inhibitors/angiotensin receptor blockers, and/or diuretics) can increase the risk of renal failure

Counseling Points

- Average diet supplies about 2 g creatine daily as well as the amino acid precursors for endogenous synthesis
- Maintain adequate hydration (at least 2000 ml of water daily)
- Avoid use in combination with caffeine and ephedra
- Products may contain an impurity from processing (dicyandiamide)

Key Point

- Best to avoid during pregnancy and lactation until safety data are available

---

Natural Supplement: Echinacea

Introduction

Echinacea is primarily use as an immune "booster" and is derived most commonly from the genus of plants known as *Asteraceae*, which includes the purple coneflower, which is the most common.

Mechanism of Action for the Drug Class

A number of polysaccharides, alkylamides, caffeic acid esters (echinacosides), and other constituents that all vary between species and plant parts possess nonspecific immunomodulatory activity; may be accounted for in part by altering cell surface binding (T-lymphocytes, macrophages) and increased cytokine production.

■ Echinacea

Brand Names

EchinaGuard, Echinaforce, Esberitox, Echinacea, various

Generic Names

Echinacea (*Echinacea purpurea, E. angustifolia, E. pallida*), black-eyed susan, coneflower, hedgehog, Indian head, purple cone flower, snakeroot

Dosage Forms

Tablets, capsules, liquid extract

Usage

- Treatment of the "common cold"*
- Prevention and treatment of minor upper respiratory infections

Dosing

- 900 mg three times daily of aerial portions of *E. purpurea* standardized to 4% phenolics

- 0.25–1 ml three times daily of a liquid extract (1:1 in 45% ethanol)
- Renal dosage adjustment: Not known

Adverse Reactions: Most Common
- GI complaints (altered taste, nausea, vomiting)
- Neurologic complaints (transient tiredness, somnolence, dizziness, headache)
- Dermatologic (allergic skin reaction, eczema)
- Other (asthma exacerbation, anaphylaxis)

Adverse Reactions: Rare/Severe/Important
- Hepatotoxicity

Major Drug Interactions
- Potential to interfere with immunomodulating agents (theoretical)

- May inhibit CYP3A4 or P-glycoprotein but expected to be low risk

Counseling Points
- Limit continuous use to 2–8 weeks
- Value for treatment may exceed that for prevention of upper respiratory infections
- Avoid use if you have a history of allergy to ragweed, daisy, sunflower, and/or chrysanthemum because they are likely to cross-react with echinacea

Key Points
- Contraindicated for patients with autoimmune diseases and/or on immunosuppressant agents
- Best to avoid during pregnancy and lactation until safety data are available

---

Natural Supplement: Feverfew

Introduction
Feverfew is one of the more commonly used herbal supplements touted for its anti-inflammatory and analgesic effects. It is sometimes favored as a natural product for migraine sufferers.

Mechanism of Action for the Drug Class
Various metabolites including parthenolide inhibit prostaglandin synthesis, platelet aggregation, and leukotriene synthesis.

■ Feverfew

Brand Names
Feverfew Extract, Herbal Sure Feverfew, Mygrafew, NuVeg Feverfew Leaf, Premium Feverfew Leaf

Generic Name
Feverfew (*Tanacetum parthenium*)

Dosage Forms
Tablets, capsules, liquid extract

Usage
- Pain and inflammation*
- Headaches, including treatment and prophylaxis of migraines*

Dosing
- 200–250 mg daily including the treatment of migraines
- Renal dosage adjustment: Not known; however, use with caution in patients with renal impairment due to expected effects on renal prostaglandins

Adverse Reactions: Most Common
- Avoid skin contact due to high potential for sensitization when contact with skin
- Transient tachycardia
- Bruising, bleeding, GI ulceration
- Abdominal pain, diarrhea

Adverse Reactions: Rare/Severe/Important
- Renal failure, hepatotoxicity

Major Drug Interactions
- Concurrent use of NSAIDs can increase risk of GI toxicities (dyspepsia, GI ulceration) and nephrotoxicity
- Antiplatelet agents and anticoagulants may increase risk of bleeding
- Caution with drugs that can negatively impact renal hemodynamics, such as diuretics, ACE inhibitors/angiotensin receptor blockers, methotrexate, lithium

Counseling Points
- Monitor for signs and symptoms of bleeding especially if using concurrent therapies such as anticoagulants, NSAIDs, and antiplatelet therapy
- Discontinue 7–10 days before elective surgery
- Monitor for any changes in renal function particularly if using concurrent NSAID therapy, ACE inhibitors, angiotensin receptor blockers, and/or diuretics

Key Points
- Avoid in patients with severe renal disease
- Avoid during pregnancy, particularly the third trimester due to inhibition of prostaglandins on fetal cardiac physiology

Natural Supplement: Garlic

Introduction

Garlic supplements, another popular botanical, is believed to have many pharmacologic effects including its use as an antiseptic, antihypertensive, antilipemic agent, and expectorant. However, it is believed that the most benefits are derived from the raw garlic clove versus commercially prepared products.

Mechanism of Action for the Drug Class

Alliins are the most active substances of garlic. Belief is that garlic alliins block adenosine triphosphate citrate lyases, an important enzymatic step in the process of converting carbohydrates to fat. Another substance in garlic known as ajoene seems to demonstrate antimicrobial properties. It is believed, however, that any pharmacologic effect with garlic is seen with the use of freshly prepared products versus commercialized capsules, tablets, and powders.

■ Garlic

Brand Names

Garlicin, Garlique, Garlic Oil, Triple Garlic, Kyolic-Branded Products, High Allicin Garlic, Odor-Free Concentrated Garlic

Generic Names

Garlic (*Allium sativum*), allium, clove garlic, poor man's treacle, stinking rose

Dosage Forms

Tablets, capsules, liquid extract, dried powder, raw garlic cloves

Usage

- Treatment of hyperlipidemia*
- High blood pressure*
- Antiseptic agent*

Dosing

- Hyperlipidemia: Total daily dose of 600–900 mg of garlic powder (standardized to 1.3% of alliin content)
- Hypertension: 200–300 mg three times daily
- Antiseptic: Fresh garlic applied to the skin as antimicrobial dressing for a few hours; prolonged contact may lead to skin irritation/burns
- Renal dosage adjustment: Not known

Adverse Reactions: Most Common

- Headache, fatigue, myalgias
- Skin reactions/burns with prolonged application of fresh garlic preparations to skin
- Dyspepsia, body odor, halitosis, lacrimation

Adverse Reactions: Rare/Severe/Important

- Increase bleeding risk, particularly when combined with antiplatelet agents and/or anticoagulants

Major Drug Interactions

- Increased bleeding risks when used with antiplatelets, NSAIDs, and anticoagulants; monitor accordingly

Counseling Points

- Increased bleeding risks when used with antiplatelets, NSAIDs, and anticoagulants; monitor accordingly
- Discontinue 7–10 days before elective surgery
- Best therapeutic results are seen with freshly prepared garlic

Key Point

- Avoid during pregnancy and lactation

Natural Supplement: Ginseng (*Panax ginseng*)

Introduction

Ginseng, a very popular natural supplement worldwide, which is used as a general tonic to improve well-being and increase energy levels.

Mechanism of Action for the Drug Class

The mature root contains numerous triterpenoid saponins (ginsenosides) of varying composition and concentration between species, as well as flavonoids and vitamins, that may contribute to central nervous system stimulation/suppression, hypertension/hypotension, immunomodulation, antioxidant and anti-inflammatory activities; these may occur through an effect on the hypothalamic–pituitary–adrenal axis and neurotransmitter pathways.

■ Ginseng

Brand Names

Ginsana, G-115, Ginseng, Various

Generic Names

Ginseng, Asian Ginseng (*Panax ginseng*), Chinese ginseng, Japanese ginseng, Korean ginseng, jintsan, red ginseng, ninjin, ren shen, seng, American ginseng (*Panax quinquefolius*), anchi ginseng, red berry, ren shen, sang, tienchi ginseng

Dosage Forms

Tablets, capsules, tinctures

Usage

- Improve well-being*
- Boost energy*
- Stress relief

Dosing

- 200–600 mg daily of root extract standardized to 4–5% ginsenoside
- Renal dosage adjustment: Not known

Adverse Reactions: Most Common

- Neurologic complaints (headache, transient nervousness, insomnia, cerebral arteritis)
- Ocular (mydriasis, disturbance of accommodation)
- Cardiovascular (hypertension, hypotension)
- Metabolic (hypoglycemia)

Adverse Reactions: Rare/Severe/Important

- Dermatologic reactions such as Stevens–Johnson syndrome, postmenopausal vaginal bleeding, mastalgia

Major Drug Interactions

- May decrease the anticoagulant effect of warfarin
- May increase bleeding risk with antiplatelet agents
- May increase effects of caffeine and products that contain natural guarana
- May increase stimulant effects when used with MAOIs

Counseling Points

- Avoid doses >3 g daily
- Take within 2 hours of a meal to avoid potential hypoglycemia
- Limit continuous use to <3 months
- "Siberian ginseng" contains no ginsenosides and is actually a different botanical, *Eleutherococcus senticosus* (eleuthera)

Key Point

- Avoid during pregnancy and lactation

Natural Supplement: Ginkgo (*Ginkgo biloba*)

Introduction

Supplements derived from *Ginkgo biloba* are popularly used by those to improve memory and cognitive function.

Mechanism of Action for the Drug Class

The leaf extract contains terpene lactones (ginkgolides, bilobalide), flavonoids, and amino acids that contribute to antiplatelet, vasodilatory, and free-radical scavenging activity to improve circulatory flow; ginkgolide B inhibits platelet activating factors.

■ Ginkgo

Brand Names

Ginkai, Ginkgold, Ginkgo, Various

Generic Names

Ginkgo (*Ginkgo biloba*), bai guo ye, fossil tree, kew tree, maidenhair tree, salisburia, yinshing

Dosage Forms

Tablets, capsules, tinctures

Usage

- Memory enhancer*
- Cerebrovascular insufficiency (dementia, memory impairment)*
- Vertigo and tinnitus
- Peripheral vascular disease (intermittent claudication)

Dosing

- 40–80 mg three times daily, of a leaf extract standardized to 22–27% flavone glycosides and 5–7% terpenes
- Renal dosage adjustment: Not known

Adverse Reactions: Most Common

- GI complaints (nausea, vomiting, diarrhea)
- Neurologic complaints (headache, dizziness, restlessness)
- Cardiovascular (palpitations)
- Hematologic (bleeding)

Adverse Reactions: Rare/Severe/Important

- Dermatologic (allergic skin reaction, Stevens–Johnson syndrome)

Major Drug Interactions

- Increases the effect of antiplatelets and anticoagulants
- Decreases the effect of antiepileptics (if excessive amounts of natural contaminant from ginkgo seeds are present)

Counseling Points

- May require at least 4 weeks and possibly 6–8 weeks of treatment for effect
- Report any skin rashes, unusual bruising, or bleeding to a healthcare professional
- Use caution if combined with other products that may possess antiplatelet or anticoagulant effects
- Discontinue 2 weeks before surgery to reduce bleeding risk
- May be taken without regard to meals or food intake

Key Point

- Avoid during pregnancy and lactation

Natural Supplement: Glucosamine

Introduction

Glucosamine, a very popular supplement for joint health, is used alone or in conjunction with chondroitin. Studies have shown mixed results on the benefits of glucosamine; however, it remains a favorite of consumers and has a relatively good safety record.

Mechanism of Action for the Drug Class

This hexosamine sugar is a building block substrate for glycoproteins, glycolipids, glycosaminoglycans, proteoglycans, and hyaluronic acid required for cartilage synthesis.

■ Glucosamine

Brand Names

Cosamin, Cosamin DS, Cosamin Protek, and many others

Generic Name

Glucosamine

Dosage Forms

Tablets, capsules, liquid extract

Usage

- Pain relief from osteoarthritis*
- Maintenance of joint function*

Dosing

- 500 mg orally three times daily
- Renal dosage adjustment: Not known

Adverse Reactions: Most Common

- GI complaints (altered taste, nausea, vomiting, constipation, flatulence, abdominal bloating, cramps, diarrhea)
- Headache
- Allergic reactions (may cross-react in patients with severe shellfish allergies)

Adverse Reactions: Rare/Severe/Important

- None reported

Major Drug Interactions

- Glucosamine may decrease sensitivity to insulin and oral antidiabetic agents (of primary concern in patients with hard to manage glycemic control/those with "brittle diabetes")
- Diuretics may increase GI side effects of glucosamine

Counseling Points

- Glucosamine sulfate has been studied more frequently than other salts
- If you have a shellfish allergy, select products carefully because the products may be either synthetic or derived from marine exoskeletons
- Multi-ingredient products containing manganese may provide doses of this mineral above the tolerable upper limit for adults (11 mg)

Natural Supplement: Kava

Introduction

Kava or kava-kava, a popular botanical for anxiety relief, is a potentially dangerous herbal supplement. Warnings from the FDA have highlighted hepatotoxicity from this product. Kava is banned from sales in the United Kingdom, Germany, Switzerland, France, Canada, and Australia due to the risk of liver damage.

Mechanism of Action for the Drug Class

Kava lactones/pyrones have centrally muscle-relaxing, anticonvulsive, and antispasmodic effects. Kava also has hypnotic, analgesic, and psychotropic properties. Kava can also inhibit cyclo-oxygenase 2.

■ Kava

Brand Names

Pharma Kava, Kava Kava Premium

Generic Names

Kava (*Piper methysticum*), kava-kava, ava, ava pepper, intoxicating pepper, tonga, kew

Dosage Forms

Capsules, tinctures, tea

Usage

- Anxiety, stress, tension, agitation*

Dosing

- Capsules of kava root extract: 150–300 mg orally twice daily
- Tincture: 30 drops with water three times daily
- Renal dosage adjustment: Not known

Adverse Reactions: Most Common

- CNS complaints of dizziness, headache
- Pupillary dilation

Adverse Reactions: Rare/Severe/Important

- Case reports of hepatotoxicity with some being irreversible and fatal
- Kava dermopathy: A reversible darkening or yellowing of the skin with whitish scaly flakes

Major Drug Interactions

- Increased bleeding risks when used with antiplatelets, NSAIDs, and anticoagulants; monitor accordingly

- In vitro inhibition of CYP 1A2, 2C9, 2C19, 3A4; caution advised when kava is used with drugs metabolized by these enzymes
- Increased CNS toxicities when used with other centrally acting agents (benzodiazepines, barbiturates, opiates, ethanol)
- May decrease effectiveness of dopaminergic agents (levodopa) used in Parkinson's disease
- Concurrent hepatotoxins are to be avoided
- MAOIs

Counseling Points
- Increased bleeding risks when used with antiplatelets, NSAIDs, and anticoagulants'; monitor accordingly

- Discontinue 7–10 days before elective surgery
- Avoid use with concurrent hepatotoxins; monitor for signs and symptoms of liver toxicity
- Food enhances absorption
- Notify physician and pharmacist if self-initiating due to numerous drug interactions
- This product should be avoided because of the risk of liver toxicity

Key Points
- Avoid during pregnancy and lactation
- Warnings of hepatotoxicity: Kava should be avoided

Natural Supplement: Melatonin

Introduction
Consumers who use melatonin do so for its effect on the sleep cycle and use it as a sleep aid. Consumers who travel use melatonin to help allay feelings of tiredness from jet lag.

Mechanism of Action for the Drug Class
This pineal gland hormone is involved in regulating several functions including the sleep–wake cycle (circadian rhythm); synthesized endogenously from serotonin.

■ Melatonin

Brand Names
Melatonex, Melatonin, Melatonin Forte, Melatonin PM Complex

Generic Name
Melatonin (N-acetyl-5-methoxytryptamine)

Dosage Forms
Tablets, capsules

Usage
- Promotion of sleep*
- Prevent symptoms of jet lag*
- Treatment of insomnia*

Dosing
- 0.3–3 mg at bedtime for sleep
- Up to 5 mg daily for 3 days before and 3 days after air travel
- Renal dosage adjustment: Not known

Adverse Reactions: Most Common
- Neurologic complaints (migraine headaches, daytime drowsiness, depression)

Adverse Reactions: Rare/Severe/Important
- Hypothermia
- Hypertension
- Retinopathy
- Seizure
- Infertility

Major Drug Interactions
- Potentially additive effects with CNS depressants

Counseling Points
- Do not drive or operate machinery or engage in other skilled activities for several hours after taking melatonin
- Use only for short durations; do not use chronically
- Select immediate-release products over sustained-release products
- Select products containing synthetic melatonin over those derived from animal pineal glands

Key Point
- Avoid during pregnancy or if trying to conceive and if lactating

Natural Supplement: Saw Palmetto

Introduction

Saw palmetto is touted for prostate health, although recent randomized prospective controlled trials have shown little benefit for this indication. Nonetheless, it remains a popular product among consumers.

Mechanism of Action for the Drug Class

Lipid fraction (fatty acids, sterols) inhibits 5-α-reductase activity and possesses antiandrogenic, antiproliferative, and anti-inflammatory properties.

■ Saw Palmetto

Brand Names

Nutrilite, PROST Active, PROST Active Plus, Sabal Select, Solaray

Generic Names

Saw palmetto (*Serenoa repens*; also *Serenoa serrulata*), American dwarf palm tree, cabbage palm, sabal fructus

Dosage Forms

Tablets, capsules

Usage

- Symptoms of benign prostatic hypertrophy (BPH)*

Dosing

- 160 mg twice daily or 320 mg daily of a liposterolic extract of ripe fruit, standardized to 85–95% fatty acids/sterols
- Renal dosage adjustment: Not known

Adverse Reactions: Most Common

- GI complaints (nausea, vomiting, constipation, diarrhea)
- Neurologic complaints (headache, insomnia, dizziness)
- Estrogenic effects

Adverse Reactions: Rare/Severe/Important

- None reported

Major Drug Interactions

- None documented

Counseling Points

- Before use, see healthcare provider to rule out prostate cancer
- May require at least 4–6 weeks and as long as 3–6 months for full effect
- Does not seem to alter prostate size; questionable benefit as demonstrated by randomized prospective controlled trials

Key Point

- Avoid during pregnancy and lactation; not intended for women

Natural Supplement: St. John's Wort

Introduction

St. John's wort is widely touted for depression and is quite popular in Europe, as well as in the United States and Canada for this indication. Clinical trials have demonstrated effectiveness as an antidepressant for mild depression versus significant cases of clinical depression.

Mechanism of Action for the Drug Class

Extract from the flower contains naphthodianthrones (hypericins), flavonoids (hyperoside), phloroglucinols (hyperforin), and other constituents that probably inhibit to some degree central serotonin, norepinephrine, dopamine, and γ-aminobutyric acid reuptake.

■ St. John's Wort

Brand Names

St. John's Wort (from various manufacturers)

Generic Names

St. John's wort (*Hypericum perforatum*), goat weed, hypericum, John's wort, Klamath weed, millepertuis, tipton weed

Dosage Forms

Tablets, capsules, liquid

Usage

- Mild to moderate depression*

Dosing

- 300 mg three times daily or 450 mg twice daily of a flower extract standardized to 0.3% dianthrones (or total hypericins), or 2–6% hyperforin
- Renal dosage adjustment: Not known

Adverse Reactions: Most Common

- GI complaints (dry mouth, nausea, vomiting, constipation, abdominal pain, bloating, diarrhea)

- Neurologic complaints (headache, dizziness, insomnia, fatigue, restlessness, anxiety, hypomania, serotonin syndrome)
- Dermatologic (allergic skin reaction, photosensitivity)
- Other (anorgasmia)

Adverse Reactions: Rare/Severe/Important
- Serotonin syndrome, hypertensive crisis

Major Drug Interactions
- Strong enzyme inducer (CYP3A4, CYP2D6, CYP1A2, P-glycoprotein) through pregnane X receptor binding; increases the clearance of benzodiazepines, cyclosporine, digoxin, estrogens, irinotecan, protease inhibitors, simvastatin, tacrolimus, theophylline, and warfarin

- Additive effects with other antidepressants
- Additive effects with other serotoninergic-acting drugs
- Increased phototoxicity with other drugs known to be photosensitizers (i.e., amiodarone, methotrexate, tetracyclines, etc.)

Counseling Points
- Requires at least 2–3 weeks of treatment for effect
- Take in the morning if you experience insomnia
- Limit sun exposure or consider using a sunscreen
- Avoid the use of alcohol

Key Point
- Avoid during pregnancy and lactation

Natural Supplement: Valerian

Introduction
Valerian in the form of teas and capsules is used as a sleep aid; however, these same sedative effects can pose a risk to those using other CNS depressants.

Mechanism of Action for the Drug Class
Valerianic acid components have been shown to decrease the degradation of γ-aminobutyric acid (GABA) with an increase of GABA at the synaptic cleft via inhibition of reuptake and an increase in secretion. This increase of available GABA may be one factor responsible for the sedative effects of valerian.

■ Valerian

Brand Names
Herbal Sure Valerian Root, NuVeg Valerian Root, Quanterra Sleep, Natural Herbal Valerian Root, Nature's Root Nighttime

Generic Names
Valerian (*Valeriana officinalis*), valerian root, capon's tail, heliotrope, vandal root

Dosage Forms
Teas/teabags, extracts, tablets, capsules

Usage
- Sleep aid*
- Insomnia caused by anxiety*
- Restlessness

Dosing
- Restlessness: 220 mg of extract three times daily
- Sleep aid: 400–900 mg 30 minutes before bedtime
- Renal dosage adjustment: Not known

Adverse Reactions: Most Common
- GI complaints (nausea, vomiting, constipation, diarrhea)
- Neurologic complaints (headache, insomnia, dizziness)

Adverse Reactions: Rare/Severe/Important
- Reports of rare hepatotoxicity

Major Drug Interactions
- Antiplatelet agents and anticoagulants: Increased risk of bleeding
- Barbiturates, benzodiazepines, ethanol, opiates: Increased CNS depression
- Hepatotoxins: Use with caution; may elevate transaminases
- Iron: Binds with iron leading to malabsorption; separate administration time by 1–2 hours
- Loperamide: Paradoxical delirium and confusion

Counseling Points
- Avoid driving or working with heavy equipment when starting therapy due to sedative effects
- Avoid use with alcohol or other sedative medications
- Monitor for signs and symptoms of hepatotoxicity (dark amber urine, skin or eye jaundice/yellowing, right upper-quadrant abdominal pain)

Key Point
- Avoid during pregnancy and lactation

Nutrients and Vitamins

Introduction

Vitamins are macronutrients essential for life. They regulate metabolism and assist in different biochemical processes such as the formation of hormones, blood cells, nervous system chemicals, and genetic material. They differ in their physiologic actions. The fat-soluble vitamins include vitamin A, vitamin D, vitamin E, and vitamin K. These are generally consumed along with fat-containing foods. The water-soluble vitamins include B vitamins and vitamin C. These cannot be stored by the body and must be consumed frequently, usually every day. The only vitamin manufactured in our bodies is vitamin D. All others must be derived from the diet. Deficiencies in vitamin intake can cause different health problems.

Dietary Supplement: β-Carotene

Mechanism of Action for the Drug Class
One of several hundred carotenoids with varying activity depending on isomer; converted in part to vitamin A (retinol) at the GI tract and may contribute some antioxidant activity.

■ β-Carotene

Brand Names
Various

Generic Names
β-Carotene, all-*trans*-β-carotene

Dosage Forms
Tablets, capsules

Usage
- Meet vitamin A requirement*
- Reduce risk of cardiovascular disease, cancer, age-related macular degeneration and cataracts*

Dosing
- No more than 20–30 mg daily
- Renal dosage adjustment: Not known

Adverse Reactions: Rare/Severe/Important
- Hepatotoxicity when used in high doses
- Carotenoderma (orange/yellow skin discoloration) at doses >300 mg daily

Major Drug Interactions
- Decreases bioavailability of other carotenoids (e.g., lutein)
- Cholestyramine, mineral oil, orlistat, and proton pump inhibitors may reduce β-carotene absorption

Counseling Point
- Dietary content of β-carotene is approximately 3 mg daily

Dietary Supplement: Calcium

Mechanism of Action for the Drug Class
Structural role in bone and teeth, as well as roles in vascular, neuromuscular, and glandular function among others.

■ Calcium

Brand Names
Calcium (Various), Cal-Lac, Caltrate, Calsorb, Citracal, Os-Cal, Tums

Generic Names
Calcium (salts: carbonate, citrate, etc.)

Dosage Forms
Tablets

Usage
- Prevent or treat calcium deficits*
- Manage osteoporosis*
- Hypertension
- Premenstrual syndrome
- Reduce risk of colon cancer

Dosing
- 500 mg of elemental calcium two to three times daily
- Age 14–18 years: 1300 mg daily; pregnant or lactating: 1300 mg daily
- Age 19–50 years: 1000 mg daily; pregnant or lactating: 1000 mg daily

- Age >50 years: 1200 mg daily
- Tolerable upper intake level: 2500 mg daily from all sources
- Renal dosage adjustment: Not known

Adverse Reactions: Most Common
- GI complaints (nausea, constipation, flatulence)

Adverse Reactions: Rare/Severe/Important
- Renal insufficiency, nephrolithiasis
- Hypercalcemia

Major Drug Interactions
- Decreases absorption of etidronate, levothyroxine, quinolones, tetracyclines, iron, magnesium, and zinc
- Increases the hypercalcemia risk of tamoxifen
- Corticosteroids decrease calcium status
- Loop diuretics increase urinary calcium loss
- Thiazide diuretics increase renal calcium reabsorption

Counseling Points
- Avoid the following sources of calcium because of potential contaminants:
  - Bone meal, dolomite, oyster shells (may be of risk in patients with severe shellfish allergy)
- Dose in terms of elemental calcium:

Calcium Salt	Elemental Calcium	Calcium (mg)/Salt (g)
Calcium carbonate	40%	400
Dibasic calcium phosphate	23%	230
Calcium citrate	21%	210
Calcium lactate	13%	130
Calcium gluconate	9%	90

- Maximize calcium absorption by dividing doses (500 mg/dose maximum), and take with meals

---

Dietary Supplement: Vitamin D

Mechanism of Action for the Drug Class
Vitamin D is essential for promoting calcium absorption in the gut and maintaining adequate serum calcium and phosphate concentrations.

■ Cholecalciferol

Brand Names
Vitamin D, D3

Generic Name
Cholecalciferol

Dosage Forms
Capsules, tablets

Usage
- Dietary supplement, treatment of vitamin D deficiency, or prophylaxis of deficiency*
- Osteoporosis prevention and treatment*

Dosing
- Age 18–50 years: 200 IU/day
- Age 51–70 years: 400 IU/day
- Elderly age >70 years: 600 IU/day

Contraindications
- Hypercalcemia; hypersensitivity

Adverse Reactions: Most Common
- None

Adverse Reactions: Rare/Severe/Important
- Hypervitaminosis D: Signs and symptoms include hypercalcemia, resulting in headache, nausea, vomiting, lethargy, confusion, sluggishness, abdominal pain, bone pain, polyuria, polydipsia, weakness, cardiac arrhythmias (e.g., QT shortening, sinus tachycardia), soft tissue calcification, calciuria, and nephrocalcinosis

Major Drug Interactions
- No known drug interactions

Counseling Point
- Take as directed

Dietary Supplement: Cyanocobalamin

Mechanism of Action for the Drug Class
The role of cyanocobalamin, or Vitamin B$_{12}$, is essential in the maintenance of cellular integrity, particularly in disease states such as anemia, pregnancy, thyrotoxicosis, malignancy, liver, neurologic, or kidney disease.

■ Cyanocobalamin

Brand Names
CaloMist, Nascobal, Twelve-Resin

Generic Names
Cyanocobalamin, vitamin B$_{12}$

Dosage Forms
Tablets, injection, lozenge, intranasal solution

Usage
- Prevention and treatment of Vitamin B$_{12}$ deficiency*
- Pernicious anemia treatment*

Dosing
- Recommended adult intake: 2.4 µg/day
- Recommended intake during pregnancy: 2.6 µg/day
- Recommended intake during lactation: 2.8 µg/day
- Vitamin B$_{12}$ deficiency dosing:
  - Intranasal:
    - Nascobal: 500 µg in one nostril once weekly
    - CaloMist: Maintenance therapy (following correction of vitamin B$_{12}$ deficiency): 25 µg in each nostril daily; if suboptimal response, 25 µg in each nostril twice daily
  - Oral: 250 µg/day
  - IM; deep SUB-Q: initial 30 µg/day for 5–10 days; maintenance: 100–200 µg/month

- Pernicious anemia: IM; deep SUB-Q: 100 µg/day for 6–7 days; if improvement noted, administer the same dose on alternating days for 7 doses, then every 3–4 days for 2–3 weeks; maintenance dosage: 100 µg/month. Alternative dosing of 1000 µg/day for 5 days followed by a maintenance dose of 500–1000 µg/month also is used.
  - For a hematologic remission/correction of pernicious anemia, maintenance doses are as follows:
    - Intranasal (Nascobal): 500 µg in one nostril once weekly
    - Oral: 1000–2000 µg/day
    - IM: deep SUB-Q: 100–1000 µg/month
- Renal dosage adjustment: None

Adverse Reactions: Most Common
- Well-tolerated; injection site reactions/redness with IM; deep SUB-Q injections

Adverse Reactions: Rare/Severe/Important
- CHF, polycythemia vera, paresthesias, pulmonary edema

Major Drug Interactions
- Chloramphenicol: May diminish the effect of cyanocobalamin
- Alcohol: Heavy use/consumption >2 weeks can impair vitamin B$_{12}$ absorption

Counseling Point
- Use exactly as prescribed

Dietary Supplement: Ergocalciferol

Mechanism of Action for the Drug Class
The role of ergocalciferol, a vitamin D analog, is essential in the maintenance of vitamin D levels, particularly in women to prevent osteoporosis and in patients with chronic kidney disease. Ergocalciferol stimulates calcium and phosphorous absorption from the small intestine and promotes secretion of calcium from bone to blood; it also promotes renal tubule resorption of phosphorous.

■ Ergocalciferol

Brand Name
Drisdol

Generic Name
Ergocalciferol

Dosage Forms
Capsules, liquid, tablets (*Note*: 1 µg = 40 international units [IU])

Usage
- Prevention and treatment of vitamin D deficiency*
- Treatment of refractory rickets
- Treatment of hypophosphatemia and hypoparathyroidism

Dosing
- Recommended adult intake (age 18–50 years): 5 µg/day
- Recommended adult intake (age 51–70 years): 10 µg/day

- Prevention and treatment of osteoporosis for adults age ≥50 years: 10 µg/day
- Vitamin D deficiency/insufficiency in patients with chronic kidney disease (CKD) (Kidney Disease Outcomes Quality Initiative guidelines for stage 3–4 CKD):
  - Serum 25-hydroxyvitamin D level <5 ng/ml: 50,000 IU/week for 12 weeks, then 50,000 international units/month
  - Serum 25-hydroxyvitamin D level 5–15 ng/ml: 50,000 IU/week for 4 weeks, then 50,000 international units/month
  - Serum 25-hydroxyvitamin D level 16–30 ng/ml: 50,000 IU/month
- Hypoparathyroidism: 625 µg to 5 mg/day orally

- Nutritional rickets and osteomalacia:
  - Adults with normal absorption: 25–125 µg/day
  - Adults with malabsorption: 250–7500 µg/day
  - Renal dosage adjustment: None

Adverse Reactions: Most Common
- Nausea, metallic taste in mouth, dry mouth

Major Drug Interactions
- None significant

Counseling Point
- Use exactly as prescribed

Key Point
- For osteoporosis, adequate calcium supplementation is required with vitamin D analog supplementation.

Dietary Supplement: Ferrous Sulfate

Mechanism of Action for the Drug Class
Ferrous sulfate is one of the most widely used iron supplements. These supplements replace the iron found in hemoglobin, myoglobin, and other enzymes.

■ Ferrous Sulfate

Brand Names
Feosol, Fer-Gen-Sol, Fer-in-Sol, Fer-Iron, Feratab, Slow-Fe

Generic Name
Ferrous sulfate

Dosage Forms
Elixir, liquid, tablets

Usage
- Prevention and treatment of iron-deficiency anemia*

Dosing
- Treatment of iron-deficiency anemia: 300 mg orally two to four times daily or 250 mg of the extended-release formulation one to two times daily
- Prophylaxis of iron deficiency: 300 mg orally daily
- Renal dosage adjustment: None

Adverse Reactions: Most Common
- GI: constipation, dark stools, GI irritation, nausea, stomach cramping, vomiting, staining of teeth with liquid preparations

Major Drug Interactions
- Antacids may decrease the absorption of iron salts; consider therapy modification
- Bisphosphonates: Oral iron salts may decrease the absorption of oral bisphosphonates
- Cefdinir: Oral iron salts may decrease concentration of cefdinir forming an insoluble cefdinir-iron complex. This may be objectively noted by a red-appearing nonbloody stool. Avoid this combination if possible, but if not, separate doses by several hours to minimize interaction.
- Dimercaprol is contraindicated to use with iron salts because it may enhance nephrotoxicity
- Fluoroquinolone antibiotics (oral); tetracycline derivatives (oral): Oral iron salts can decrease the absorption of these antibiotics; separate doses by 2–4 hours to avoid this interaction
- H2-receptor antagonists may decrease the absorption of iron salts
- Levodopa; methyldopa: Oral iron salts may decrease absorption of levodopa/methyldopa; separate doses by 2–4 hours to lessen this interaction
- Levothyroxine: Oral iron salts can decrease the absorption of levothyroxine; separate doses by 2–4 hours to avoid this interaction
- Pancrelipase: Oral iron salts can decrease the absorption of pancrelipase; separate doses by 2–4 hours to avoid this interaction
- Phosphate supplements: Oral iron salts can decrease the absorption of these supplements; separate doses by 2–4 hours to avoid this interaction
- Foods: Particularly grains, dietary fiber, tea, coffee, eggs, milk, and wines with tannins may decrease oral iron salt absorption. Counsel patients to take on empty stomach if possible.

Counseling Points

- Use exactly as prescribed
- Keep out of reach of children; iron toxicity is one of the leading accidental drug poisonings seen in young children
- Stool may turn black; this is important to recognize, particularly when you are on anticoagulants and/or antiplatelet agents. Be wary that black stool can also be an indication of blood in stool. Contact physician if this occurs while taking anticoagulants or anti-platelet agents with iron supplements.
- Take between meals for maximal absorption; try to take on empty stomach for maximal absorption. Do not take with milk or antacids.
- If constipation occurs, try increasing fluids and foods with fruit and fiber. If >3–4 days, contact physician.

Key Points

- The elemental iron content of ferrous sulfate is 20%; 324 mg of ferrous sulfate tablet contains 65 mg of elemental iron. Therefore, with special-formulated preparations (exsiccated) such as Feosol, a 200-mg tablet contains 65 mg of elemental iron and Slow-Fe, an oral exsiccated and time-released tablet; 50 mg of elemental iron is contained in a 160 mg tablet.
- For oral solutions and elixirs, prescriptions should never be written in only volume (milliliters) because different concentrations of iron exist; use dosages in milligrams
- Use with caution with patients receiving multiple blood transfusions to prevent accidental iron overload/toxicity

---

Dietary Supplement: Folic Acid

Mechanism of Action for the Drug Class

Folic acid is necessary for the formation of numerous enzymes and coenzymes in many metabolic systems, particularly in the formation of DNA and RNA bases (purines and pyrimidines). It is also required for the maintenance of red blood cell production.

■ Folic Acid

Brand Names

Folvite, Folacin-800 (OTC)

Generic Name

Folic acid

Dosage Forms

Tablet, injectable

Usage

- Treatment of megaloblastic (macrocytic) anemia due to folic acid deficiency*
- Antenatal dietary supplement to prevent fetal neural tube defects*
- Decrease homocystine levels

Dosing for Each Indication

- For treatment of folic acid deficiency:
  - Dose: 0.4 mg daily
- For prevention of fetal neural tube defects in pregnant women:
  - Dose: 0.4–0.8 mg daily. Women at high risk should receive 4 mg daily.

Adverse Reactions

- Rare

Major Drug Interactions

Drugs Affecting Folic Acid

- Methotrexate, trimethoprim, chloramphenicol, phenytoin, and phenobarbital (decreased folic acid effectiveness)

Folic Acid's Effect on Other Drugs

- Phenytoin, phenobarbital, primidone (folic acid decreases the effect of these medications)

Contraindications

- Treatment with folic acid in other megaloblastic anemias (pernicious anemia and vitamin B_{12} deficiency) without proper diagnosis can mask these anemias and lead to progression that can include irreversible nerve damage

Counseling Point

- Take folic acid replacement only with the recommendation of a physician

Key Point

- Decreases the incidence of fetal neural tube defects >50%

Dietary Supplement: Vitamin C

Mechanism of Action for the Drug Class

Essential cofactor in numerous biochemical reactions, including the indirect provision of electrons to enzymes, which require prosthetic metal ions in reduced form for their activity; an antioxidant in aqueous environments and is a cofactor in carnitine, neurotransmitter, and collagen synthesis; exists in both reduced and oxidized forms.

■ Vitamin C

Brand Names

Ascorbate-C, C Aspa Scorb, Ester-C

Generic Names

Vitamin C, L-Ascorbic acid

Dosage Forms

Tablets, chewable tablets, capsules, powder

Usage

- Improves wound healing*
- Reduces symptoms of the common cold (unproven; anecdotal)*
- Prevents and treats scurvy
- Improves dietary iron absorption

Dosing

- 90 mg daily (men); 75 mg daily (women) is the RDA
- Increase RDA by 35 mg in smokers
- Renal dosage adjustment: Lower doses recommended in renal insufficiency

Adverse Reactions: Most Common

- GI complaints (nausea, abdominal cramps, flatulence, diarrhea)

Adverse Reactions: Rare/Severe/Important

- Renal consequences (hyperoxaluria, risk of nephrolithiasis)

Major Drug Interactions

- Increases bioavailability of co-trimoxazole
- Increases clearance of estradiol/levonorgestrel
- Decreases effect of warfarin
- Aspirin, ethanol reduce tissue saturation of vitamin C
- Oral contraceptives, tobacco smoke exposure increase clearance of vitamin C

Counseling Points

- Intestinal absorption and renal reabsorption are saturable processes, so doses >200 mg should be divided to limit GI discomfort
- Tolerable upper intake level set at 2000 mg daily from all sources
- Chronic use of chewable vitamin C products may increase the risk of dental erosions and caries
- No difference in bioavailability or activity exists between "natural" and "synthetic" vitamin C

Key Points

- High daily doses may interfere with laboratory tests but may be assay-dependent:
  - False increase (serum aspartate aminotransferase, bilirubin, creatinine, carbamazepine)
  - False decrease (serum lactate dehydrogenase, uric acid, vitamin B_{12}, theophylline)
  - False negative (guaiac test)
- Use with caution in patients with glucose-6-phosphate dehydrogenase deficiency
- For pregnant women, daily limits from all sources should be no greater than 2000 mg of vitamin C

Dietary Supplement: Vitamin E

Mechanism of Action for the Drug Class

Protects cell membrane (polyunsaturated fatty acids) from oxidative damage, inhibits proliferation of smooth muscle, and decreases adhesion of platelets, leukocytes, and endothelial cells.

■ Vitamin E

Brand Name

Not applicable

Generic Names

Vitamin E, tocopherols (α, β, γ, δ), tocotrienols (α, β, γ, δ)

Dosage Forms

Tablets, capsules (various isomers including all-*racemic* [formerly *d,l-*] α-tocopherol, and RRR [formerly *d-*] α-tocopherol)

Usage

- Vitamin E deficiency*
- Prevention of cardiovascular disease morbidity and mortality (not labeled/approved)*
- Slow down progression of neurologic disorders (e.g., dementia, Parkinson's disease [not labeled/approved])

Dosing

- 15 mg daily of α-tocopherol is the RDA
- Tolerable upper intake level set at 1000 mg daily from all α-tocopherol sources
- Renal dosage adjustment: None

Adverse Reactions: Most Common

- GI upset

Adverse Reactions: Rare/Severe/Important

- Increased risk of bleeding and hemorrhagic stroke
- Thrombocytopenia

Major Drug Interactions

- Increases effect of warfarin, antiplatelet agents, insulin, and digoxin
- Cholestyramine, orlistat, and mineral oil decrease vitamin E absorption
- Fish oil increases vitamin E requirements

Counseling Point

- Take as prescribed

Key Points

- The predominant form of vitamin E in the diet is γ-tocopherol; in the body it is α-tocopherol; select a product containing both forms
- Bioavailability is enhanced in the presence of food containing some dietary fat
- Use a water-miscible formulation in patients with malabsorptive disorders
- Although IUs are no longer recognized as a dosing unit for vitamin E, it is still found in product labeling; this requires conversion to milligram α-tocopherol for comparison to dosing recommendations:
  - mg = IU all-*rac*-α-tocopherol as acetate/succinate ÷ 2.2
  - mg = IU RRR-α-tocopherol as acetate/succinate ÷ 1.5

Review Questions

1. Which herbal supplement is touted for migraine relief, mainly because it possesses pharmacologic properties similar to nonsteroidal anti-inflammatory drugs (NSAIDs)?
   A. St. John's Wort
   B. Chondroitin
   C. Feverfew
   D. Valerian

2. Ubiquinone is also an alternative name for what dietary supplement?
   A. Coenzyme-Q
   B. Creatine
   C. Glucosamine
   D. Chondroitin

3. A popular herbal supplement used as an immune system booster and derived from the purple coneflower is
   A. Valerian
   B. Feverfew
   C. Echinacea
   D. Digitalis

4. Kyolic-branded products contain what natural supplement?
   A. Garlic
   B. Tocopherol
   C. Asian ginseng
   D. Siberian ginseng

5. Gingko biloba is popularly used to
   A. Treat mild to moderate depression
   B. Increase memory
   C. Increase energy
   D. All of the above

6. Patients with severe shellfish/crustacean allergy may have to use caution or avoid which natural supplement?
   A. Ginseng
   B. Glucosamine
   C. Chondroitin
   D. Ava pepper

7. Warnings regarding what serious adverse effect is associated with the use of kava?
   A. Liver failure
   B. Seizure
   C. Aplastic anemia
   D. Sterility in males

8. *Hypericum perforatum* is better known as
   A. St. John's wort
   B. Feverfew
   C. Valerian
   D. Ginseng

9. Significant interactions with St. John's wort include
   A. Induction of cyclosporine metabolism
   B. The potential of serotonin syndrome with antidepressants
   C. Increased phototoxicity when used with a drug like amiodarone
   D. All of the above

10. A botanical used as a sleep aid often dosed as a tea, is best described as
    A. Melatonin
    B. Valerian
    C. Creatine
    D. Gingko biloba

11. The following oral supplements can decrease the effectiveness of oral fluoroquinolones and tetracyclines except
    A. Calcium
    B. Ferrous sulfate
    C. Zinc
    D. Vitamin B_{12}

12. Patients with pernicious anemia require what vital supplement?
    A. Vitamin A
    B. Vitamin B_{12}
    C. Vitamin C
    D. Vitamin K

13. 10 μg of ergocalciferol is equivalent to how many IUs of ergocalciferol?
    A. 100 IU
    B. 400 IUs
    C. 50,000 IUs
    D. Cannot determine

14. A black stool may be a side effect of what dietary supplement?
    A. Ferrous sulfate
    B. Calcium chloride
    C. Tannic acid
    D. Vitamin C

15. Tocopherol is a synonymous term associated with
    A. Vitamin D
    B. Vitamin C
    C. Vitamin E
    D. Riboflavin

CHAPTER 1

1. A	6. A	11. B
2. A	7. C	12. B
3. D	8. A	13. A
4. D	9. D	14. D
5. A	10. A	15. B

CHAPTER 2

1. C	6. B	11. D
2. B	7. C	12. B
3. D	8. C	13. C
4. A	9. A	14. B
5. D	10. C	15. C

CHAPTER 3

1. D	6. B	11. A
2. C	7. B	12. C
3. C	8. A	13. B
4. D	9. D	14. B
5. D	10. C	15. D

CHAPTER 4

1. B	6. A	11. B
2. D	7. C	12. B
3. B	8. D	13. A
4. A	9. D	14. D
5. C	10. A	15. C

CHAPTER 5

1. A	6. B	11. B
2. D	7. D	12. A
3. C	8. D	13. C
4. B	9. C	14. B
5. D	10. D	15. C

CHAPTER 6

1. A	6. B	11. D
2. B	7. C	12. A
3. B	8. C	13. B
4. A	9. A	14. D
5. B	10. A	15. C

CHAPTER 7

1. D	6. A	11. D
2. B	7. D	12. A
3. B	8. B	13. D
4. D	9. B	14. B
5. B	10. B	15. D

CHAPTER 8

1. A	6. D	11. A
2. D	7. D	12. D
3. D	8. A	13. B
4. C	9. D	14. D
5. B	10. B	15. B

CHAPTER 9

1. A	6. B	11. C
2. B	7. B	12. C
3. D	8. A	13. A
4. C	9. D	14. A
5. A	10. A	15. D

CHAPTER 10

1. A	6. B	11. D
2. A	7. A	12. A
3. B	8. D	13. D
4. C	9. D	14. A
5. A	10. B	15. B

CHAPTER 11

1. D	6. D	11. C
2. D	7. C	12. A
3. C	8. D	13. D
4. D	9. B	14. D
5. A	10. D	15. C

CHAPTER 12

1. D	6. B	11. D
2. A	7. A	12. B
3. A	8. C	13. B
4. A	9. D	14. A
5. D	10. D	15. C

CHAPTER 13

1. D	6. D	11. C
2. C	7. A	12. B
3. A	8. A	13. A
4. B	9. D	14. D
5. C	10. D	15. C

CHAPTER 14

1. C	6. A	11. B
2. B	7. C	12. C
3. D	8. D	13. A
4. A	9. B	14. B
5. B	10. D	15. C

CHAPTER 15

1. C	6. B	11. D
2. A	7. A	12. B
3. C	8. A	13. B
4. A	9. D	14. A
5. B	10. B	15. C

kava, 223–224
melatonin, 224
saw palmetto, 225
St. John's wort, 225–226
valerian, 226
Nature's Root Nighttime. *See* valerian
nausea and vomiting, 139
chemotherapy-induced, 127, 135
postoperative, 127
radiation-induced, 127
neck cancer. *See* head/neck cancer
nefazodone, 90–91
Neisseria meningitides, asymptomatic carriers of, 25
neomycin, 176
neomycin-polymyxin B, 24
neoplastic diseases, 123–124
NeoProfen. *See* ibuprofen
Neoral. *See* cyclosporine
Neosporin. *See* gramicidin; neomycin; neomycin-
polymyxin B; polymyxin B sulfate
nephrotic syndrome, in children, 49–50
nervous system diseases, 123–124
Neulasta. *See* pegfilgrastim
Neupogen. *See* filgrastim
neural tube defect prevention, 231
neuroblastoma, 49–51, 55–56
neuroendocrine tumors, 51–52
neurogenic bladder, 172
Neurontin. *See* gabapentin
neuropathic pain, 2, 86, 88, 95
neutropenia
febrile, 37–38
in HIV, 144
Nexium. *See* esomeprazole
niacin, 154–155
niacin deficiency. *See* pellagra
Niacin-Time. *See* niacin
Niacor (IR). *See* niacin
Niaspan ER (Rx). *See* niacin
NicoDerm CQ. *See* nicotine
Nicorette. *See* nicotine
nicotine, 83, 169–170
withdrawal, 62–63, 169
nicotinic acid, 154–155
Nicotrol Inhaler. *See* nicotine
Nicotrol NS. *See* nicotine
Nicotrol OTC. *See* nicotine
Nifediac CC. *See* nifedipine
Nifedical XL. *See* nifedipine
nifedipine, 72
Niravam. *See* alprazolam
nitrates, 74
nitrofuran, 37
nitrofurantoin, 37
nitroglycerin, 74
nitroimidazole, 34
Nitrostat. *See* nitroglycerin
Nizoral. *See* ketoconazole
NNRTI. *See* nonnucleoside reverse
transcriptase inhibitor
nonbenzodiazepine, 82–83, 103–104
non-Hodgkin lymphoma, 49–50, 53–56
B-cell, 57

nonnucleoside reverse transcriptase inhibitor
(NNRTI), 43–44
nonsteroidal anti-inflammatory analgesics, 10–13
nonsteroidal anti-inflammatory selective
COX-2 inhibitor, 9–10
norethindrone, 121
ethinyl estradiol and, 118–121
norgestimate
ethinyl estradiol and, 118–121
nortriptyline, 96
Norvasc. *See* amlodipine
Norvir. *See* ritonavir
Novadex. *See* tamoxifen
Novolin 70/30. *See* 70% NPH and 30%
regular insulin mixture
Novolin N. *See* NPH, insulin
Novolin R. *See* regular, insulin
NovoLog. *See* aspart, insulin
NovoLog Mix 70/30. *See* 70% intermediate-
acting insulin aspart suspension and
30% rapid-acting aspart insulin solution
NPH, insulin, 17–18
70% NPH and 30% regular insulin mixture, 18
NRTI. *See* nucleoside/nucleotide reverse
transcriptase inhibitor
NSCLC. *See* lung cancer, non-small cell
Nu Veg Feverfew Leaf. *See* feverfew
Nu Veg Valerian Root. *See* valerian
nucleoside/nucleotide reverse transcriptase
inhibitor (NRTI), 41–43
Nuprin. *See* ibuprofen
nutrients, 217, 227
Nutrilite. *See* saw palmetto
nystatin, 38

obsessive–compulsive disorder (OCD), 92, 93, 94
obstructive sleep apnea/hypopnea syndrome, 111
Ocuflox. *See* ofloxacin
ocular herpes simplex infection, 40–41
Odor-Free Concentrated Garlic. *See* garlic
ofloxacin, 177
olanzapine, 98–99
Olux. *See* clobetasol propionate
omega-3 fatty acids, 156
omeprazole, 137
ondansetron, 127–128
Onsolis. *See* fentanyl
onychomycosis, 39
ophthalmia neonatorum, 177
ophthalmic products
administration of, 175
β-adrenergic blocking agents, 179–180
antibiotics, 175–178
prostaglandin agonist, 178–179
opiate addiction, detoxification from, 4–5
oral contraceptives
combined
biphasic, 120
monophasic, 118–119, 120
triphasic, 120, 121
progestin-only, 121
oral lesions, 212, 213
oral lichen planus, 211

oral mucosal inflammation, 210
Oramorph. *See* morphine
organ transplant
prevent rejection of, 167, 168
oropharyngeal cavity
Candida infections of, 38–39
Ortho Tri-Cyclen. *See* oral contraceptives,
combined
Ortho-Cyclen. *See* ethinyl estradiol
combinations
Ortho-Novum 7/7/7. *See* oral contraceptives,
combined
Os-Cal. *See* calcium
osteoarthritis, 9–13, 142, 218, 223
osteogenic sarcoma, 55
osteomyelitis, 29
osteoporosis, 114–118, 121–122, 227, 228
osteosarcoma, 54, 55–56
ovarian cancer, 49–53, 55–56, 58–59
overactive bladder agents, 171–172
oxcarbazepine, 86
oxybutynin, 171–172
oxycodone, 6
oxycodone/acetaminophen, 8
OxyContin. *See* oxycodone
OxyIR. *See* oxycodone
oxymetazoline, 198
Oxytrol. *See* oxybutynin

Pacerone. *See* amiodarone
paclitaxel, 59
Paget's disease, 114–115
pain, 105, 142, 203, 218, 220
acute, 9–10
cancer and, 62–63
low back, 108
mild, 1
mild to moderate, 8–9, 11–13
moderate, 6–7, 8
moderate to severe, 2, 3–4, 5, 6, 8
neuropathic, 2, 86, 88, 95
in postherpetic neuralgia, 84, 88, 203
severe, 3, 4–5, 62–63
Pamelor. *See* nortriptyline
Pamprin IB. *See* ibuprofen
panax ginseng, 221–222
pancreatic cancer, 51–53
panic disorders, 69–70, 81, 92, 93, 94, 103
pantoprazole, 137–138
Paraplatin-AQ. *See* carboplatin
Parcopa. *See* carbidopa
Parkinson disease, 69–70, 162, 218
paroxetine, 94
paroxysmal supraventricular tachycardias, 70–71
patent ductus arteriosus, 11–12
Paxil. *See* paroxetine
Paxil CR. *See* paroxetine
PBPC. *See* peripheral blood progenitor cell
PCOS. *See* polycystic ovarian syndrome
PCP. *See Pneumocystis jiroveci* pneumonia
pegfilgrastim, 144–145
pellagra, 154
pelvic inflammatory disease, 28, 34

Rheumatrex. *See* methotrexate

rhinitis, allergic/nonallergic, 183, 185, 186, 196, 199

Rhinocort Aqua. *See* budesonide

rickets, 229

rickettsialpox, 36

rifampin, 25

Riomet. *See* Metformin

risedronate, 114–115

Risperdal. *See* risperidone

Risperdal-M. *See* risperidone

risperidone, 99–100

Ritalin. *See* methylphenidate

Ritalin LA. *See* methylphenidate

Ritalin SR. *See* methylphenidate

ritonavir, 44–45

Rituxan. *See* rituximab

rituximab, 57

Robaxin. *See* methocarbamol

Robitussin. *See* guaifenesin

Robitussin DM. *See* guaifenesin

Rocephin. *See* ceftriaxone

Rocky Mountain spotted fever, 36

Rolaids. *See* calcium carbonate

ropinirole, 102

rosacea, 34

rosiglitazone, 21

rosuvastatin, 151

Roxanol. *See* morphine

Roxicet. *See* oxycodone/acetaminophen

Roxicodone. *See* oxycodone

Sabal Select Solaray. *See* saw palmetto

salmeterol, 192

    fluticasone and, 190

Sandimmune. *See* cyclosporine

Sarafem. *See* fluoxetine

sarcomas, 55–56

    bone, 50–51

    dermatofibrosarcoma protuberans, 56–57

    Ewing, 49–50

    Kaposi, 59

    osteogenic, 55

    osteosarcoma, 55–56

    rhabdomyosarcoma, 49–50

    soft tissue, 50–51, 58–59

saw palmetto, 225

saxagliptin, 16

schizophrenia, 69–70, 98, 99, 100, 139

SCN. *See* severe chronic neutropenia

scurvy, 232

Seasonale. *See* ethinyl estradiol combinations

seborrheic dermatitis, 207

sedative-hypnotic agents, 185, 186

    benzodiazepine, 102–103

    nighttime, 91

    nonbenzodiazepine, 103–104

    preoperative/procedural, 82

seizures, 81–89

selective estrogen receptor modulators, 121–122

selective mutism, 93

selective serotonin reuptake inhibitors, 92–95

Septra. *See* trimethoprim/sulfamethoxazole

Serevent. *See* salmeterol

Seroquel. *See* quetiapine

serotonin-norepinephrine reuptake inhibitors, 91–92

sertraline, 94–95

Serzone. *See* nefazodone

severe chronic neutropenia (SCN), 144

sex hormones (estrogens, progestins, estrogen and progestin combinations, estrogen and androgen combinations), 116–118

shift-work sleep disorder, 111

shingles. *See* herpes zoster

sildenafil, 167

simethicone, 131

simvastatin, 151

Sinemet. *See* carbidopa

Sinemet CR. *See* carbidopa

Sinequan. *See* doxepin

Singulair. *See* montelukast

sinusitis, 198

sitagliptin, 16

sitosterolemia, homozygous, 155

Skelaxin. *See* metaxalone

skeletal muscle relaxants, 82, 104–108

skin

    cleanser for, 206

    infections of, 24–36

    irritations, 212

    lesions, infected, 205

sleep, 224

    aids, 226

    disorders, 185

Slo-Niacin. *See* niacin

Slow-Fe. *See* ferrous sulfate

Slow-K. *See* potassium chloride

smoking cessation aids, 90, 108, 169–171. *See also* nicotine

    nicotine, 169–170

    partial nicotinic agonist, 108–109

    varenicline, 170–171

social phobia, 81, 84

soft tissue infections, 28–30, 36

soft tissue sarcomas, 50–51, 58–59

solar keratoses, 52

Solu-Medrol. *See* methylprednisolone

Soma. *See* carisoprodol

Sorine. *See* sotalol

sotalol, 68

Sotret. *See* isotretinoin

sour stomach, 133

Spiriva. *See* tiotropium

spironolactone, 75

splenic marginal zone lymphoma, 57

Sporanox. *See* itraconazole

St. John's wort, 225–226

statins. *See* HMG-CoA reductase inhibitors

Stavzor. *See* valproate/divalproex

stem cell immobilization, 49–50

stimulants, 109–111

stomach cancer, 52

streptococcal infections, 27

stress, 223

    relief of, 222

stress-induced ulcers, 134, 135

stroke, 141, 148

Sublimaze. *See* fentanyl

substance withdrawal. *See* alcohol; heroin withdrawal; nicotine

sulfonylureas, 19–20

sumatriptan, 79–80

supraventricular arrhythmias, 67–68

supraventricular tachycardias, paroxysmal, 70–71

surgical prophylaxis, 28

Sustiva. *See* efavirenz

swelling, chronic, 123–124

Symbicort. *See* budesonide

Synthroid. *See* levothyroxine sodium

syphilis, 32

systemic autoimmune diseases, 57

systemic embolization, 141

systemic herpes simplex infection, 40–41

systemic lupus erythematosus, 49–50, 161

tacrolimus, 168

tadalafil, 167

Tagamet. *See* cimetidine

tamoxifen, 113

tamsulosin, 62

targeted therapy, antineoplastics, 56–58

taxanes, 58–59

Taxol. *See* paclitaxel

Taxotere. *See* docetaxel

Taztia XT. *See* diltiazem

tears

    increase production of, 167

Tegretol. *See* carbamazepine

Tegretol XR. *See* carbamazepine

temazepam, 103

Temovate. *See* clobetasol propionate

temporomandibular joint disorder, 105

tenofovir, 42–43

Tenormin. *See* atenolol

tension, 223

tension/muscle contraction headaches, 108, 139

    butalbital with caffeine and acetaminophen, 1–2

Terazol. *See* terconazole

terazosin, 62

terconazole, 208

testicular cancer, 49–50, 55–56

tetanus, supportive therapy in, 107

tetracyclines, 36

theophylline, 200

Therapeutic Lifestyle Changes (TLCs), 151

thiazide diuretics, 75–76

thiazolidinediones, 20–21

Thrive. *See* nicotine

thromboembolic complications, 141, 148

thrombolytics, 148–149

thrombosis, 146

thrombotic events, 143

thyroid cancer, 50–51